HEALTH PROMOTING PRACTICE

Also by Angela Scriven:

Angela Scriven (ed.), *Alliances in Health Promotion: Theory and Practice**

Angela Scriven and Judy Orme (eds), *Health Promotion: Professional Perspectives*, second edition*

Angela Scriven and Sebastian Garman (eds), *Promoting Health: Global Perspectives**

* Also published by Palgrave Macmillan

Health Promoting Practice

The Contribution of Nurses and Allied Health Professionals

edited by

Angela Scriven

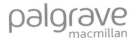

First published in 2005 by
PALGRAVE MACMILLAN
Houndmills, Basingstoke, Hampshire RG21 6XS and
175 Fifth Avenue, New York, N.Y. 10010
Companies and representatives throughout the world.

PALGRAVE MACMILLAN is the global academic imprint of the Palgrave
Macmillan division of St. Martin's Press, LLC and of Palgrave Macmillan Ltd.
Macmillan® is a registered trademark in the United States, United Kingdom
and other countries. Palgrave is a registered trademark in the European
Union and other countries.

ISBN-13: 978–1–4039–3410–9 hardback
ISBN-10: 1–4039–3410–X hardback
ISBN-13: 978–1–4039–3411–6 paperback
ISBN-10: 1–4039–3411–8 paperback

This book is printed on paper suitable for recycling and made from fully
managed and sustained forest sources.

A catalogue record for this book is available from the British Library.

10 9 8 7 6 5 4 3 2 1
14 13 12 11 10 09 08 07 06 05

Printed and bound in China

Contents

PART II

PART III

Contents   vii

List of Figures and Tables

Figures

Tables

Notes on Contributors

Jo Adams is Lecturer in Occupational Therapy at the School of Health Professions and Rehabilitation Sciences at the University of Southampton. Clinically she has worked as an occupational therapist in physical rehabilitation in community, hospital and voluntary organisations in the United Kingdom, America, Canada and Uganda. Her research interests include community rehabilitation and housing for individuals with severe disability and she has published her rheumatology research in both national and international journals.

Claire Anderson is Director of the Centre for Pharmacy, Health and Society in the School of Pharmaceutical Sciences, University of Nottingham. She is on the board of the College of Pharmacy Practice. Her major research interest is about the role of community pharmacists in improving the health of the public. She is also interested in pharmacy practice enhancement; pharmacy education; prescribing of and use of medicines; health, medicines and the Internet, pharmaceutical care and self-care.

Miriam Armstrong is Chief Executive of the charity PharmacyHealthLink. She trained and worked as a dentist, researcher and NHS manager before running the national initiative Health at Work in the NHS. As Chief Executive of PharmacyHealthLink she now works closely with the Department of Health, major health professional and public health organisations to promote the health of the public through pharmacies. She has been managing editor and co-author of a large number of professional and public information health materials.

Stephen Ashford was previously course leader for the MSc in Neurorehabilitation at Brunel University. He is currently clinical specialist in physiotherapy and research physiotherapist at the Regional Rehabilitation Unit, Northwick Park Hospital, London. His key area of clinical expertise is the rehabilitation and management of brain injured adults. Research interests include management of complex neurological disability, spasticity management and physical management approaches. His current research is in the field of spasticity management intervention with a particular focus on botulinum toxin as an adjunct to therapy intervention.

Helen Ashton is Associate Lecturer for the MSc in Health Studies at Bath Spa University College. She has been teaching in the continuing professional education of health professionals and associated with diabetes nursing and education for over 20 years. As a registered nurse, she maintains her clinical links through her involvement with diabetes clinics for young persons. Her recent research has been with members of the local diabetes team in Bath focussed on patients' self-management of their diabetes.

Anita Atwal is Occupational Therapy Lecturer at Brunel University. She has published and presented both nationally and internationally. She completed a PhD examining issues surrounding discharge planning and teamwork. Her research interests centre upon interprofessional working, discharge planning, and older people in care homes and acute healthcare. She is currently co-editing a book for occupational therapy undergraduates on older people.

Alison Blenkinsopp is Professor of the Practice of Pharmacy, Department of Medicines Management, Keele University. Her main research area is primary care and the wider role of community pharmacists. She has a particular interest in patients' perspective on medicine use. She has published widely for both academic and health service audiences.

Alan Borthwick is Lecturer in Podiatry at the School of Health Professions and Rehabilitation Sciences of the University of Southampton. He worked as a clinician and manager before pursuing an academic career 18 years ago, attaining a professional fellowship, a certificate in teaching practice, an MSc in behavioural biology and a PhD in the sociology of the professions. He has published widely in the area of healthcare professionalisation and presented his research across the UK, Europe and Canada. His current research interests focus upon the changing nature of interprofessional relationships and access to services within the context of healthcare modernisation.

Karen Bunning is Senior Lecturer in Speech and Language Therapy at the School of Allied Health Professions at the University of East Anglia, where she is employed to develop a new degree programme in speech and language therapy. Her current research involves looking at communicative access and inclusion for people with severe learning disabilities and multiple impairments, and developing interventions to improve social participation.

Lorraine De Souza is Fellow of the Chartered Society of Physiotherapy and Professor of Rehabilitation at Brunel University. She has been involved in clinical practice and research in multiple sclerosis for 20 years and continues to have a strong and active interest in the field. She has published widely, at international level, papers and book contributions focussed on the assessment, care, management and physiotherapy treatment for people with MS. Her recent research on professionally guided self-management in MS has been used by the National Institute for Clinical Excellence (NICE) as evidence for new national guidelines for the management of MS. Professor De Souza is currently Chair of the MS Professional Network, an international organisation devoted to the development, identification and dissemination of best practice in MS care.

Christine Fox is Senior Lecturer in Nutrition and Dietetics at the Universtiy of Plymouth. She has 20 years' experience working as a public health dietitian in a number of settings including research, academia, the food industry and government. Her research explored the occupational emergence of dietitians working in the community, and she has contributed to the strategic development of community dietetics to address the public health agenda. She was involved in the Department of Health's Five-a-Day Pilot Projects and the South West Schools' Healthier Tuck Shops Project for the Food in Schools Programme.

Sally French is Senior Lecturer in the Department of Allied Health Professions at the University of Hertfordshire. She is also an Associate Lecturer at the Open University. She has a background in physiotherapy but for many years has taught psychology and sociology applied to health, illness and disability to health and social care students.

Priscilla Harries is the Course Leader for the MSc in Occupational Therapy at Brunel University. She has published and presented, both nationally and internationally, on the role of occupational therapists in anorexia nervosa prevention and treatment. She is currently involved in the development of research projects on eating disorders for the National Association of Occupational Therapists. Her research interests also include the mental health needs of women, priorities in service provisions, and expertise development.

Veronica Henshall is Head of Orthoptics at the Royal Albert Edward Infirmary in Wigan. She has been involved with clinical teaching and research over the past ten years and lectures on the undergraduate communication module for the School of Health Sciences at the University of Liverpool. She is currently involved in researching the area of oral contraceptives and their ocular effects.

Sally Hinton is the National Coordinator for the BACR (British Association of Cardiac Rehabilitation) Phase IV Exercise Instructor Training module. She has many years experience in cardiac rehabilitation both in lecturing and in developing and delivering services. She completed an MSc in Health Promotion at Brunel University with research in patients' compliance with exercise after cardiac rehabilitation. She continues to help to develop and promote the physiotherapist's role in cardiac rehabilitation and is involved in postgraduate training within this field.

Lorely Ide is Researcher and Lecturer in the Centre of Rehabilitation Research at Brunel University. She has been involved in research in physiotherapy since the early 1980s and has undertaken research into carers of people with neurological disease. Over the last ten years she has been lecturing at Brunel and has been working on studies of multiple sclerosis.

Jenni Jones is Lecturer in Physiotherapy at Brunel University specialising in Cardiopulmonary Medicine. She has experience in cardiac rehabilitation ranging from co-coordinating the physiotherapy service at Harefield Hospital to co-coordinating the physical activity component of EUROACTION, a large

European-wide research project in cardiac prevention and rehabilitation, based at Imperial College, London. She is the current Chair of the Association of Chartered Physiotherapists in Cardiac Rehabilitation (ACPICR) and is actively involved in its activities to develop Phase III exercise training for physiotherapists.

Melanie Jones has been a Research Officer in the School of Health Science at the University of Wales Swansea since 1996. Her first degree was in Social Anthropology. She subsequently completed her doctoral thesis, which is an ethnographic study of users' experiences of complementary therapies. Her research work in her current post has included ethnographic work, systematic reviews, policy evaluations and research in healthcare ethics. Her research interests are in medical anthropology and theories of embodiment.

James Law is currently Professor and Head of Department in the Department of Language and Communication Science, City University, London. He has been principal investigator on a number of funded research projects. In 1998 he completed a systematic review funded by the Health Technology Assessment programme of the National Health Service in 1998 into interventions for language delayed children. He has since led a team looking at the effective collaboration between education and health services in provision for children with speech and language needs in England and Wales and has also recently completed a study evaluating early years provision for the charity I CAN. He has recently led a project looking at promoting the communication skills of primary care professionals working with the communication disabled and is also currently working on a project setting the language baseline in the national Sure Start programme. He has edited and written a number of texts: Law, J. (ed.) (1992) *The Early Identification of Children with Language Impairment*, London: Chapman and Hall; Law, J. and Elias, J. (1996) *Trouble Talking – a Guide for Parents of Children with Speech and Language Difficulties*, London: Jessica Kingsley; Chiat, S., Law, J. and Marshall, J. (1997) *Language Disorders in Children and Adults: Psycholinguistic Approaches to Therapy*, London: Whurr; and Law, J., Parkinson, A. and Tamnhe, R. (2000) *Communication Difficulties in Childhood*, Oxford: Radcliffe.

Ruth Lewis is Policy and Research Officer at the NHS Confederation. She was previously Assistant to the Chief Executive at the charity PharmacyHealthLink and a graduate of the NHS Management Training Scheme.

Jill Lloyd is Physiotherapy Lecturer at Brunel University. She is responsible for the organisation of the clinical education of physiotherapy students and teaches some musculoskeletal elements on the undergraduate course. She has worked extensively in rheumatology in hospitals in West London. She is the Vice President of Health Professionals in Rheumatology in the European League against Rheumatism (EULAR) and a former Chair of the Rheumatic Care Association of Chartered Physiotherapists (RCACP). Publications include contributing to and co-editing with Carol Davis (1999) *Rheumatological Physiotherapy*, London: Mosby.

Michelle Morris is Head of Speech and Language Therapy Services in Salford, Greater Manchester. She is the Department of Health Network Advisor for Speech and Language Therapy and is a member of the Professional Development Board at the Royal Collage of Speech and Language Therapists. She is currently developing a programme to build public health capacity for Allied Health Professionals (AHPs). Her research is centred on the identification of the opportunities and barriers to AHPs working in a public health way. She is interested in developing Speech and Language Therapy services which promote a health and wellbeing model and which reduce the inequalities experienced by disadvantaged communities.

Claudius Neophytou is Researcher and Lecturer in the Centre of Rehabilitation Research at Brunel University. He has a background in health psychology and expertise in qualitative research. His early research, while at Bath University, investigated men's and women's experience of obesity within Western society. More recently he has finished working on a study of carers of people with multiple sclerosis and he is currently investigating the needs of electrically powered wheelchair users.

Susan Nancarrow is Senior Research Fellow and Senior Lecturer in the Faculty of Health and Social Care at Sheffield Hallam University. She trained as a podiatrist in Australia and worked in a variety of settings, ranging from Aboriginal health services to community and private practice. She completed a PhD examining issues of health service accountability at the Australian National University before moving to the United Kingdom. Her research interests centre upon healthcare workforce development issues, including analyses of professional role boundary dynamics and the emergence of new worker roles in the healthcare arena.

Sally Pearce trained as an occupational therapist at the University of Southampton and has subsequently worked in the acute sector in the NHS within Rheumatology and Trauma specialities. For the last four years she has been clinical lead for community rehabilitation within Portsmouth and South East Hampshire. She has a particular interest in the psychological aspects of physical functioning and rehabilitation.

Jill Rodgers is a partner in In Balance Healthcare UK. She has worked in diabetes nursing and education for ten years and has published widely in diabetes related journals. She has helped the concept of empowerment become an accepted part of diabetes care in the United Kingdom, and currently runs workshops for health professionals around empowerment and consultation styles. She is a visiting Senior Clinical Lecturer at the University of Warwick.

Fiona Rowe is Lecturer in Orthoptics at the University of Liverpool and a research associate at Warrington Hospital. She has been involved with teaching and research for over ten years and has published widely, including her textbook (2004) *Clinical Orthoptics*, second edition, Oxford: Blackwell. She is currently research-active in a number of neuro-ophthalmology areas, binocular vision and visual field assessment and driving. She is Chair of the British Orthoptic Society Professional Development Committee and represents the British Orthoptic Society on a number of national bodies.

Paul Scott graduated in neurobiology and taught in Lesotho before returning to take a Masters in Dietetics. His work as a hospital dietitian was followed by a career move to health promotion, working with local partners on food strategy and a variety of practical projects such as food co-ops, cook and taste sessions and farmers' markets. Currently, he is nearing the completion of a Master of Public Health degree and working as a trainee Specialist in Public Health on the South West Regional public health training scheme.

Lynn Sayer is Programme Leader for the Community Health Nursing Courses at Brunel University. She is a registered nurse, health visitor and qualified district nurse who has been teaching in community nurse education for 18 years. She leads a range of undergraduate and postgraduate professional nursing related courses. Her research interests are in the areas of multiprofessional education, mentorship and practice teaching.

Angela Scriven is Course Leader for the MSc in Health Promotion and Public Health at Brunel University. She has been teaching and researching in the field of health promotion for over 20 years and has published widely including the edited books (1998) *Alliances in Health Promotion: Theory and Practice*, Basingstoke: Palgrave Macmillan; (2001) *Health Promotion: Professional Perspectives*, Basingstoke: Palgrave Macmillan (co-edited with Judy Orme); and (2005) *Promoting Health: Global Perspectives*, Basingstoke: Palgrave Macmillan (co-edited with Sebastian Garman). Her research is centred on the relationship between health promotion policy and practice within specific contexts.

John Swain is Professor of Disability and Inclusion in the Faculty of Health, Social Work and Education at the University of Northumbria and an Associate Lecturer at the Open University. He has written and researched extensively in the field of disability studies.

Thelma Sumsion is Director of the School of Occupational Therapy at the University of Western Ontario in London, Ontario, Canada. She has been investigating client centred practice since the early 1980s and has several publications to her credit including the edited text (1999) *Client-centred Practice in Occupational Therapy: a Guide to Implementation*, Edinburgh: Churchill Livingstone. Her research continues to focus on client centred practice with a current interest in the opportunities for and barriers to the application of this approach in mental health settings.

Jane Thomas is Senior Lecturer in Education Studies at the School of Health Science, University of Wales, Swansea. She has nursing, midwifery and health visiting experience and a longstanding interest in child and school health. Her research interests include school nursing, community care, professional ethics and curriculum evaluation. She was involved in the foundation of the MSc in Health Promotion at Swansea and sustains an active involvement with the programme.

Julia Verne is Director of the South West Public Health Observatory, Acting Director of the South West Cancer Intelligence Service and Consultant in Public Health Medicine at the South West Regional Public Health Group. The latter post includes a substantial health promotion component including regional responsibility for promoting healthy eating. In addition to a qualification in Medicine, she has an MSc and PhD in Epidemiology and is a Fellow of the Faculty of Public Health Medicine. She has had a varied career, including being a Consultant in Public Health Medicine responsible for the delivery of a district health promotion service, policy development at the Department of Health, and collaborative multiagency work at local level.

Paul Wainwright is Reader in the School of Health Science at the University of Wales, Swansea. He trained as a general nurse in Southampton, gained an MSc in Nursing at the University of Manchester and a PhD at the University of Wales. His research interests include the nature of professional practice, the content of professional roles and the relationships between the various roles and work of healthcare professionals. He helped found the MSc in Health Promotion in Swansea, and was the lead investigator in a review of the evidence of effectiveness of school nurses in health promotion.

Janet Weeks is an experienced health visitor and has held part-time lecturing posts on the Masters in Healthcare Practice and the Masters in Healthcare Management at Bath Spa University College, running modules on clinical audit and on care transfer/hospital discharge. She has a long established interest in the health promotion role of nurses and has researched the role of palliative care in promoting wellbeing and quality of life in people with terminal illness. An emerging research interest is the development of the public health role of health visitors and their contribution to reducing inequalities in health through partnership working with communities and other agencies.

Dean Whitehead is Senior Lecturer. At the time of writing he was actively involved in the planning and delivery of Health Promotion and Health Policy programmes and modules at the University of Plymouth, UK. Dean has since taken up a similar role and post at Massey University in New Zealand. He is a prolific publisher in recent years and is especially interested in the conceptual development of health promotion and health education theory and practice. His research favours the use of action research methods and is centred upon health promotion and health education practice within the acute clinical environment.

Ann Wilcock is an eminent occupational therapist with an international reputation. She has been employed in occupational therapy education in Australia for the last 25 years and has also held visiting professorial appointments in the United Kingdom. She is currently Professor of Occupational Therapy at Deakin University. She has published widely but is perhaps best known for her two-volume history of occupational therapy (2001) *A Journey from Self Health to Prescription*, and (2002) *A Journey from Prescription to Self Health*, London: College of Occupational Therapists.

Acknowledgements

I would like to acknowledge and thank all the contributors for their enthusiasm and support for this text and all those who have helped with the development of ideas in individual chapters. A special word of thanks goes to Bethan Rylance for her highly efficient support and assistance in finalising the manuscript and to Jon Reed and Magenta Lampson at Palgrave Macmillan for their encouragement throughout.

List of Acronyms

ACPICR	Association of Chartered Physiotherapists Interested in Cardiac Rehabilitation
AHPs	Allied Health Professionals
AHPwSI	Allied Health Professionals with Special Interests
AIMH(UK)	Association of Infant Mental Health UK
AR	Action Research
BDA	British Dietetic Association
BHF	British Heart Foundation
BMI	Body Mass Index
CAOT	Canadian Association of Occupational Therapists
CAT	Cognitive Analytical Therapy
CBT	Cognitive Behaviour Therapy
CETHV	Council for the Education and Training of Health Visitors
CHD	Coronary Heart Disease
CNG	Community Nutrition Group
CNS	Central Nervous System
COMA	Committee on the Medical Aspects of Food Policy
COT	College of Occupational Therapists
CPHVA	Community Practitioner and Health Visitors Association
CSP	Chartered Society of Physiotherapy
CT	Cognitive Therapy
CVD	Cardiovascular Disease
DfEE	Department for Education and Employment
DfES	Department for Education and Science

DoH	Department of Health
DSP	Diabetes Specialist Podiatrists
EDNOS	Eating Disorders Not Otherwise Specified
EHC	Emergency Hormonal Contraception
EULAR	European League Against Rheumatism
FPH	Faculty of Public Health
GAS	Goal Attainment Scaling
GP	General Practitioner
HDA	Health Development Agency
HEA	Health Education Authority
HImP	Health Improvement Programmes
HPH	Health Promoting Hospitals
HVA	Health Visitors Association
ICD	International Classification of Diseases
ICF	International Classification of Functioning, Disability and Health
ICIDH	International Classification of Impairments, Disabilities and Handicaps
IPT	Interpersonal Psychotherapy
MCA	Medicines Control Agency
MET	Motivational Enhancement Therapies
MI	Myocardial Infarction
MS	Multiple Sclerosis
NACNE	National Advisory Committee on Nutrition Education
NHS	National Health Service
NICE	National Institute for Clinical Excellence
NMC	Nursing and Midwifery Council
NOS	National Osteoporosis Society
NSF	National Service Frameworks
NZGG	New Zealand Guideline Group
OA	Osteoarthritis

PALS	Patient Advice and Liaison Service
PAR	Participatory Action Research
PCT	Primary Care Trust
PGD	Patient Group Directions
PNF	Proprioceptive Neuromuscular Facilitation
POM	Prescription Only Medicine
PRUs	Pupil Referral Units
RA	Rheumatoid Arthritis
RCACP	Rheumatic Care Association of Chartered Physiotherapists
RCN	Royal College of Nursing
RPSGB	Royal Pharmaceutical Society of Great Britain
SCP	Society for Chiropodists and Podiatrists
SEBC	Stages of Exercise Behaviour Change
SHEPS	The Society of Health Education and Promotion Specialists
SIGN	Scottish Intercollegiate Guidelines Network
SLT	Speech and Language Therapy
SWPHO	South West Public Health Observatory
UKCC	United Kingdom Central Council
WHO	World Health Organisation
WHOQOL	World Health Organisation Quality of Life

Foreword

This book occupies an important niche in health promotion literature. It presents an overview of professional activities in contemporary health promotion at a time when critical reflection is more pertinent than ever.

We are on the cusp of the twentieth anniversary of the Ottawa Charter for Health Promotion. In 2005 in Bangkok the World Health Organisation will lead a re-examination of this document, and by the time this book is in many readers' hands, a Bangkok Charter on health promotion will have been adopted. At the International Union for Health Promotion and Education's global conference in Vancouver in 2007, both Charters will again be in the spotlight.

The fact that there is ongoing discussion of the need for a new directive indicates how the Ottawa Charter continues to have significance, despite the remarkable developments since its adoption 20 years ago. Indeed, the best test of the Bangkok Charter's impact will be the degree of attention it receives in 2025, when the young readers of this book have aged into the vanguard of health promotion leadership.

That health promotion is contemporaneous is indubitable. Yet it is not merely a theoretical debate. It is clear that the high level political machinations that culminate in health promotion Charters and Declarations have significance for the day-to-day work of health professionals.

It is evident that health promotion provides common ground for many health professionals, which enhances the quality and effectiveness of cross-discipline teamwork. Education in health promotion stimulates and enables dialogue, respect, and eagerness for collaboration, regardless of discipline-specific training. It ensures a high regard for the principles of empowerment and participation. It instils appreciation for the expertise of non-health professionals. It creates commitment to community based solutions, and to action in community settings. Health promotion's conferences, continuing education offerings, journals and newsletters help maintain the bonds forged in early training.

What relevance do health promotion's high level political processes, and Charters and Declarations, have within this? The answer is that if health promotion is to deliver in the ways mentioned, it must have mechanisms of action, it must have infrastructure, and it must have visibility in education, in practice, and in policy arenas. The existence of these essential elements should not be taken for granted. There is an attractive logic that, since health promotion has relevance to all public health work, it should be diffused in health care systems. To the contrary, health promotion's distinctiveness requires diligent preservation, in no small part because of its almost unique bridge building capability.

The Charters and Declarations ensure that health promotion remains vital, and isn't taken for granted, by providing periodic illumination with critical debate. Two outcomes of debate that can be safely anticipated are affirmation of health promotion's foundational values, and agreement on the need for ever more innovative health promotion strategies and more effective collaboration in our rapidly changing times.

An overview such as this book provides is therefore not only timely, but reflects the spirit of debate that is the very core of health promotion itself.

Maurice B. Mittelmark
President, International Union for Health
Promotion and Education
Professor and Director, International Graduate
Programme in Health Promotion
University of Bergen
February 2005

Health Promoting Practice: a Context and Overview

ANGELA SCRIVEN

Both health and health promotion are contested and imprecise terms. The Ottawa Charter, regarded by many as a seminal document on health promotion, defined the term loosely as the process of enabling people to increase control over and improve their health. The Charter accompanied this definition with a number of fundamental principles that have been influential in informing professional practice in the promotion of health over the past two decades. Health, whilst it continues to be a disputed concept, is generally considered within the health promotion literature to be a positive multidimensional concept emphasising social and personal resources as well as physical capacities (see Chapter 1 for further discussion of the Ottawa Charter and the term health promotion). Within the context of these definitions it can be seen that members of Allied Health Professions (AHPs) and nurses have much to contribute in enabling and empowering individuals and groups to increase control over and improve their health and wellbeing. They have important skills in advocacy and mediation and many are in appropriate positions to create supportive environments, be proactive in promoting healthy public policy, form multiprofessional health coalitions and work towards strengthening community action.

Evidence based health promoting practice

Health promotion within the broader framework of public health is generally considered to be more effective when comprehensive approaches based on sound evidence are adopted. The current emphasis on evidence based practice is a positive attempt to improve the quality and cost-effectiveness of health promoting interventions. There is at this time considerable debate about the nature of evidence in health promotion and what the appropriate methods are for measuring efficiency and effectiveness. It is beyond the scope of this text to present these debate in full, but the authors contributing to this text have drawn on evidence, where it is available, to support their accounts of practice.

Multiprofessional health promoting practice

Many of the recent public health policy directives, both within the UK and internationally, have encouraged partnership working and collaboration involving multiagency and multiprofessional working. These calls for intersectoral action are based on a number of arguments. It is generally recognised that health and illness are created and influenced by multiple factors, many outside of the parameters of health service policy. Health improvement therefore, requires collaboration between statutory, voluntary and private sector organisations, with efficiency and effectiveness aided when duplication of effect is avoided and service transition is as seamless as possible. It is hoped that this text, in exploring the wide range of health promoting professional activities that nurses and AHPs engage in, will not only inform practice within professional boundaries, but also encourage those working for health improvement to engage in multiprofessional teamwork. Many of the authors' accounts of practice in this text deal directly with multiprofessional action. See for example, Chapter 19 where Scott et al. make an assessment of the potential and possible tensions for dietitians working in multidisciplinary partnership across professional boundaries, and Chapter 5 where Thomas et al. discuss the ways school nurses can work effectively with other professional groups. Whilst each chapter deals with specific professional case studies, therefore, the authors demonstrate how multiprofessional action is vital to health development and offer examples of how this happens in practice (for detailed coverage of interprofessional working, see Scriven, 1998).

The organisation of the volume

The contents of this book are centred on the health promoting practice of nurses and allied health professionals. Chapters provide professional overviews and case studies of specific practice. It is not a textbook on how to promote health, but rather a reader that details the contribution of a range of important professional disciplines to health improvement and forms a companion text to *Health Promotion: Professional Perspectives* (Scriven and Orme, 2001). The book is divided into four parts, each with a discrete perspective: Part I Nursing, Part II Occupational Therapy, Part III Physiotherapy and Part IV Other Allied Health Professionals. Parts I, II and III begin with an overview chapter that explores the contexts and cultures in which the specific professional group function and outlines both the constraints on and potential for a health promoting role. These general overviews are followed by chapters that chronicle in the form of case studies of practice, examples of health promoting action in the specific profession under consideration. Part IV presents a broader representation of the health promotion and public health contribution of a wide range of AHPs, including podiatrists, speech and language therapists, dieticians, pharmacists and orthoptists. Not all health promoting practice within nursing and the allied health professions can be covered in one small volume. The selection of chapters, however, clearly demonstrates the important health promoting roles and functions of these professional groups.

The promotion of health and wellbeing is an important aspect of public health practice, with health promotion having evolved into an extremely broad range of complex approaches undertaken by a large number of diverse professional groups, both nationally and internationally (see Scriven and Garman, 2005, for a global perspective on health promotion). The book begins with a chapter that offers a critical introduction to some of the fundamental principles and methodologies that inform practitioners in the promotion of health. National and World Health Organisation (WHO) policy imperatives, such as the Ottawa Charter, will form the context for this introduction. The principle of empowerment is given particular attention as it is utilised by many contributors in the book to describe their health promoting practice.

The culture, context and progress of health promotion in nursing

Nurses have potentially a significant role in the multidisciplinary health promotion arena. The first part of the book explores this role from different nursing specialist fields and identifies a range of ways in which specialist remits afford the opportunity to promote health. Whitehead begins with an overview chapter highlighting the culture, context and progress of health promotion in nursing. There are several key arguments. The first is that most nursing disciplines have failed in their attempts to adopt a consistent and effective health promotion role. The second argument is that many nurses' health promoting practice remains firmly entrenched within a traditional preventative health education framework and is in need of a radical overhaul. Linked to this is the assertion that traditionally nurses view individualistic and behaviourally orientated *empowerment* as the mainstay of health promotion activity, whilst not fully understanding the process. Whitehead suggests that failure of nurses to take up the challenge of the more radical methodology advocated by some health promoters is because their remit is insufficiently flexible to allow this to happen. The chapter ends with tentative but nevertheless positive indications that nursing disciplines are ready to claim a more prominent health promotion position alongside other health professional groups.

Some of the arguments above reappear in Chapter 3, where Weeks et al. critically assess the health promoting role of health visitors, members of the community nursing group (now carrying the title of public health nurses) that Whitehead identifies as having most potential for promoting health. Weeks et al. make the case that health promotion has long been a central tenet of health visiting but it is often an adjunct rather than a synergistic aspect of their role. The reason given for this situation is inflexible remits that restricts the role of health visitors to young families, at an individual level, with little opportunity for engagement with broader, more radical health promotion initiatives. The authors suggest that the new public health agenda will result in more opportunity to engage in participatory community development and empowerment approaches that address significant issues, such as health inequalities and social exclusion. These emerging new health promoting functions, it is argued, will require health visitors to develop new skills, forge new partnerships and work across professional boundaries to effect and sustain health gain in individuals, groups and communities.

The authors of Chapter 4, Ashton and Rodgers, also echo the earlier arguments of Whitehead by suggesting that there has been a heavy reliance on health education in diabetes nursing. They recommend the adoption of an empowerment process to promote the health of people with diabetes, which they argue is substantially different from the traditional, health education compliance oriented approach. The chapter describes the elements of an empowerment model of behavioural change, a critique of the concept, and the challenges facing diabetes nurses wishing to implement this philosophy in their health promoting practice.

Chapter 5 explores the potential contribution of school nursing to the promotion of health, with a critical examination of current and historical aspects of their role. The authors present school nursing as an evolving nursing discipline and identify the issues that have inhibited full involvement in the promotion of health in the education sector, including fragmentation and a lack of coordination of roles and functions. Like other authors in this section, Thomas et al. end with a rallying call, urging school nurses to meet the challenges of a proactive and more radical health promoting function.

In the final chapter in Part I, Whitehead presents an innovative and comprehensive hospital nurse initiated and led health promotion strategy based on preventative osteoporosis service provision. The argument is reiterated that there has been a domination of health education in the hospital nursing field, at the expense of broader, more holistic health promotion activities, a situation regarded as surprising given the health promoting hospital initiatives. The case study, however, offers an interesting example of what can be achieved through adopting health promotion principles of participation, collaboration and multiprofessional partnerships in hospital nursing settings. The chapter ends with a note of encouragement to hospital nurses, who have the size and scope in institutional health service arenas to make themselves instrumental in developing broad and wide reaching health promotion strategies.

Promoting health through occupational therapy

Over the last two decades there has been a growing international interest by some associations of occupational therapy and their respective members in the contribution that occupational therapists can make to the multidisciplinary field of health promotion. More recently the College of Occupational Therapy (COT) in the United Kingdom has recommended that occupational therapists take a more proactive stance in the health promotion arena and have advocated the Ottawa Charter principles to inform this professional development (see Scriven and Atwal, 2004 for a detailed discussion of this initiative).

The overview to Part II of the book is written by Wilcock, who has been highly proactive at an international level in identifying the opportunities for and the barriers to the adoption of a primary health promotion professional remit by occupational therapists. Wilcock debates the actual and potential health promotion role of occupational therapy and provides strong arguments for the profession to move towards a primary health promoting agenda. Her main proposition is that occupational therapists must extend their functions beyond the amelioration of illness and become directly involved with the promotion of optimal states of health in line with more radical and primary health promotion methodologies.

Sumsion, in the second chapter of Part II, establishes the links between client centred practice and health promotion, which she argues are both integral components of occupational therapy practice. Issues of partnerships, communication, choice, power and empowerment are examined in the context of both their relevance to health promotion and to occupational therapy. Sumsion provides information that will enable occupational therapists and other healthcare workers to understand the principles of a client centred health promoting approach.

Some of Sumsion's arguments are continued in Chapter 9 where the premise presented by Atwal is that inequalities in power can impact upon communication and the outcome of the discharge process. The discussion identifies a set of tensions in the health promotion approach to discharge planning, between individual autonomy and client participation and organisational efficiency. In a similar argument to the one used in the Wilcock chapter, Atwal suggests that the dominance of the medical profession has resulted in occupational therapists being less powerful partners in health promotion arenas, and in particular in the discharge planning forums. The chapter identifies significant secondary and tertiary health promotion roles for occupational therapists in a healthy discharge process.

In the next chapter, Harries outlines the enabling role that occupational therapists can play in promoting the health of people with eating disorders. As one of the providers of psychological therapies, occupational therapists have a significant secondary health promotion role. Harries proposes that meaningful occupational engagement can be utilised as a tool for primary health promoting initiatives in this area. In particular, individuals' self-worth can be fostered through occupational challenges that are well matched to individuals' occupational capacity, promoting autonomy and self-efficacy and reducing some of the risk factors that can lead to the development of eating disorders.

As an interesting contrast, Adams and Pearce begin their chapter by arguing that occupational therapists are more inclined to address physical symptoms rather than psychological symptoms when working with people with rheumatoid arthritis (RA). The authors maintain that occupational therapists have much to offer in enabling active coping styles and initiating positive strategies that encourage the individual with RA to take responsibility for and control of their symptoms. The chapter promotes a psychosocial model of care that employs health promotion principles to improve individual autonomy and clearly demonstrates how occupational therapists can undertake an effective tertiary health promotion role.

Culture and context for promoting health through physiotherapy practice

Part III of the text is devoted to physiotherapy and begins with the contention by French and Swain in their overview chapter that physiotherapy has been dominated by doctors and largely taken a biomedical orientation to patient and client care. Their discussion of this issue identifies a number of barriers to physiotherapists adopting a more holistic and proactive health promoting role. Issues such as the domination of the medical rather than the social sciences in the undergraduate curriculum and the lack of clinical interest groups in health promotion within physiotherapy are seen as significant barrier. Recommendations are made about how physiotherapists can develop a more proactive health promoting role.

In the next chapter Ashford illustrates how recent changes to neurorehabilitation have resulted in physiotherapists adopting heath promoting principles by emphasising the importance of client empowerment and participation in the rehabilitation process. The need for the physiotherapist to promote health and independence both in the rehabilitation environment and beyond is identified.

Jones and Hinton also offer an example of the empowering role of physiotherapists, this time in a cardiac rehabilitation setting. The authors examine how the cardiac rehabilitation programme supports important lifestyle behaviour modifications, aiming to empower the family as a whole to make these changes and be able to maintain them in the long term.

De Souza et al. examine the broader health promoting role of the physiotherapist in the long-term management of multiple sclerosis (MS). A self-help model of care that places the person with MS and their carers at the centre of decision making and managing change in their lives is seen as crucial. This health promoting approach underpins the successful empowerment of individuals in developing self-help strategies.

The education of the person with arthritis and their family in self-management strategies is an important secondary health promoting role undertaken by the physiotherapist and is examined by Lloyd in the final chapter of this part of the book. A full discussion of the health promotion interventions that can be used is considered in the light of the nature of the arthritis, the resources available and the functional deficits of the person with arthritis.

The health promotion contribution of other Allied Health Professionals

The current UK government health policy agenda emphasises interprofessional collaboration and the breaking down of traditional professional boundaries, a growth in Allied Health Professions' scope of practice and an expansion in roles relating to the promotion of health. The final part of the book offers insights in to the specific roles and functions of a wider group of Allied Health Professionals. There is a clear impression given of the diverse range of health promoting practice undertaken by the Allied Health Professionals and of the need to work in partnerships across a wide range of professional boundaries.

Part IV begins with a chapter that focuses on the profession of podiatry. The role development within this profession has been significant. Borthwick and Nancarrow outline the emerging specialist focus and the reshaping of the therapeutic role in the context of NHS modernisation and the multidisciplinary public health arena, identifying areas where more health promoting functions are being established.

In Chapter 18 Law et al. demonstrate how speech and language therapists are involved in primary, secondary and tertiary health promotion across the whole lifespan. They argue that the key to appropriate health promotion is a cohesive team approach and the clear delivery of non-contradictory messages. The chapter explores the central role of communication to health promotion and the particular challenges that this poses to professionals working with people with communication disabilities.

The authors of Chapter 19 propose that the barriers to healthy eating need to be overcome through empowerment of individuals and communities. Whilst they discuss the health promotion role of the dietitian with individuals with established medical needs, Scott et al. argue for effective collaborative health promoting partnerships and for greater integration of health promotion practice between dieticians, nutritionists, health visitors, health promotion specialists and other health professionals to promote better nutrition of the population as a whole.

The role of community pharmacists in promoting and maintaining the health of the communities they serve is now well established. The chapter by Armstrong et al. presents evidence to demonstrate that community pharmacists make a positive contribution to health improvement in activities linked to key public health targets such as smoking cessation, coronary heart disease (CHD), the supply of emergency contraception, immunisation, and drug misuse services. The authors end by recommending that pharmacists broaden their health promoting endeavours to a more proactive role within the wider population.

In the final chapter of the book, Rowe and Henshall argue that whilst orthoptists address specialist orthoptic areas of ocular alignment and movement, and associated vision defects, their expanded role offers health promoting opportunities with patients with visual field abnormalities, cataract, glaucoma, stroke and neurological rehabilitation, specific literacy difficulties and low vision impairment.

Conclusions on the health promoting role of nurses and Allied Health Professionals

The text does not pretend to offer a full insight into the contribution that nurses and Allied Health Professionals can make to health promotion. It sets out, however, to illustrate that the professional groups around which the book is based offer a significant and expanding contribution to the promotion of health. The accounts of practice demonstrate both professional opportunities and some of the inhibiting factors that constrain health promotion activity. What must also be remembered is that health promotion, like other aspects of work within the health and social care professions, is normally achieved through multisectoral action in partnership or alliance working. Many chapters focus directly on this.

There are a number of conclusions that can be drawn from across the contributions in this book. The first is that historically the bioscientific model has tended to dominate practice in nursing and in the Allied Health Professions and creates a tension and a major inhibiting factor for more radical participation in health promotion initiatives. There is an indication that health education dominates as an approach and on occasion the use of the term empowerment indicates that there needs to be more critical understanding of this complex process. Whilst there is recognition by all the authors of the potential for their profession to promote the health and wellbeing of individuals and groups, some professional groups appear to be more advanced in both their conceptual understanding and commitment to a health promotion function. There are clearly aspects that must be attended to if nurses and Allied Health Professionals are to establish a strong primary health promotion identity. It is apparent from this book that the obstacles to overcome are the inflexibility of professional remits and, for some groups, the lack of training in health promotion.

There would seem to be many opportunities for nurses and AHPs to engage in more radical and synergistic health promotion activities, within the public health role that the government envisages for these professions. The specialist skills and unique access of these professionals to a wide range of population groups offers them real potential for health promotion, both within professional boundaries and through strong collaborative partnerships for health. Despite the evident barriers to overcome before nurses and AHPs are fully capable of fulfilling their health promoting ambitions, the accounts of practice that make up this book demonstrate a serious commitment and valuable contributions to the promotion of health.

References

Scriven, A. (ed.) (1998) *Alliances in Health Promotion: Theory and Practice.* Basingstoke: Palgrave Macmillan.

Scriven, A. and Atwal, A. (2004) Occupational therapists as primary health promoters: opportunities and barriers. *British Journal of Occupational Therapy* 27 (10): 424–9.

Scriven, A. and Garman, S. (eds) (2005) *Promoting Health: Global Perspectives.* Basingstoke: Palgrave Macmillan.

Scriven, A. and Orme, J. (eds) (2001) *Health Promotion: Professional Perspectives.* Basingstoke: Palgrave Macmillan.

CHAPTER 1

Promoting Health: Perspectives, Policies, Principles, Practice

ANGELA SCRIVEN

The health professions occupy an interconnected world where multiprofessional action is commonly regarded as a prerequisite to the achievement of health improvement. One area of practice that has been significant in pulling together different professional groups under the same banner is health promotion (Scriven, 1998; Scriven and Orme, 2001). With the emergence in the United Kingdom (UK) of the new public health agenda, building multiprofessional understanding and capabilities in the promotion of health is now seen as crucial. Accordingly, the overall purpose of this text is to provide insights into health promotion as a field of activity, with the function of this opening chapter being to introduce some important health promotion perspectives, policies and principles and assess the implications of these for practice. This assessment will provide the background for the remaining chapters that chronicle specific examples of nursing and Allied Health Professions (AHPs) health promoting endeavour.

Perspectives on the origins and meaning of health promotion

Health promotion is a fairly recent idiom, used for the first time in the mid 1970s (Lalonde, 1974), although it is accepted that the objective of promoting health predates the explicit use of the expression (Macdonald, 1998; Webster and French, 2002). Whilst there are a number of different accounts of the first use of the term, see Green and Kreuter (1991) for one of these, the most pertinent and creative explanation of the origins of health promotion as a field of activity is offered by Green and Frankish (2002: 322). They describe in poetic terms how health promotion arose from the fertile delta produced by the converging streams of health education, the self-care movement, public

1

health, social and preventative medicine, and the women's movement. Green and Frankish maintain that health promotion was created from the community development and participatory approaches to public health that have been a feature of work in low-income countries and subsequently commandeered by high-income countries in Europe, North America and Australasia to alleviate health service cost pressures. Many other authors acknowledge these tangled roots of health promotion (Nutbeam, 2002; Scriven and Garman, 2005), but none so vividly as Seedhouse (2004: 27) who accuses health promotion of being a magpie profession that has accumulated a stockpile of adopted techniques, models and goals.

An important catalyst for the development of health promotion has been the surpassing of communicable diseases by non-communicable diseases as the key cause of morbidity and mortality globally (Yach et al., 2005) and the epidemi-ological links that are now firmly established between noncommunicable diseases and lifestyles (Department of Health (DoH), 1999, 2004a, 2004b; House of Commons Health Committee, 2004). The challenge of both pre-venting and reducing the prevalence of noncommunicable diseases resulted in the notion of refocussing upstream (McKinley, 1979). The McKinley analogy proved to be convincing arguments for the development of health promotion, articulating the need and the desire for preventative approaches to be adopted that target the general population. Whilst preventative goals have tended to dominate policy and practice over the 30 years since its inception, a shared understanding of the meaning and purpose of health promotion continues to be elusive (Cribb and Duncan, 2002; Laverack, 2004). A radical position and summing up of key issues relating to the problems associated with a lack of a clear definition can be found in Seedhouse (2004: 28–32). Seedhouse is tenacious in putting the case that the meaning of health promotion remains murky, that there is a perpetual theoretical fog and that the often quoted Ottawa Charter definition of health promotion (taken from World Health Organisation (WHO), 1986) offers infinite scope and purpose and as a conse-quence is meaningless. This last point reiterates the argument put by Tannahill (1985) some 20 years earlier, when he asserted that health promotion had so many meanings it had become meaningless.

These claims are legitimate. Shared meaning is fundamentally important to professional unity and identity and currently there is no universally agreed description of health promotion as a term or as a field of professional activity. This is due in part to the diversity of disciplinary and ideological perspectives that have influenced the evolution of health promotion, resulting in conflict-ing conceptualisations and what some regard as a paradigm struggle over philosophical assumptions (Falk Raphael, 1999). The close association of health promotion with medicine and public health, for example, has given rise to disease reduction objectives, with disease prevention and public health often used in an interchangeable way with the term health promotion (DoH, 2001a). The equally strong links between health promotion and the social sciences (Bunton and MacDonald, 2002) have resulted in it being celebrated as a social movement (Mittelmark, 2005) addressing broad determinants of health, with empowerment as a primary goal (Laverack, 2004). Health promotion has also been viewed as a mechanism for controlling populations (Nettleton and Bunton, 1995). All of the above ideological disciplinary influences are apparent in the multiplicity of approaches to heath promotion discussed later in the chapter.

There is little doubt that promoting health is a political activity, with significant ethical dilemmas (Cribb and Duncan, 2002), conflicting values and potential ambiguity endemic in practice. The complexities of these issues are one reason why there is still an apparent lack of an agreed meaning. Over the 30 years since the term was first penned, definitions have ranged from the very general, such as the Ottawa Charter version castigated by Seedhouse above, which describes health promotion as a process of enabling people to exert control over and improve their health (WHO, 1986) to the highly individual and/or specific, such as Tones (2001) who argues that health promotion is the radical militant wing of public health and is essentially made up of two approaches, healthy public policy and health education.

Whilst it remains impossible to provide a precise and universally accepted definition of health promotion, there is some consensus in the literature about what it entails as an endeavour. The term refers to a multiprofessional, holistic field of overlapping strategies (Tannahill, 1985) at primary, secondary, tertiary and quaternary levels encompassing behavioural, health education, community development, empowerment, preventative and protective approaches undertaken in a range of settings alongside the environmental, legal, fiscal and other policy measures designed to advance health (Jones, 2000; Katz et al., 2000).

Primary, secondary, tertiary and quaternary health promotion

The four different levels of health promotion mentioned above (see also Table 1.1) are important in understanding the breadth of action. Primary health promotion would reflect McKinley's (1979) vision of upstream, preventative activity, targeting the general population with the aim of averting ill health and disability. Approaches used in primary health promotion are diverse and might range from health education to legislative, fiscal and policy measures (see Chapters 19 and 20 for examples of primary health promotion).

Secondary health promotion is directed at individuals or population groups where health damaging activity has already occurred. Health promotion at this level might involve behavioural and empowerment approaches, such as dietitians running weight loss programmes with obese patients or a physiotherapist enabling a patient to rehabilitate following a coronary heart attack. The purpose here would be to change health damaging habits and increase health enhancing behaviour to prevent ill health moving to a chronic or irreversible

Table 1.1   Levels of health promotion

Level	Purpose	Example
Primary	Promoting the health of the general population to maintain health, prevent health damaging behaviour, prevent ill health and improve quality of life	School nurses engaged in sex education in schools, to prevent sexually transmitted diseases and teenage pregnancies and improve relationship skills
Secondary	Promoting the health of individuals or groups where health damaging behaviour has already occurred, to change behaviour and prevent health moving to a chronic or irreversible stage	Dietitians working with obese patients to support weight loss and a return to a healthy BMI
Tertiary	Promoting the health of those with chronic conditions or a disability to enhance quality of life and potential for healthy living	Physiotherapists working with patients with arthritis to improve functional ability and quality of life
Quaternary	Promoting the emotional, social and physical health and wellbeing of the terminally ill	Hospice nurses working to improve the quality of life of terminally ill patients

Sources: Using ideas from Ewles and Simnett (2003): 29 and Hancock (2001)

stage and, where possible, to restore people to their former state of health (see Chapter 10 and Chapter 14 for examples of secondary health promotion).

Tertiary health promotion aims to enable individuals or groups who have chronic conditions or are disabled to maximise their potential for healthy living. This might involve podiatrists working with diabetes patients to prevent amputations (Chapter 17) or physiotherapists enabling MS sufferers to enhance their wellbeing and quality of life (Chapter 15) or diabetes nurses empowering patients to self manage (Chapter 4).

Quaternary health promotion concentrates on facilitating optimal states of empowerment and emotional, social and physical wellbeing during a terminal stage. Whilst there are no direct examples of this level of health promotion in this text, many Allied Health Professionals and nurses would have a remit for promoting health at this level.

The contribution of health promotion to public health

There are strong arguments pointing to the centrality of health promotion to public health, due in part to its contribution to the development of thought and theory in an evolving social model of health (Bunton and MacDonald, 2002: 9; Nutbeam, 2002). The rejection of a disease orientated medical or pathogenic model of health differentiates health promotion from the more medically orientated aspects of public health and is crucial in understanding health promotion practice. Health promotion involves distinctive methodologies based on a positive, salutogenic (Antonovsky, 1996) interpretation, with health seen as an holistic concept incorporating wellbeing and involving more than the absence of disease or disability (hence the notion that health can be promoted at both tertiary and quaternary levels) (see Tones and Green, 2004: 8–13 for further analysis of these points).

There is a growing body of evidence to demonstrate that health promotion results in improved public health outcomes and has a significant role in tackling the wider determinants of health (International Union of Health Promotion and Health Education [IUHPE], 1999). Nonetheless, there is still much to do in convincing policy makers and the public health fraternity of the distinctive value of health promotion (Scriven, 2002, 2003; Scott-Samuel, 2003; Scriven, 2004) and ensuring that the evidence base is rigorous (Watson and Platt, 2000; Peersman and Oakley, 2001).

The health promotion policy environment

It is understandable why some assert that the current policy environment in the UK is highly conducive to the promotion of health (Parish, 2001; Nutbeam, 2003). The second strategy for improving the health of the population in England (DoH, 1999) (also reflected in the late 1990s by similar public health strategies in Wales, Scotland and Northern Ireland) shifted attention from the strong emphasis on individual lifestyles of the earlier strategy (DoH, 1992) to the reduction of health inequalities through the removal of social or environmental barriers to health. This indicated a move away from individual lifestyle approaches that had dominated health promotion for the previous three decades (for the historical context of public health policy see Baggott, 2000; Peersman, 2001; Webster and French, 2003). One contradictory element however, which has been replicated in the new public health white paper for England (DoH, 2004b) was the setting of targets for the reduction in the morbidity and mortality rates linked to cancers, accidents, mental illness and cardiovascular diseases, demonstrating that tackling non-communicable disease and disability remains a key public health objective.

Health promotion is also firmly embedded in other policies. The NHS Plan (DoH, 2000a), for example, and the National Service Frameworks (such as the DoH, 2000b) have extended the roles of nurses and therapists, whilst Shifting the Balance of Power (DoH, 2001b) in creating Primary Care Trusts has provided new opportunities for multidisciplinary health promotion partnership working at a local level.

UK policies have been strongly influenced by international health promotion declarations. One such document, the Ottawa Charter (WHO, 1986) is regarded as seminal in the evolution of health promotion (Scriven, 2005; Scriven and Garman, 2005). Important elements of the Charter were prioritising the social model of health, targeting of the wider determinants, particularly health inequalities, and the linking of the achievement of health with structural adjustment brought about through political, economic and social change. These priorities indicate that the attainment of health is not just the business of those professionals who work within the health and social services, but that significant measures to improve health must be taken outside these sectors and are the responsibility of politicians and planners. Those directly engaged in health promotion are encouraged to act as *advocates*, ensuring the conditions favourable to health are in place, as *enablers* to facilitate people to achieve their fullest health potential and to overcome health inequalities and finally as *mediators*, to arbitrate between differing interests in society for the pursuit of health.

The charter recommended five health promotion actions, which have proved highly influential. The first focuses on *building healthy public policy* in all sectors and at all levels, encouraging coordinated action to ensure health, income and social policies foster greater equity through legislative, fiscal, taxation and organisational change. The second action concerns *creating supportive environments*, providing a template for a socio ecological approach to health and the principle of reciprocal maintenance with an emphasis on individual and community responsibility. The third recommendation centres on *strengthening community action*, establishing participatory community development processes that aim to empower communities to take ownership and control of their own health. The fourth action involves *developing personal skills* that enable control to be exercised over health, to make choices conducive to health and to cope with chronic illness and injuries. The final action is concerned with *reorienting health services*, resulting in the health sector moving in a health promotion direction, beyond its responsibility for providing clinical and curative services towards a healthcare system that contributes to the pursuit of health. This changing mandate has seen the development of collaborative health partnerships across sectors and disciplines, and a refocusing on the individual as a participant in health decisions.

The principles and the agendas established in Ottawa and developed subsequently in Adelaide (WHO, 1988) (healthy public policies) Sundvall (WHO, 1991) (supportive environments) and Jakarta (1997) (partnerships) are now firmly embedded in both UK, including the new white paper for England (DoH, 2004b) and international policy directives, and have been reflected in a wide range of initiatives, such as Health For All (WHO, 1998) and the settings approach to health promotion.

Health promoting principles and practice

Since Ottawa, health promotion has evolved into a multi professional field of activity undertaken across a wide range of sectors and settings, both nationally and internationally. A feature of health promotion in the UK has been the establishment of a specialised form of provision, mainly delivered through the NHS. These health promotion specialists, to use a generic term, have a full-time health promotion remit that embrace the Ottawa principles. As a group they are associated with anti authoritarian, community development approaches rooted in a social model of health and an empowering philosophy (Kelly and Charlton, 1992) with an emphasis on the wider determinants of health. Prioritising the wider determinants is critical. Many authors from Black et al. (1980), Whitehead (1992) to Acheson (1998) and Graham (2000) have noted that health is largely determined by economic and environmental conditions. These determinants are untouched by a narrow health education approach that has dominated the work of some professional groups (see Part I, Chapter 2 of this book for further discussion of this point in relation to nursing practice).

The Society of Health Education and Promotion Specialist (SHEPS) established the principles and philosophy that they believe should guide health promotion practice (SHEPS, 2002) much of which has relevance to nurses and AHP practitioners. In particular, they advocate the involvement of service users and the general population as equal partners in the development of health, with participation and empowerment as paramount goals.

Approaches used to promote health

Entire books are devoted to the approaches, models, principles and theories employed in health promotion (for excellent examples see Ewles and Simnett, 2003; Nutbeam and Harris, 2003; Tones and Green, 2004). It is only possible in this opening chapter to offer a very brief overview.

Approaches tend to span a spectrum from authoritarian top-down to participatory bottom–up modes, and from a focus on individuals to targeting the whole population (see Figure 1.1).

Chapters 2, 7 and 12 of this book suggest that nurses and Allied Health Professionals have a strong association with authoritarian approaches targeting individuals or small groups, with interventions that fall in to the top left-hand segment of Figure 1.1. There are other chapters in this book, however, which illustrate a significant emphasis on participatory, client-centred, empowerment approaches. The Ottawa Charter established the conditions for empowerment to become a key philosophical tenet for health promotion, but it remains a complex term often used as a catchword (Jones, 2000), making its position as a guiding principle problematic. In essence, empowerment is a process that provides the means for individual or groups to develop the capacity of choice (Labonte, 2004) and become more involved in, able to take control of and make decisions about personal or community health and wellbeing. How empowerment is facilitated in practice is generally lacking in empirical insight (see Tones, 1995, 2001; Labonte, 1996; Raeburn and Rootman, 1998; Laverack, 2004, for influential work in this area).

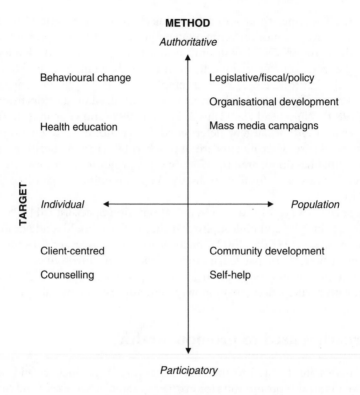

METHOD

Authoritative

Behavioural change   Legislative/fiscal/policy

                                      Organisational development

Health education   Mass media campaigns

Individual ←——————————————————→ *Population*

Client-centred   Community development

Counselling   Self-help

Participatory

Figure 1.1   Health promotion approaches

Source: Adapted from Beattie (1991)

Empowerment in practice

In an attempt to apply empowerment to practice, some authors have identified and isolated what they consider to be the requisites of individual empowerment and the key characteristics of what might constitute an empowered person (see Scriven and Stiddard, 2003 for a fuller discussion of this point). Some authors approach empowerment from a psychological perspective. Gutierrez (1990), for example, distinguishes key conditions as increasing self-efficacy, developing group consciousness, reducing self-blame and assuming personal responsibility for change. This interpretation concentrates on self-evaluation, internal thought and perception. Using a sociological standpoint Weeden and Weiss (1993) define empowerment in terms of ways of feeling, ways of thinking and ways of behaving, whereas Stein (1997) identifies personal factors and categorises them into those of an internal/psychological nature and those that are situation/social factors.

Table 1.2 Personal development linked
to empowerment

Personal characteristic	Area of enhancement
Psychological perception	Self-esteem Self-efficacy Internal locus of control
Cognitive development	Health information Critical consciousness
Life skills	Decision making Assertiveness Interpersonal skills

From the literature, including the examples outlined very briefly above, it is possible to draw three main threads specific to the personal factors and competencies that health professionals would need to develop when aiming to empower individuals or groups (see Table 1.2).

The first is psychological perception that involves enhancing self-esteem, self-efficacy and internal locus of control. The second relates to cognitive development and would involve increasing awareness of health information and a political dimension through the raising of a critical consciousness. Finally, the acquisition of skills, such as decision making, assertiveness and interpersonal skills is regarded as fundamentally important to achieving an empowered state. Clearly the personal characteristics and competencies outlined above are part of a dynamic and complex mesh of interrelating issues that determine health action, analysed in detail by Tones and Green (2004: 75–105). Tones (2001: 16) has also argued that empowerment must be seen as more than just an ideological commitment and provides a breakdown of the role of the health professional in an empowering encounter, which includes communication, motivation and the facilitation of decision making and the provision of support. For nurses and AHPs, this would involve empowering processes being incorporated seamlessly in all health promotion encounters and also acknowledging that external determinants relating to power and control will influence client or community progress towards empowerment.

Linking health promotion approaches

To be truly effective, a comprehensive range of health promoting action is vital. In smoking prevention, for example, a combination of approaches might involve health education (educating young people on the health risks of smoking, developing assertiveness skills so that they have the ability to resist pressure to smoke), individual empowerment (building self-esteem and internal locus of control), community development (communities lobbying for a ban on billboard advertising close to schools and for a ban on smoking on

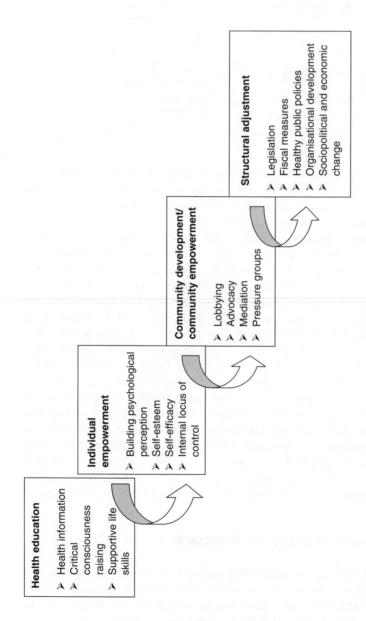

Health education

∧ Health information
∧ Critical
  consciousness
  raising
∧ Supportive life
  skills

Individual empowerment

∧ Building psychological
  perception
∧ Self-esteem
∧ Self-efficacy
∧ Internal locus of
  control

Community development/ community empowerment

∧ Lobbying
∧ Advocacy
∧ Mediation
∧ Pressure groups

Structural adjustment

∧ Legislation
∧ Fiscal measures
∧ Healthy public policies
∧ Organisational development
∧ Sociopolitical and economic
  change

Figure 1.2 Relationship between key health promotion approaches

public transport) and structural adjustment (taxation on cigarettes, legislation connected with advertising).

Health promotion approaches are not autonomous. In a comprehensive methodology as outlined above, the relationship between approaches is central (see Figure 1.2).

Health education is essential to empowerment. It would be difficult for individuals or communities to be empowered without health information or critical consciousness raising or having developed supportive life skills. *Individual empowerment* facilitates *community development* and *community empowerment*. The mediation, advocacy, lobbying and pressure groups that are some of the key features of community empowerment are necessary to bring about *structural adjustment* in the form of legislative outcomes or fiscal measures and so on.

Critiquing health promotion approaches

The early dominance of a preventative upstream philosophy discussed earlier has encouraged a lifestyle perspective that has resulted in a significant disciplinary influence of the behavioural and social sciences in shaping approaches to health promotion practice (Bunton and Macdonald, 2002; Scriven and Garman, 2005). Consequently, the social, environmental and structural conditions that strongly determine morbidity and mortality rates (Marmot and Wilkinson, 1999) have been less instrumental in influencing the nature of professional health promoting practice over the past three decades. The domination of lifestyle approaches has provoked a number of sociopolitical critiques of health promotion, including structural, surveillance and consumption critiques (see Nettleton and Bunton, 1995) and feminist critiques (Daykin and Naidoo, 1995). It is crucial that nurses and AHPs are reflective and critical of their own practice, develop ethical insights and sound understanding of these sociopolitical critiques, in order to extend their health promoting capabilities.

The contribution of nurses and AHP to health promotion practice

Recent UK government directive insists that health services must evolve from dealing with acute problems through more effective control of chronic conditions to promoting the maintenance of good health (DoH, 2004b; Wanless, 2004). What this and other policy directive are demanding is for those working in a health service to adopt a primary health promoting role.

AHPs are also being asked to identify how they can contribute to improving people's health (East, 2004) including how they might tackle current public health targets, particularly obesity, smoking and sexually transmitted infections. East (2004) asserts that all AHPs have a role in promoting public health and argues that more effort and investment must go into boosting the number of AHPs and other professionals who can be involved in primary preventative activities. Wynne (2004) supports and advances this view by suggesting that AHPs could also be more proactive in tackling the wider determinants of health and health inequalities.

The further integration of health promotion into the remits of nurses and Allied Health Professionals seems like an astute strategy, as they have great frequency and duration of contact with the clients in their care and they are also perceived as credible sources of health promotion by patients (Nagel et al., 1999). However, there is much to overcome in advancing this approach. In a health service environment of limited resources and significant throughput targets, it is often difficult to move to an upstream position where promoting health takes precedence over curing disease.

Some authors both within and outside this book believe that the potential for health promotion has been largely underutilised and unrecognised in both nursing and in the Allied Health Professions. Law et al., for example, in Chapter 18 argue that AHPs have not been explicitly associated with health promotion not because of any lack of involvement in the area, merely that their activity has tended to be construed as clinical, working with the patient to alleviate the effects of illness or disability rather than promoting health and wellbeing in the population in general. In an attempt to redress this balance the broad range of health promotional activities carried out by the Allied Health Professions has recently been described, emphasising their central role in the promotion of health and wellbeing (DoH, 2003).

The report on obesity (House of Commons Health Committee, 2004) is an appropriate example of the important role that nurses and AHPs could take in achieving the health goals relating to this significant public health issue. AHPs and nurses have particular skills, knowledge and personal contact with patients that place them in a very strong position to drive health promotion initiatives to tackle obesity across the NHS. Pearson (2004) argues that AHPs are not only ideally placed but also have a responsibility to promote healthy eating and exercise in a multidisciplinary approach, and calls for physiotherapists, occupational therapist and dietitians and podiatrists to work closely together to deliver health promotion approaches. These nurse/AHP multidisciplinary partnerships can be wide ranging. An example of an exercise activity and healthy eating health promotion activity for people with learning disabilities recently established in Dorset (AHP Bulletin, 2004) has dietitians involved in menu planning, physiotherapists developing exercise programmes, nursing staff monitoring changes in medication needs as a result of lifestyle changes, occupational therapists involved in prescribing activity, podiatrists ensuring footwear and care do not limit activity, and speech and language therapists helping with communication strategies.

In concluding, it is important to acknowledge that in order to promote health effectively a critical and reflective stance must be taken. Practitioners need to be aware of the conflicting conceptualisations of health and health promotion and the competing judgments on the determinant of health. They need to have developed an understanding of the body of theory relating to health behaviour and health promotion in general and the ethical and political dimensions associated with health promoting activities. This chapter has only been able to introduce some of the more general issues relating to health promoting practice, but in the course of doing this has referenced other important literature in the field. A key focus has been questions around coherently defining heath promotion and understanding some of the complex principles that influence practice, such as empowerment. Health promotion has matured and is now a national and global objective embedded in many policy statements. Whilst no one particular group owns health promotion, for nurses and Allied Health Professionals it is seen as part of established and broadening professional remits. The chapters that follow identify just some of the contribution that AHPs and nurses can make to the promotion of health and demonstrate that whilst there may not be a universally agreed meaning, their health promoting endeavours are both worthwhile and extensive.

References

Acheson, D. (1998) *Independent Inquiry into Inequalities in Health Report.* London: The Stationery Office.

AHP Bulletin (2004) www.dh.gov/uk/publicationsandstatistics/bulletins/alliedhealthprofessionalbulletin/ Issued 26 June.

Antonovsky, A. (1996) The salutogenic model as a theory to guide health promotion. *Health Promotion Internationa,* **11** (1): 11–18.

Baggott, R. (2000) *Public Health: Policy and Politics.* Basingstoke: Palgrave Macmillan.

Beattie, A. (1991) Knowledge and control in health promotion: a test case for social policy and social theory. In Gabe, J., Calnan, M. and Bury, M. (eds) *The Sociology of the Health Service.* London: Routledge.

Black, D., Morris, J., Smith, C. and Townsend, P. (1980) *The Black Report.* London: Penguin.

Bunton, R. and Macdonald, G. (eds) (2002) *Health Promotion: Disciplines, Diversity and developments,* second edition. London: Routledge.

Cribb, A. and Duncan, P. (2002) *Health Promotion and Professional Ethics.* Oxford: Blackwell Science.

Daykin, N. and Naidoo, J. (1995) Feminist critiques of health promotion. In Bunton, R., Nettleton, S. and Burrows, R. (eds) *The Sociology of Health Promotion: Critical Analysis of Consumption, Lifestyle and Risk.* London: Routledge.

Department of Health (1992) *The Health of the Nation.* London: HMSO.

Department of Health (1999) *Saving Lives: Our Healthier Nation.* London: The Stationery Office.

Department of Health (2000a) *The NHS Plan. A Plan for Investment. A Plan for Reform.* London: The Stationery Office.

Department of Health (2000b) *National Service Framework for Coronary Heart Disease.* London: The Stationery Office.

Department of Health (2001a) *The Report of the Chief Medical Officer's Project to Strengthen the Public Health Function.* London: The Stationery Office.

Department of Health (2001b) *Shifting the Balance of Power within The NHS: Securing Delivery.* London: The Stationery Office.

Department of Health (2003) *Ten Key Roles for Allied Health Professionals.* London: Department of Health Publications.

Department of Health (2004a) *Choosing Health? A Consultation on Action to Improve People's Health.* London: HMSO.

Department of Health (2004b) *Choosing Health: Making Healthier Choices Easier.* London: The Stationery Office.

East, K. (2004) Public health consultation. *AHP Bulletin.* London: DoH.

Ewles, L. and Simnett, I. (2003) *Promoting Health: a Practical Guide.* Edinburgh: Baillière Tindall.

Falk Raphael, A. (1999) The politics of health promotion: influences on public health promoting nursing practice in Ontario, Canada from Nightingale to Nineties. *Advances in Nursing Science* **22** (1): 23–39.

Graham, H. (ed.) (2000) *Understanding Health Inequalities.* Buckingham: Open University Press.

Green, L. W. and Frankish, J. C. (2002) Health promotion, health education and disease prevention. In *Critical Issues in Global Health.* San Francisco: Jossey-Bass.

Green, L. W. and Kreuter, M. (1991) *Health Promotion Planning: an Educational and Environmental Approach.* Mountain View, CA: Mayfield.

Gutierrez, L. M. (1990) Working with women of colour, an empowerment perspective. *Social Work* **35** (2): 149–53.

Hancock, T. (2001) Healthy people in healthy communities in a healthy world: the science art and politics of public health in the 21st century. Paper presented at the launch of the OU School of Health and Social Welfare Health Promotion and Public Health Research Group, 12 September. Milton Keynes: The Open University.

House of Commons Health Committee (2004) *Obesity: Third Report of Session 2003–2004.* London: The Stationery Office.

International Union of Health Promotion and Health Education (1999) *The Evidence of Health Promotion Effectiveness: Shaping Public Health in a New Europe.* Brussels/Luxembourg: ECSC-EC-EAEC.

Jones, L. (2000) Promoting health: everybody's business? In Katz, J., Peberdy, A. and Douglas, J. (eds) *Promoting Health: Knowledge and Practice.* Basingstoke: Macmillan (nowPalgrave Macmillan)/Open University.

Katz, J., Peberdy, A. and Douglas, J. (2000) *Promoting Health: Knowledge and Practice.* Basingstoke: Palgrave Macmillan in association with the Open University.

Kelly, M. and Charlton, B. (1992) Health promotion: time for a new philosophy? *British Journal of General Practice* June, 223–4.

Labonte, R. (1996) Measurement and practice, power issues in quality of life, health promotion and empowerment. In Renwick, R., Brown, I. and Nagler, M. (eds) *Quality of Life in Health Promotion and Rehabilitation, Conceptual Approaches, Issues and Applications.* London: Sage.

Labonte, R. (2004) Foreword. In *Health Promotion Practice: Power and Empowerment.* London: Sage.

Lalonde, M. (1974) *A New Perspective on the Health of Canadians.* Ottawa: Information Canada.

Laverack, G. (2004) *Health Promotion Practice: Power and Empowerment.* London: Sage.

Macdonald, T. H. (1998) *Rethinking Health Promotion: A Global Approach.* London: Routledge.

Marmot, M. and Wilkinson, R. (1999) *Social Determinants of Health*. Oxford: Oxford University Press.

McKinley, J. B. (1979) A case for refocusing upstream: the political economy of health. In Javco, E. G. (ed.) *Patients, Physicians and Illness*. Basingstoke: Macmillan (now Palgrave Macmillan).

Mittelmark, M. (2005) Global health promotion: challenges and opportunities. In Scriven, A. and Garman, S. (eds) *Promoting Health: Global Issues and Perspectives*. Basingstoke: Palgrave Macmillan.

Nagel, A., Schofield, M. and Redman, S. (1999) Australian nurses' smoking behaviour, knowledge and attitudes towards providing smoking cessation care to their patients. *Health Promotion International* **14** (2): 133–44.

Nettleton, S. and Bunton, R. (1995) Sociological critiques of health promotion. In Bunton, R. Nettleton, S. and Burrows, R. (eds) *The Sociology of Health Promotion: Critical Analysis of Consumption, Lifestyle and Risk*. London: Routledge.

Nutbeam, D. (2002) Foreword. In Bunton, R. and Macdonald, G. (eds) *Health Promotion: Disciplines, Diversity and Development*, second edition. London: Routledge.

Nutbeam, D. (2003) Keynote address given at a one day SHEPS conference *Health Promotion Specialists' Needs in Meeting the Public Health Agenda*, 1 April. London: Avonmouth House.

Nutbeam, D. and Harris, E. (2003) *Theory in a Nutshell: a Guide to Health Promotion Theory*, second edition. Sydney: McGraw-Hill.

Parish, R. (2001) Future research priorities and the role of the Health Development Agency. Paper presented at the launch of the OU School of Health and Social Welfare Health Promotion and Public Health Research Group, 12 September. Milton Keynes: The Open University.

Pearson, D. (2004) www.dh.gov/uk/publicationsandstatistics/bulletins/alliedhealth professionalbulletin/ Issued 26 June

Peersman, G. (2001) Promoting health: principles of practice and evaluation. In *Using Research for Effective Health Promotion*. Buckingham: Open University Press.

Peersman, G. and Oakley, A. (2001) Learning from research. In Oliver, S. and Peersman, G. (eds) *Using Research for Effective Health Promotion*. Buckingham: Open University Press.

Raeburn, J. and Rootman, I. (1998) *People Centred Health Promotion*. New York: Wiley.

Scott-Samuel, A. (2003) Specialist health promotion – can we save it before they destroy it? *Public Health News* 8 December.

Scriven, A. (1998) *Alliances in Health Promotion: Theory and Practice*. Basingstoke: Palgrave (now Palgrave Macmillan).

Scriven, A. (2002) *Report of the Survey into the Impact of Recent National Health Policies on Specialist Health Promotion Services in England*. London: Brunel University.

Scriven, A. (2003) Health promotion specialists and the multi disciplinary public health agenda: implications for postgraduate education. *Health Education Journal* **62** (2): 153–69.

Scriven, A. (2004) Health promotion specialists and their position in the multidisciplinary public health workforce in England. Presentation at the 18th World Conference on Health Promotion and Health Education, Melbourne, Australia.

Scriven, A. (2005) Promoting health: a global context and rationale. In Scriven, A. and Garman, S. (eds) *Promoting Health: Global Issues and Perspectives*. Basingstoke: Palgrave Macmillan.

Scriven, A. and Garman, S. (eds) (2005) *Promoting Health: Global Issues and Perspectives*. Basingstoke: Palgrave Macmillan.

Scriven, A. and Orme, J. (eds) (2001) *Health Promotion: Professional Perspectives*. Basingstoke: Palgrave Macmillan.

Scriven, A. and Stiddard, L. (2003) Empowering schools: translating principles into practice. *Health Education* 103 (2): 110–19.

Seedhouse, D. (2004) *Health Promotion: Philosophy, Prejudice and Practice*, second edition. Chichester: Wiley.

Society of Health Education and Promotion Specialists (2002) *Health Promotion in Transition, Paper 5: Principles and Philosophy*. Birmingham: SHEPS.

Stein, J. (1997) *Empowerment and Women's Health: Theory, Methods and Practice*. London: Zed Books.

Tannahill, A. (1985) What is health promotion? *Health Education Journal* 44: 167–8.

Tones, K. (1995) Health education as empowerment. In *Health Promotion Today*. London: Health Education Authority.

Tones, K. (2001) Health promotion: the empowerment imperative. In Scriven, A. and Orme, J. (eds) *Health Promotion: Professional Perspectives*. Basingstoke: Palgrave Macmillan.

Tones, K. and Green, J. (2004) *Health Promotion: Planning and Strategies*. London: Sage.

Wanless, D. (2004) *Securing Good Health for the Whole Population: Final Report*. London: HMSO.

Watson, J. and Platt, S. (2000) Connecting policy and practice; the challenge of health promotion research. In Watson, J. and Platt, S. (eds) *Researching Health Promotion*. London: Routledge.

Webster, C. and French, J. (2003) The cycle of conflict: the history of the public health promotion movements. In Adams, L., Amos, M. and Munro, J. (eds) *Promoting Health: Politics and Practice*. London: Sage.

Weeden, L. and Weiss, E. (1993) Women's empowerment and reproductive health programs: an evaluation paradigm. Presentation at the Annual Meeting of the Population Association of America, Cincinnati, OH. New York: Centre for Population and Family Health, Columbia University.

Whitehead, M. (1992) *The Health Divide*. London: Penguin.

World Health Organisation (1986) *Ottawa Charter for Health Promotion*. Geneva: WHO.

World Health Organisation (1988) *The Adelaide Recommendations*. Geneva: WHO.

World Health Organisation (1991) *Sundvall Statement on Supportive Environments for Health*. Geneva: WHO.

World Health Organisation (1997) *The Jakarta Declaration on Health Promotion in the 21st Century*. Geneva: WHO.

World Health Organisation (1998) *Health for All in the 21st Century* (A51/5). Geneva: WHO.

Wynne, A. (2004) Public health consultation. *AHP Bulletin*. London: DoH.

Yach, D., Beaglehole, R. and Hawkes, C. (2005) Globalisation and noncommunicable diseases. In Scriven, A. and Garman, S. (eds) *Promoting Health: Global Issues and Perspectives*. Basingstoke: Palgrave Macmillan.

PART I

NURSES' CONTRIBUTION TO THE PROMOTION OF HEALTH

CHAPTER 2

The Culture, Context and Progress of Health Promotion in Nursing

DEAN WHITEHEAD

For the last few decades, United Kingdom (UK) and global agencies have sought to highlight the importance of health promotion as a mainstay and primary driver for health service activity and reform. Today, there is a realisation that health promotion and health policy agendas govern facets of *all* health professional practice, regardless of setting or discipline. Therefore recent health service reforms in the UK, and especially those related to public health interventions, dictate that all health professional groups have a vested and specific duty to implement effective health promotion reform as a fundamental part of their practice.

For nearly a quarter of a century nursing has been heralded, from both within and outside its ranks, as the health profession most likely to spearhead a concerted health promotion reform programme within healthcare services. For instance, UK national governing bodies such as the Department of Health (DoH), Royal College of Nursing (RCN) and the United Kingdom Central Council (UKCC), now the Nursing and Midwifery Council (NMC), and international bodies have implored nurses to take on a more active health promotion role (United Kingdom Central Council, 1986; World Health Organisation (WHO), 1986; Royal College of Nursing, 1988; Department of Health and Human Services, 1991; Department of Health, 1997, 1998; National Health Service Executive, 1998; WHO, 2000). The contradictory reality, however, is that for the major part of this period nursing has failed to seize upon this opportunity and at best, only paid lip service to the presented opportunities. Thus health promotion progress and reform has been notably slow in nursing over the last 20 years. Instead nurses have, for the most part, remained firmly entrenched within the ritualised and traditional frameworks of limited and limiting health education practices. This is despite the fact that moving away from a limited and reductionist medical model of disease prevention, towards a far broader and multidimensional approach to health

19

promotion, is seen as the appropriate way forward for nursing (Liimatainen et al., 2001). This part of the book aims to put forward explanations for this state of affairs in nursing, clarify its actual and potential contribution to the important field of health promotion and its subdisciplines, and speculate on what the future holds for health promotion and nursing.

What is health promotion and how does it apply to nursing?

Health promotion has a radical wing that promises fundamental reform of health structures within communities and society as a whole (see Chapter 1 for a fuller analysis of health promotion as a contested field of activity). It has a primary concern with empowering citizens to take control of their health through methods such as community development, political advocacy, formulating integrated health strategies and social marketing (Webster and French, 2002). The changes in the health promotion literature over the last decade or so, have seen the balance shift from individual empowerment programmes to the emphasis being placed on health policy driven initiatives that work through the processes of social examination, modification and collective social action. Indeed, Rawson (2002) argues that sociopolitically orientated community development approaches are now the most authentic and ideal form of health promotion practice. Similarly, McMurray (1999: 262) indicates that the most significant shift in conceptualisation and emphasis for health promotion has been from teaching people how to manage their health, the individual and behavioural orientation, to a more socially embedded methodology that capitalises on the inherent capacity of community members to establish their own goals, strategies and priorities for health, through a socioecological, community development approach to community health.

Of course, this does not preclude individual empowerment strategies or fail to acknowledge their usefulness, but it does make the crucial distinction between individual and community empowerment. Therefore according to Wallerstein (1992: 200), health promotion in the community context is a social action process that promotes participation of people, organisations and communities towards the goals of increased individual and community control, political efficacy, improved quality of life and social justice.

Health promotion strategies are frequently based on the premise that the health of the individual is intertwined with the collective societal health of the communities that they live in and are served by. Health promotion strategies can therefore be necessarily and inherently politically based, politically driven and politically expedient activities. Accordingly, the recent health promotion literature stresses the sociopolitical nature of health promotion far more than has been the case in the past, further emphasising the broader determinants of health such as ecological, cultural, economic and environmental factors within an environmental engineering process. The desired outcomes of health promotion activity, according to Whitehead (2004) can be summarised as:

1. The need and desire to develop and implement community driven health reform based on social action, social cohesion and social capital.
2. The willingness of communities to become empowered and self-reliant with regard to determining collective health needs and priorities.
3. The attainment of health gain as a fundamental priority and a shared social objective of community.
4. The active formulation and development of public health policy driven by communities as it applies to those communities.

Using the health promotion context outlined above, the role and function of the nurse is acknowledged in health promotion activities but assumes that their intervention is only likely to be a transitional phase, designed to facilitate personal support and set up necessary resources for community based reform. Most individuals are powerless on their own to influence the overall health of their own communities and therefore need to be collectively motivated, mobilised and empowered towards the political means to address and overcome structural dilemmas and inequalities. Therefore, one goal of health promotion is the facilitation of a concerted social empowerment that creates full and organised community participation and ultimate self-reliance (Yeo, 1993: 233). It is in the early stages of community development where nurses can be most active and visible. They do so particularly through political processes such as critical consciousness raising, agenda setting, lobbying and social education programmes (Whitehead, 2003). Effective health promotion also assumes of the health professional that they are themselves autonomous, empowered, politically motivated, able to move freely in and out of health service arenas and able to collaborate at both a multiprofessional and multiagency level. If this is not the case, nurses may need to view their practices in a different light. For instance, Macdonald (1998) argues that many health professionals are not in a position to empower clients and instead offer *impowerment*. In this context, empowerment is facilitated through a client's own endeavours without reference to an authority, while *impowerment* is power conferred on clients by someone in authority. In reality, many nurses are often only in a position to act and engage in *impowering* practices.

The context of health promotion, as it has been applied to nursing in the past, is in need of a radical overhaul. Morgan and Marsh (1998) state that, although the concept of health promotion in nursing has evolved, its definition still remains too broad. The old way of looking at health promotion in nursing meant viewing individualistic and behaviourally orientated *empowerment* as the mainstay of health promotion activity. Particularly at a political level, Robinson and Hill (1998) argue that this individualistic orientation is a major obstacle to nursing related health promotion practice. Nonetheless, an increasing number of conceptual examples bring the nursing literature in line with the more recent and radical sociopolitical agenda of health promotion

(Hagedorn, 1995; Rush, 1997; Morgan and Marsh, 1998; Norton, 1998; Robinson and Hill, 1998; Shields and Lyndsey, 1998; Whitehead, 2001a, 2003). The problem for health promotion in nursing is that, although conceptually and contextually it is well defined and delineated within its literature, this clarity is rarely manifested in practice. This situation has led to a certain tension for health promotion activities in nursing practice.

The tension facing health promotion in nursing

To date, it is fair to say that most nurses have adopted a relatively limited traditional health education stance, rather than a progressive and broad ranging health promotion role. This traditional health education activity has remained firmly entrenched within biomedically orientated frameworks of service delivery that advocate the adoption of reductionist, mechanistic, individualistic and allopathic health programme activities. Thus many nurses still work within the narrowly defined behavioural change frameworks of traditional health education practice that do not readily lend themselves to the broader ranging health promotion strategies previously mentioned. Compounding this, the last decade or so has witnessed calls for a further increase in the amount of preventative health education activity that nurses undertake (Whitehead, 2001c) rather than a more active health promotion role. This follows on from Dines' (1994: 225) conclusion of a decade ago that the health education work of nurses was a constrained activity logically limited in its impact. It has subsequently taken until now for most nurses to get to grips with the recent necessary determinants of health education practices, with the broader determinants and expectations of a health promotion role put to one side. In the meantime, health promotion has advanced at a rapid pace meaning that the current health education practices of nurses are now compared against those of a more progressive health promotion paradigm, where they fare more unfavourably.

The fact that nurses continue to contextually confuse the terms health education and health promotion remains a major tension in nursing practice. The two paradigms are commonly referred to interchangeably within nursing texts. In many cases, no discernable difference is qualified, suggesting that some practitioners are oblivious to the fact that health education and health promotion are interrelated but are not interdependent. Notable examples of this can be seen in the recent nursing literature. For instance, Caelli et al. (2003) put forward the case for a decision support system for health promotion in nursing. The proposed system, however, clearly has little to do with health promotion and everything to do with traditional, reductionist and behavioural health education processes. This continuing practice of interchanging paradigms, rather than a clear delineation of terms and approaches, is damaging for nursing and its perpetuation will present a significant barrier to reform.

The above stated situations have created an uneasy tension between health education and health promotion practice in nursing and raised questions about the ability of nurses to move from a health education ethos towards a broader health promotion paradigm (Morgan and Marsh, 1998; Piper and Brown, 1998; Whitehead, 2001a). Falk Rafael (1999) suggests that such tension has resulted in a situation where nurses are actively excluded from health promotion work by other health professional groups, are devalued as an ancillary medical service and are consequently invisible in the world of health promotion. Nursing curricula have compounded this problem by continuing to deliver programmes where the main emphasis lies predominantly on disease centred health education action at the expense of sociopolitical models of health (Macleod-Clark and Maben, 1998; Poskiparta et al., 2000; Liimatainen et al., 2001; Whitehead, 2002).

What does or should a health promoting nurse do?

While it is difficult to argue that the state of health education and health promotion activity in nursing is anywhere near as healthy as it could be, at least there is some evidence that effective practice prevails. A number of examples of effective nurse led health education strategies are available in the nursing related literature (Haddock and Burrows, 1997; Galvin et al., 2000; Hoyer and Horvat, 2000; Thassri et al., 2000; Twinn, 2001; Bolman et al., 2002; Whitehead et al., 2004), albeit they are mainly examples of biomedically orientated interventions. Several of these examples identify the more progressive types of health education activity that border on wider ranging health promotion strategies. It is, however, certainly more difficult to find specific examples of effective nurse led health promotion programmes (Huyhn et al., 2000; Westbrook and Schultz, 2000; Choudhry et al., 2002). These examples, however, do constitute the beginnings of a useful baseline to denote current activities in nursing and serve as templates for future studies, particularly in the case of the health promotion examples.

It is noted that the examples of effective health related programme activities cited above occur in a variety of practice settings and also represent a relevant mix of both health education and health promotion activities. While this account advocates a concerted push towards broader health promotion strategies in nursing, it also realistically acknowledges the place of effective health education alongside. It is important to note that an effective health promoting nurse acknowledges the wider sociopolitical determinants of a client's community based health while, at the same time, valuing the individual's autonomy at the core of clinical practice (Robinson and Hill, 1998). On the other hand, a good health educating nurse is one who acknowledges that health education programmes can only be effective if they are enhanced by the supportive environment offered within a healthy public policy framework (Norton, 1998). Therefore effective health education programmes are those that are conducted in the context of overall health planning and in conjunction with a range of health promotion activities (Dougherty, 1993).

What many nurses fail to realise is that biomedically orientated health education practices do not necessarily preclude active and broader health promotion activity, but a different mindset is needed to counter such thinking. Dew (2001), for instance, highlights the position of various derivatives of the medical model and, in particular, the personal integrity model. This model allows the medically orientated practitioner to reject the position of a normative treatment status and allow clients to pursue and fulfil their own health potential. It represents a more humanistic and empowering alternative to the rigid imposition of the more commonplace medical scientific integrity model. True health education activities must be voluntaristic, create understanding, provide skills for rational choices and assist clients in clarifying their values as well as respect and contribute to the autonomy of the client (Tones, 2002; see also Chapter 4 in this part for empowerment approaches that reflect these principles). Health education activities are most limiting and restrictive when they are seen to adopt the non-educational techniques of coercing clients into adopting expert driven medically approved behaviours. Nettleton (1996) draws on the concepts of risk, surveillance and the rational self to establish a new paradigm in medicine that acts in turn as a critical analysis of health promotion. Similarly, some authors have described the emergence of a psychosocial environmental epidemiological model of medical practice that facilitates a move away from the ontological dualism inherent in the mainstream medicalisation debates (Nettleton, 1996; Scott, 1999). This goes some way to accommodate a constructivist, postpositivist approach to a development of the health promotion knowledge that is needed in nursing (Labonte et al., 1999).

One of the biggest hurdles that both the health educating and the health promoting nurse, and yet one of the more obvious opportunities for reform, relates to the notion of settings based health promotion. Whereas up until quite recently it could be argued that there was little difference in the way that nurses understood or conducted their health related programmes, regardless of whether they worked in institutional or community settings, recent evidence suggests that a clear division is fast emerging in favour of community based, primary healthcare related health promotion interventions. This is working alongside a more general trend towards health priority based on a population based approach. It is an area that, regardless of setting or discipline, nurses need to espouse. As Harrison (2002: 164–5) argues, population health is really an outcome of emergent capacity arising from the effects of health related social, economic and cultural activity and investment and needs concerted, sophisticated and integrated political action to bring about change. As such, it requires professionals concerned with public health, including nurses, to engage with the politics of systems and organisations.

The value of settings based health promotion is not in separating and delineating settings but in recognising their connections, particularly through the notions of whole community, population based health, public health and seamless health services. In effect, hospital, community and all other settings are duty bound to work together towards the same health related goals.

The emergence of the WHO sponsored Health Promoting Hospitals (HPH) movement and the realisation of the Public Health Hospital (PHH) concept have changed the form of health promotion in recent years (WHO, 1990, 1991, 1997). Hospitals should no longer act or be tolerated as isolated institutions that are culturally and administratively separated from their surrounding communities. In the run up to the public and primary healthcare reforms that look to place healthcare services in the heart of communities, the concept of seamless services is a priority. Many hospitals are now required to pursue a notable shift from their focus on an acute based curative service function towards the delivery of their health services across the whole health and social care continuum. As resources and priority shift from institutional and curative based service delivery, towards community driven preventative social action and cohesion, hospitals are compelled to demonstrate similar shifts and therefore so too are the health professionals (and particularly nurses) employed within them. The HPH movement, as an adjunct to this reform, incorporates the principles of capacity building and organisational change, as part of a concerted reorientation of service delivery that promotes health within and outside a hospital's physical boundaries.

Although hospitals are considered by some to be the high temples of sick care, the extensive resources that they command mean that even a small shift of focus has the potential to bring with it an increase in resources dedicated to organisational health promotion and resultant health benefits to the surrounding community (Johnson and Baum, 2001). Pelikan et al. (1997: 25) cogently portrays a health promoting hospital as using episodes of acute illness or injury as windows of opportunity to promote health, for instance by providing or organising rehabilitation, and empowering patients to make better use of primary healthcare services. By networking with the relevant local services and associations, the HPH builds alliances for continuous care and health promotion, thus becoming a robust agent for health development in the community.

Not until this type of reform is driven and supported by nurses and nursing bodies can they begin to witness a concerted health promotion reform strategy within seamless health service delivery.

The future for health promotion in nursing

Nursing is, by the nature of its size and close client contact alone, the most relevant professional body to initiate and implement health promotion activity across a wide range of health service settings and disciplines. Size alone though, as nurses have repeatedly demonstrated over the years, is no predictor of engagement or success in health promotion. A concerted and consistent commitment on the part of all nurses to initiate and determine a relevant and appropriate health promotion and health policy agenda is the only guarantee of successful reform and participation. This is not, however, a singular path that is talked about here. It is a collaborative path of equal partnership with all relevant stakeholders, particularly the lay public and health service clients, accompanied by a clear, passionate, collective and universal nursing voice and vote. Whitehead (2001c) has, however, already highlighted the considerable barriers that nurses face in their attempts to apply collaborative activities in their health promotion practice. Nurses will need to make expansive inroads into unfamiliar territories if they wish to impact on wide ranging health promotion reform and stake a valid claim to determine their own unique health agenda. Harrison (2002: 175) highlights the sort of health promotion shift that is required.

The health development professions, particularly nurses, must ally themselves with civic society in the development of systems of health governance at each level of social and economic administration. They must network their knowledge and skills across all levels, systems, sectors and professions. They must politically intervene within the social machinery of the state and within all forms of social organisation and systems where decisions are made and resources allocated. They must join in the wider social project of sustainable human development at every level, from local to global.

Broad health promotion reform in nursing will involve the adoption of a radically different mindset for practice. It will mean developing a range of diverse and innovative activities and approaches that are unfamiliar to many nurses, as a vehicle for leaving behind many of the rigid and ritualistic practices that are currently commonplace. This will involve specific yet unfamiliar activities, such as influencing media advocacy initiatives as a means of critical consciousness raising for political and social change (Chapman and Lupton, 1994; Holder and Treno, 1997; Whitehead, 2000). The emergence of evolving empirical methods for conducting and evaluating health promotion research will place further demands on nurses. Many health promoters are now championing the use of action research as a particularly valid method for implementing and evaluating whole system, health promoting organisational reform. It is seen by many as a method that fulfils both the enabling and the empowering goals of health promotion, as well as the principles of participatory learning that underpin preventative health education approaches (Green et al., 1996; Wilkinson et al., 1997; WHO, 1998; Tones, 2000; National Co-ordinating Centre for NHS Service Delivery and Organisation Research & Development, 2001; National Health Service South West Regional Office, 2002; Whitehead et al., 2003). Reassuringly for nursing based studies, action research is rapidly becoming well established and accepted as a legitimate research approach.

Considering the scope and opportunity that nurses have to implement innovative and effective health promotion practice, it is somewhat perplexing that they have often been particularly hesitant to embrace health promotion reform. On the whole, nurses remain unmoved by the call of various national and global agencies for active engagement in broad health promotion programmes. Nurses are urged to universally initiate and adopt a far more proactive health promotion role. Many nurses have demonstrated their ability to take on an active and successful health education role, so why not realistically expect this role to extend further into the realms of wider reaching health promotion reform? Nursing now has little choice in the matter. If nurses continue to fail to affect health promotion reform these agendas will, instead, be forced upon them and they will be subsumed into health related strategies that are of other people's making. As stated previously, some studies are beginning to surface in the nursing literature that suggest a very gradual evolution towards health promotion strategies that directly impact on the sociopolitical, cultural and economic environment of communities (see Choudhry et al., 2000; Huyhn et al., 2000; Westbrook and Schultz, 2000). This book represents a part of that broadening ethos and it is reassuring to know that many of its readers will be nurses who are beginning to take an active interest in health promotion reform.

While health service reform has dictated that health professionals have had to become more socially accountable and transparent, the place of health promotion is now to the fore. More nurses will be aware of this fact than in the past. An escalating number of nurses are striving to reject the traditions of a past passive role as they realise the value of determining and implementing their own health agendas, rather than being at the behest of others. This said, from the available evidence in context, nursing's health promotion practice still remains sporadic, piecemeal and localised. The global health challenge remains and there is still a lot more work to be done at the national and local levels. Until nursing can demonstrate that it is moving beyond pockets of effective health promotion activity towards sustained and universal activity, its overall effectiveness will remain more limited than it should be.

References

Bolman, C., de Vries, H. and van Breukelen, G. (2002) Evaluation of a nurse managed minimal contact smoking cessation intervention for cardiac patients. *Health Education Research* **17:** 99–116.

Caelli, K., Downie, J. and Caelli, T. (2003) Towards a decision support system for health promotion in nursing. *Journal of Advanced Nursing* **43:** 170–80.

Chapman, S. and Lupton, D. (1994) *The Fight for Public Health: Principles and Practice of Media Advocacy*. London: BMJ Publishing.

Choudhry, U. K., Jandu, S., Mahal, J., Singh, R., Sohi-Pabla, H. and Mutta, B. (2002) Health promotion and participatory action research with South Asian women. *Journal of Nursing Scholarship* **34:** 75–81.

Department of Health (1997) *The New NHS: Modern, Dependable*. London: The Stationery Office.

Department of Health (1998) *Our Healthier Nation: a Contract for Health*. London: The Stationery Office.

Department of Health and Human Services (1991) *Healthy People 2000: National Health Promotion and Disease Prevention Objectives*. Publication no. [PHS] 91-50213. Washington, DC: DHSS.

Dew, K. (2001) Modes of practice and models of science in medicine. *Health* **5:** 93–111.

28   *Health Promoting Practice*

Dines, A. (1994) What changes in health behaviour might nurses logically expect from their health education work? *Journal of Advanced Nursing* **20**: 219–26.

Dougherty, C. J. (1993) Bad faith and victim blaming: the limits of health promotion. *Healthcare Analysis* **1**: 111–19.

Falk Rafael, A. R. (1999) The politics of health promotion: influences in public health promoting nursing practice in Ontario, Canada from Nightingale to the nineties. *Advances in Nursing Science* **22** (1): 23–39.

Galvin, K., Webb, C. and Hillier, V. (2000) The outcome of a nurse led health education programme for patients with peripheral vascular disease who smoke: assessment using attitudinal variables. *Clinical Effectiveness in Nursing* **4**: 54–66.

Green, L. W., O'Neill, M., Westphal, M. and Morisky, D. (1996) The challenges of participatory action research for health promotion. *Promotion et Education* **3** (4): 3–5.

Haddock, J. and Burrows, C. (1997) The role of the nurse in health promotion: an evaluation of a smoking cessation programme in surgical pre-admission clinics. *Journal of Advanced Nursing* **26**: 1098–1110.

Hagedorn, S. (1995) The politics of caring: the role of activism in primary care. *Advances in Nursing Science* **17**: 1–11.

Harrison, D. (2002) Health promotion and politics. In Bunton, R. and Macdonald, G. (eds) *Health Promotion: Disciplines, Diversity and Developments*, second edition. London: Routledge.

Holder, H. D. and Treno, A. J. (1997) Media advocacy in community prevention: news as a means to advance policy change. *Addiction* **92**: 189–200.

Hoyer, S. and Horvat, L. (2000) Successful breast feeding as a result of a health education programme for mothers. *Journal of Advanced Nursing* **32**: 1158–67.

Huyhn, K., Kosmyna, B., Lea, H., Munch, K. R., Reynolds, H. S., Specht, C., Tinker, E. C., Yee, A. J. and French, L. R. (2000) Creating an adolescent health promotion: a community partnership between university nursing students and an inner-city High School. *Nursing and Healthcare Perspectives* **21**: 122–6.

Johnson, A. and Baum, F. (2001) Health promotion hospitals: a typology of different organisational approaches to health promotion. *Health Promotion International* **16**: 281–7.

Labonte, R., Feather, J. and Hills, M. (1999) A story/dialogue method for health promotion knowledge development and evaluation. *Health Education Research* **14**: 39–50.

Liimatainen, L., Poskiparta, M., Sjogren, A., Kettunen, T. and Karhila, P. (2001) Investigating student nurses' constructions of health promotion in nursing education. *Health Education Research* **16**: 33–48.

Macdonald, T. H. (1998) *Rethinking Health Promotion: a Global Approach*. London: Routledge.

Macleod-Clark, J. and Maben, J. (1998) Health promotion: perceptions of Project 2000 educated nurses. *Health Education Research* **13** (2): 185–96.

McMurray, A. (1999) *Community Health and Wellness: A Sociological Approach*. Sydney: Harcourt.

Morgan, I. S. and Marsh, G. W. (1998) Historic and future health promotion contexts for nursing. *Image – Journal of Nursing Scholarship* **30**: 379–83.

National Co-ordinating Centre for NHS Service Delivery and Organisation Research & Development (2001) *Managing Change in the NHS: Organisational Change – a Review for Healthcare Managers, Professionals and Researchers*. London: NCCSDO.

National Health Service Executive (1998) *A Consultation on a Strategy for Nursing, Midwifery and Health Visiting*. Health Service Circular 1998/045. London: NHSE.

National Health Service South West Regional Office (2002) *Our Healthier Nation: Improving the Competence of the Workforce in Health Promotion – Practice Placements as Learning Environments*. Bristol: NHS-SWRO.

Nettleton, S. (1996) Women and the new paradigm of health and medicine. *Critical Social Policy* 16: 33–53.

Norton, L. (1998) Health promotion and health education: what role should the nurse adopt in practice? *Journal of Advanced Nursing* 28: 1269–75.

Pelikan, J., Lobnig, H. and Krajic, K. (1997) Health promoting hospitals. *World Health* 3: 24–5.

Piper, S. M. and Brown, P. A. (1998) The theory and practice of health education applied to nursing: a bi-polar approach. *Journal of Advanced Nursing* 27: 383–9.

Poskiparta, M., Liimatainen, L. and Sjogren, A. (2000) Health promotion in the curricula and teaching of two polytechnics in Finland. *Nurse Education Today* 20: 629–37.

Rawson, D. (2002) Health promotion theory and its rationale construction: lessons from the philosophy of science. In Bunton, R. and Macdonald, G. (eds) *Health Promotion: Disciplines, Diversity and Developments*, second edition. London: Routledge.

Robinson, S. and Hill, Y. (1998) The health promoting nurse. *Journal of Clinical Nursing* 7: 232–8.

Royal College of Nursing (1988) *The Health Challenge*. London: RCN.

Rush, K. L. (1997) Health promotion ideology and nursing education. *Journal of Advanced Nursing* 25: 1292–8.

Scott, A. L. (1999) Paradoxes of holism: some problems in developing an anti-oppressive medical practice. *Health* 3: 131–49.

Shields, L. E. and Lindsey, A. E. (1998) Community health promotion nursing practice. *Advances in Nursing Science* 20: 23–36.

Thassri, J., Kala, N., Chusington, L., Phongthanasarn, J., Boonsrirat, S. and Jirojwong, S. (2000) The development and evaluation of a health education programme for pregnant women in a regional hospital, southern Thailand. *Journal of Advanced Nursing* 32: 1450–8.

Tones, K. (2002) Editorial – reveille for radicals: the paramount purpose of health education? *Health Education Research* 17: 1–5.

Twinn, S. (2001) The evaluation of the effectiveness of health education interventions in clinical practice: a continuing methodological challenge. *Journal of Advanced Nursing* 34: 230–7.

United Kingdom Central Council for Nursing, Midwifery & Health Visiting (1986) *Project 2000: a New Preparation for Practice*. London: UKCC.

Wallerstein, N. (1992) Powerlessness, empowerment and health: implications for health promotion programmes. *American Journal of Health Promotion* 6: 197–205.

Webster, C. and French, J. (2002) The cycle of conflict: the history of the public health and health promotion movements. In Adams, L., Amos, M. and Munro, J. (eds) *Promoting Health: Politics & Practice*. London: Sage.

Westbrook, L. O. and Schultz, P. R. (2000) From theory to practice: community health nursing in a public health neighbourhood team. *Advances in Nursing Science* 23: 50–61.

Whitehead, D. (2000) Using mass media within health-promoting practice: a nursing perspective. *Journal of Advanced Nursing* 32: 807–16.

Whitehead, D. (2001a) Health education, behavioural change and social psychology: nursing's contribution to health promotion? *Journal of Advanced Nursing* 34: 822–32.

Whitehead, D. (2001b) A social-cognitive model for health promotion/health education practice. *Journal of Advanced Nursing* 36: 417–25.

Whitehead, D. (2001c) Applying collaborative practice to health promotion. *Nursing Standard* 15 (20): 33–7.

Whitehead, D. (2002) The health promotional role of a pre-registration student cohort in the UK: a grounded-theory study. *Nurse Education in Practice* 2: 197–207.

Whitehead, D. (2003) Incorporating socio-political health promotion activities in nursing practice. *Journal of Clinical Nursing* 12: 668–77.

Whitehead, D. (2004) A concept analysis of health promotion and health education: advancing and maturing the concepts. *Journal of Advanced Nursing* 47 (4): 311–20.

Whitehead, D., Keast, J., Montgomery, V. and Hayman, S. (2004) A preventative health education programme in a hospital based osteoporosis service: a multi-professional participatory action research study. *Journal of Advanced Nursing* 47 (1): 15–24.

Whitehead, D., Taket, A. and Smith, P. (2003) Action research in health promotion. *Health Education Journal* 62: 5–22.

Wilkinson, E., Elander, E. and Woolaway, M. (1997) Exploring the use of action research to stimulate and evaluate workplace health promotion. *Health Education Journal* 56: 188–98.

World Health Organisation (1986) *Ottawa Charter for Health Promotion*. Geneva: WHO.

World Health Organisation (1990) Initiation of International Network of Health Promoting Hospitals. WHO-EURO Workshop. Vienna: WHO.

World Health Organisation (1991) *The Budapest Declaration of Health Promoting Hospitals*. Copenhagen: WHO.

World Health Organisation (1997) *The Vienna Recommendations on Health Promoting Hospitals*. Copenhagen: WHO.

World Health Organisation (1998) *Health Promotion Evaluation: Recommendation to Policymakers*. Report of the WHO European Working Group on Health Promotion. Copenhagen: WHO.

Yeo, M. (1993) Toward an ethic of empowerment for health promotion. *Health Promotion International* 8: 225–35.

CHAPTER 3

The Health Promoting Role of Health Visitors: Adjunct or Synergy?

JANET WEEKS, ANGELA SCRIVEN AND LYNN SAYER

Health visitors have long been encouraged to incorporate health promotion as a central precept permeating all levels of professional action (Council for the Education and Training of Health Visitors [CETHV], 1977). This would suggest that there is a synergy between health visiting practice and health promotion. For those working in primary care, however, the demands of caseload routines involving universal developmental screening of infants and children from birth to five years of age have resulted in health promotion being viewed by some as an adjunct, with only minor engagement in broader health promotion approaches and interventions (Department of Health (DoH), 2001). This chapter will critically examine the impact of recent health policy changes on the health visiting service in the United Kingdom (UK) and determine the opportunities and potential barriers to developing a more synergistic relationship between health visiting practice and health promotion.

Health visitors in the UK are trained nurses who have completed community focussed professional development at undergraduate or postgraduate degree level. The majority of health visitors are attached to a general practitioner (GP) surgery or assigned to a geographical area, with responsibility for a caseload of families with children under the age of five years. However, some are also employed to work with older persons, some have specific community development roles, whilst others work in specialist areas such as child protection, children with special needs, or with the homeless or traveller groups. Regardless of the nature of their remits, there are common principles that govern the practice of all health visitors.

The principles of health visiting

Cowley (2003) has recently summed up the distinctive purpose of health visiting as an unsolicited public health service based on the provision of health promotion and preventive care to families and communities. This description, and others (see CETHV, 1977: 9) assigns importance to health promotion as an aspect of health visitor functions, with a number of principles influencing practice. These principles are multifaceted and include the search for and iden- tification of health needs, facilitation of health enhancing activities and the shaping of health policies. The Health Visitors Association (HVA), who also described health visiting as empowering individuals, families and communities to take responsibility for health, endorsed these broader dimensions of health visiting practice (HVA, 1985). The position of health promotion as a central precept of health visiting remains remarkably durable with reassessments of the health visiting principles reaffirming the importance of the health promoting function (Twinn and Cowley, 1992; Cowley, 2003).

The influence of health promotion's fundamental principles in health visit- ing practice has been the focus of research and evaluation. Kendal (1993) and Machen (1996) investigated interactions between health visitors and clients in the context of health promoting practice. Their results were mixed. Kendal's findings indicated a directive and controlling aspects of health visitors' work with clients that failed to encourage a participatory approach in the health pro- moting interventions. The health visitors in this study perceived themselves as experts, who offered unsolicited advice without acknowledging the clients' own health knowledge (Kendall, 1993). Machen (1996) however, concluded that there was a high level of satisfaction with the facilitative approach of health visitors amongst the women who participated in her study. These women appreciated the responsive and sensitive nature of health visitors and felt empowered by this approach.

More recent studies have explored the health promoting nature and rele- vance of health visiting work to contemporary mothers (see, for example, Normandale, 2001; McHugh and Luker, 2002; St Aubyn and Perkins, 2003). Such studies continue to show mixed client reactions to the health promoting aspects of health visiting practice.

Whilst there is no clear evidence that the health promoting principles embedded in health visiting practice are effective, they remain highly relevant to the current public health agenda. Health visitors have a central role to play as part of the multidisciplinary public health workforce in promoting and maintaining good health in families and communities (Wanless, 2004).

Implications for health visiting of recent NHS policy changes

With the publication of the second national strategy for health in England *Saving Lives: Our Healthier Nation* (DoH, 1999a) the UK government emphasised the need to target the fundamental but complex, social, economic and environmental determinants of ill health, in order to improve the health of disadvantaged members of society. The main ideas underpinning this and other recent policy initiatives are that health professionals should work towards the reduction of health inequalities and the empowerment of individuals, families and communities to improve their own health through needs led public health and community development activities. In accordance with these ideas and health goals, health visitors were encouraged to develop a family centred public health role working with target populations to improve health and tackle health inequality. These themes were briefly revisited in the policy document *Making a Difference: Strengthening the Nursing, Midwifery and Health Visiting Contribution to Health and Healthcare* (DoH, 1999b), where it was recognised that the development of new and innovative ways of working can be constrained by structural barriers within the health service. Nonetheless, the significant role of health visitors is now being recognised by government in policy documents and they are deemed sufficiently important to contribute to the public health work of the new Primary Care Trusts (PCTs) at both a strategic and operational level (Home Office, 1998; DoH 1999a; Dalziel, 2003).

The publication of the *Health Visitor Practice Development Resource Pack* (DoH, 2001) offered health visitors and their managers a framework to develop an innovative public health role. There has been a renewed emphasis on the need to work towards local and national health priorities, particularly the National Service Frameworks (NSF), by operating across professional and agency boundaries. These new roles have been further expanded (DoH, 2002) to incorporate core functions of public health, health protection and promotion designed to improve health and to reduce inequalities.

With public health seen as the art and science of preventing disease, promoting health and prolonging life (Acheson, 1998), health visitors must seize the opportunity to be more creative in searching for approaches to improve the health of their local communities. However, the opportunities available to them in the future will depend on the direction taken by health visiting professional practice. This will become clearer when the completed National Service Framework for Children and the results of the consultation from the Green Paper *Every Child Matters* (Department for Education and Science [DfES], 2003) are published.

Health promotion or public health: which way for health visitors?

Whilst many are currently using in an interchangeable way the terms public health and health promotion (Scriven, 2002), health promotion has highly distinctive principles and methodologies that differentiate it from the more generic concept of public health (see Chapter 1 of this text for a further discourse on this issue). Some argue that health promotion is the militant wing of public health (see Tones, 2001 and Chapter 1 of this text). Whitehead (this text, Chapter 2) also considers health promotion as a radical activity that is not regularly undertaken by nurses of all disciplines, including health visitors, because they confuse health education with health promotion, and are constrained by work patterns that are biomedical and task orientated.

Poulton (2003) has identified two strands emerging from the literature that examines the many definitions of public health. One strand links the health promotional and preventive dimension in the spheres of behavioural sciences, biomedicine and epidemiology. The second strand focusses health promotion on organised social and political efforts, creating a health promoting perspective linked to social justice and social inclusion. It is this second strand that has incorporated many of the Ottawa Charter (World Health Organisation [WHO], 1986) principles that are discussed by Scriven in detail in Chapter 1 of this book. Unifying the two strands in practice, Poulton suggests, is problematic as they are based on different philosophical approaches. Health visitors are perhaps exceptional amongst nurses in the community orientated work they perform and because of this are perhaps more likely to be able to embrace health promotion from both the biomedical, behavioural science and social strands.

Empowerment approaches would be strongly associated with the social inclusion goals of the second strand discussed above. It is a process debated elsewhere in this text (see Chapters 1, 4 and 13, for example) and is a health promoting principle that is often associated with health visiting. However, Macdonald (1998) and Whithead in Chapter 2 of this book argue that many health professionals are only able to engage in impowerment activities, which implies that those in a position of authority, such as health visitors, confer power on clients. Despite capacity and remit constraints, health visitors are perhaps better placed than other nursing colleagues to undertake more pioneering and radical health promotion activities that move beyond impowerment to include more empowering outcomes.

Wright (2001) presents an interesting assessment of the many opportunities and challenges that recent health reforms pose to community nurses in general, including district and specialist nurses working within the community sector. Since Wright wrote her chapter the public health agenda has moved on and there is little doubt that the new public health strategies in the UK are creating further challenges and opportunities for health promotion through the health visiting service.

Challenges to health promoting practice

The ability to embrace novel practice is constrained by barriers that have already prevented many health visitors engaging in the enhanced functions outlined in the policy directives discussed earlier. One obstacle is that some practitioners have remained confined to a traditional health visiting surveillance role prevalent from the 1980s, a role driven by the need to undertake the developmental screening of the children on their caseload. This obstacle was recently removed (Hall and Elliman, 2003) with routine screening procedures now limited to a core universal programme, but with additional services targeted to those children who need them. The removal of this function has caused some anxieties amongst those professions concerned with the health and wellbeing of children. Both health visitors and parents have argued that the routine contacts with parents and preschool children have been the means by which developmental, health, behavioural, social or child protection problems have been identified (Smith, 2004). Hall and Elliman (2003) acknowledge such anxieties in their summary of the principles and objectives of the new and limited universal screening programme.

For the majority of health visitors engaged with families and children under the age of five years, however, the demands of a caseload, child protection work and the necessity of constant, routine and universal developmental screening of children have been a key factor in limiting the scope of their health promotion and public health work (DoH, 2001: 15; Normandale, 2001).

Cowley (2002) has argued that the health promoting principles of health visiting have also been constrained by the contract culture and internal market management ethos of the NHS in the 1980s and 1990s. She maintains that it is this culture that has led to the health visiting service being confined to rigid, task orientated and routine work patterns that are now being discouraged by the current government, with new ways of working outlined in the *Health Visitor Practice Development Resource Pack* (DoH, 2001). This document, however, predates the fourth edition of the *Health for All Children* report (Hall and Elliman, 2003) and does not identify which aspects of routine health visiting should be discarded in favour of the new approach. Cowley (2002) argues that whilst there has been no robust research into the prevailing management culture and activities of organisations that employ health visitors, professional reports indicate that restrictive work patterns remain, despite examples that demonstrate attempts to engage in innovative practice.

In a recent small study, Smith (2004) researched the views of health visitors towards their developing public health role. He found that practitioners recognised that work practices needed to change in line with demographic changes and government imperatives. There was uncertainty amongst health visitors about how they could develop an additional public health role when they were so constrained by the demands of busy caseloads outlined above. They felt that this could only be successfully resolved by strong local leadership, a clear vision of a family centred public health role, and a connection to public health policy and practice through dialogue between practitioners, local public health departments and other stakeholders. Smith also cites concerns raised by the House of Commons Select Committee on Health (2001) about the level of resources in health visiting and the capacity for undertaking this wider public health role.

Opportunities for health promoting practice

The new family centred public health role of health visitors has been described as a continuum (DoH, 2001: 13) with several main health promoting elements. This entails working with individuals and families, facilitating group work, community development, and leading and coordinating public health programmes at a community level, whilst working towards local and national public health priorities. A daunting remit, with questions arising relating to whether workforce capacity and capability is currently sufficient to service such enhanced roles (Wright, 2001). It is important to critically examine a few of the opportunities for health promoting practice within these key elements of health visiting work.

Working with individuals and families

Whilst it appears that working with individuals and families will remain a core function of health visiting work, there is scope for engaging in different and more innovative ways to help the growth and development of children, using the evidence now emerging from an unexpected source, neuroscience. Research into brain development during the 1990s that used improved neuroimaging techniques has resulted in a global body of evidence that indicates how genetic predisposition, interacting with early experience, has a direct impact on the developing brain (see Pally, 1997; Perry, 1997; Balbernie, 1999; Eliot, 1999; Winkler, 1999). There are also robust research studies from the fields of psychology and psychotherapy, linked to the research from neuroscience, that indicate the importance for the optimum development of a child, of a warm, and nurturing environment with an emotionally available caregiver (Buchanan and Hudson, 2000; Shonkoff and Phillips, 2000). Hall and Elliman (2003) argue that there is an interest amongst health visitors and parents who have access to this knowledge, and suggest such insights have the potential to improve the social circumstances in which children develop and grow. Interest in the field of infant mental health has grown in the early years of this century with the publication of specific journals, the development of the Association of Infant Mental Health UK and of conferences and education programmes, all of which are accessible to health visitors.

In a response to the government agenda challenging health visitors to participate in primary prevention (DoH, 2003), Lowenhoff (2004) suggests that the evidence from neuroscience and related fields, that supports the need to work with parents and carers to ensure sensitive responses to infant needs and secure attachment, is being largely ignored. She advocates a proactive, liberal and universal approach that supports all families in the first year of their child's life. Lowenhoff's thesis is that an investment in sensitive, early interventions that promote optimal brain growth and development, might help health professionals to prevent the unmanageable and costly problems that currently confront society, such as antisocial behaviour, crime, domestic violence and social exclusion. Indeed, Shaftoe and Walker (2000) believe that health visitors have a key role in the primary prevention of crime, in the early stages of child development when behaviour traits are beginning to form. They argue that intensive and supportive interventions with families with children can enable positive and appropriate parenting. This would be a radical role for health visitors and would fit Poulton's (2003) social justice strand of public health discussed earlier in this chapter.

It was acknowledged by Acheson (1998) that recommendations to improve the health of and reduce health inequalities in women of child bearing age, pregnant women and young children would have the most impact on the health of current and future generations. The role of health visitors in supporting families has been deemed as vital (Ministerial Group on the Family, 1998). However, there is concern that the government agenda to change traditional ways of working and extend the clinical role of nurses and health visitors in primary care will dilute the specialist and health promotion skills of health visitors (Coombes, 2003).

Hall and Elliman (2003: 70) review the efficacy of early interventions in a number of community wide programmes and have shown that good outcomes in improving the health and development of children have been achieved. However, they also acknowledge that these programmes are expensive and whilst the UK government's flagship programme to tackle child poverty and health inequalities, Sure Start, has received substantial short term funding there are concerns about the sustainability of the project. Moreover, Lowenhoff (2004) has estimated that Sure Start will only benefit a quarter of the population of children living in poverty.

Health visitor training usually involves the management of behaviour problems. However a purely behavioural approach where a parent is taught techniques in order to manage their child's behaviour does not always succeed. One approach initiated in Solihull, by a child psychologist and psychotherapist working in partnership with health visitors in that area, uses concepts derived from psychotherapy, containment and reciprocity, to underpin behaviour management (Douglas, 1999). In her early evaluation of the approach, Douglas describes how intense feelings and anxieties of parents can induce feelings of helplessness when faced with their child's behaviour. In addition, some families are unable to manage the normal developmental processes of childhood because parent and child are not in tune with each other emotionally. Once trained in this approach (Douglas, 2001), health visitors can utilise the concept of *containment* (Bion, 1959) to help restore parental capacity to think and then be receptive to ideas on how to manage their child's behaviour. An understanding of the concept of reciprocity (Brazelton et al., 1974) enables health visitors to observe communication and interaction between parent and child, deduce the level of reciprocity between them and if necessary, help the parent to be more sensitive to the child's emotional needs.

Evaluation has shown that those health visitors trained in the Solihull approach were more consistent and effective in their approach to behaviour problems, reported greater emphasis on an holistic assessment and had greater understanding of how difficulties developed (Douglas and Ginty, 2001). Many health visitors also expressed greater job satisfaction and more confidence in their skills in empowering parents to overcome the challenging behaviour of their young children. Douglas (1999: 19) argues that by attending to contain-ment and reciprocity first, behaviour management becomes an option rather than the starting point of a health visitor intervention. Indeed, Douglas and Ginty (2001: 222) claim that the approach can empower parents to find their own solutions. Therefore, this is an approach that moves away from seeing health visitors as experts in behaviour management directing parents to change their parenting styles, to one that works in health promoting partnership with parents.

   Whilst the current public health agenda (DoH, 2001) is encouraging health visitors to expand into non-traditional areas, there is, ironically, this growing body of evidence that suggests that more health visiting time should be spent working directly with parents. A review of the effectiveness of home visiting (Elkan et al., 2000), a traditional component of health visiting work, has shown it to be effective in improving a range of maternal and child psychoso-cial and health outcomes in North American studies.

Group work

Facilitating group work is a feature of much health visiting with involvement in antenatal, postnatal, parenting and a variety of support groups. Results of a small study (St Aubyn and Perkins, 2003) indicate that some women value par-ticipation in such groups for the sharing of problems and information, and the opportunities for social networking. Two examples of innovative group work facilitated by health visitors have been shown to promote the emotional health of families.

   The first involved health visitors in Stockport facilitating antenatal sessions to engage parents-to-be in preparation for parenthood, rather than just for labour and delivery (Deakin, 2002). These sessions aimed to promote the emotional health of both parents and baby at a crucial time in their lives. A theoretical framework based on the concepts of reciprocity (Brazelton et al., 1974) and emotional intelligence (Goleman, 1995) formed the basis of the work with spe-cific emphasis on the three dimensions of empathy, motivation and social skills. The participants are encouraged to discuss and share ideas about the needs and communication skills of very young babies, and then focus on parental support systems and problem solving skills. These topics are introduced by using video extracts of a baby's in utero environment and the immediate postnatal period, as well as photographs of babies displaying various emotional states, in order to stimulate discussion amongst the participants. At the time of writing, this proj-ect was in its infancy and there was no final evaluation. Informal feedback from the participants indicated that parents felt more attuned to the needs of their baby and how the baby communicated these needs (Deakin, 2002).

   The second example was based on an effort, also in Stockport, to provide a non-clinical service to people with mild to moderate depression. This involved a programme of creative activities based on an exercise on prescription initiative and called *Arts on Prescription* (Huxley, 1997). Huxley cites a number of sources (see Oliver et al., 1996) that showed a number of positive outcomes for people who participated in creative activities. They were more able to engage in social relationships and friendships, had enhanced self-esteem, sense of purpose, social skills and improved quality of life. His evaluation concluded that the mental health of people who participated in the scheme had not deteriorated and for many had improved, and they were also able to take part in more social and leisure activity. A pilot study of a similar service was later developed for women suffering from postnatal depression, also in Stockport, with health visitor support (Tyldesley and Rigby, undated). The authors also recorded positive outcomes for the participants, similar to those reported by Huxley.

Health visitors' remit with mothers and babies brings them into direct contact with the estimated 10 to 20 per cent of women who are affected by depression following childbirth (O'Hara and Swain, 1996; for further details of postnatal depression see Murray and Cooper, 1997). In response to the lack of services for such women, the Stockport project has been replicated in Somerset (Green and Weeks, 2004). A brief description of this programme may serve to illustrate some pertinent issues. The project is a partnership between the health visiting team, a local arts charity and the funding body, the local authority Adult and Community Education department. The programme is currently half way through the first pilot year, therefore has not yet been fully evaluated. However, it offers local women the chance to participate in weekly art sessions each school term, facilitated by an artist and with the health visitor in a supportive capacity. Creche facilities and art materials for up to ten women at one time are provided in the safe environment of newly refurbished studio space, run by the art charity. During the planning of this project, two local women who were suffering from postnatal depression, and the PCT manager of the Patient, Advice and Liaison Service (PALS) were consulted, to ensure that the aims, objectives and running of the groups would be sensitive to the needs of the women. Participants have also been invited to be part of the steering group for the same reason and to help plan future services. Their input is proving invaluable.

Through evaluation, informal feedback from all of the participants, and some local GPs, positive outcomes commensurate with the Stockport model has so far been recorded (Green and Weeks, 2004). As well as improving self-esteem, confidence and social networks for most of the women, there is a sense that many of the women have felt empowered by the experience. An assessment of the ongoing needs of women with postnatal depression is being formulated with their input, with a view to planning a similar art programme and other support services around the PCT area.

This programme fulfils a number of criteria that health visitors must address in order to meet the government's public health agenda. These include a multiagency partnership approach to address health needs, needs assessment, user involvement in the planning of services and working towards evidence based practice (DoH, 2001). Such work also has the potential to contribute towards the PCT's work in the NSF for Mental Health (Department of Health, 1999c).

Community development

This third dimension of public health practice in health visiting is more problematic for the profession as a whole. As previously mentioned, some health visitors have a specific remit to work in community development. For others, the drive to engage whole communities in a comprehensive needs assessment, planning and implementing new services across professional boundaries, and empowering community groups, in order to reduce health inequalities, will have huge implications in terms of resources, health visiting time and personal energy. Health visitors who have successfully engaged in such work all report a number of successful health and social outcomes for children and adults, in the communities that they serve (see Daniel, 1999; Henderson, 2000; Gooding, 2003).

Two approaches to community development in health visiting have emerged. The first is that of health visitors working without a caseload to manage, whose full commitment is focussed on working collectively with members of a community in community led, democratic processes of action, empowerment and participation (Labonte, 1998). An excellent example of community development work using this approach is the Ore Valley community project. Started by a health visitor in Hastings working with members of the community, the project expanded to involve other statutory and voluntary agencies. The result was to change an estate marked by high levels of need and multiple deprivation into a community displaying a sense of pride in its environment. The project won a Queen's Nursing Institute Award for innovation and ably demonstrates the power of health visitors to promote health through their community development work (Appleby and Sayer, 2001). However, practitioners taking this approach can be poorly supported by PCT management structures and suffer the vagaries of short term funding streams and inadequate resources.

The second approach, which is becoming more popular, is for health visitors to hold caseloads alongside undertaking community development work. Research shows that health visitors in such situations often feel constrained by the demands and priorities of their caseloads (Dalziel and McLachlan, 2000). However, there are significant advantages as practitioners can use their existing knowledge of the area, their relationships with other professionals and their access to groups within the community, all established from their caseload working (Dalziel, 2002). Many practice based examples of both approaches are detailed in the Community Practitioner and Health Visitor Association (CPHVA) publication *Joined Up Working: Community Development in Primary Care* (CPHVA, 1999).

Public health programmes at community level

This last health visiting public health remit has several components. The DoH (2001: 13) suggests that these involve leading and coordinating health needs assessment and public health programmes, implementing National Service Frameworks (NSFs) and Health Improvement Programmes (HImPs), PCT liaison, leading multidisciplinary teams, working to public health objectives, planning local interagency working and, of course, evaluating services and projects. Some of these components have been alluded to in this chapter. However, as PCTs start the process of reorganising their health visiting service and that of other community practitioners in response to this government imperative, it will take time before health visitors are proactive in this domain. Nevertheless, an example that encapsulates the individual, group and community development health promotion opportunities and meets all the criteria for public health programmes at community level, is the Sure Start programme.

The Sure Start programme for deprived areas in the UK has been designed to tackle the roots of disadvantage and inequity and is a complex community initiative (Department for Education and Employment (DfEE), 1999). It will have involved a high level of government funding of £1.4 billion over five years, and has four main objectives which include improving social and emotional development, improving health, improving children's ability to learn and strengthening families and communities. Houston (2003b) argues that the programme will also highlight the plight of deprived families outside the postcode boundary of Sure Start, as they will see improved services but will not be able to access them. In order to help such families outside Sure Start areas, Houston (2003a) urges health visitors and other workers to be proactive about using some of the new ways of working that are emanating from the programme. This will be challenging for health visitors unless they are fully motivated to change working practices and are enabled to do so by their employing Trusts.

The four examples of health visitors' public health enhanced remit discussed above demonstrate that there are many opportunities for health visitors to engage in more radical and synergistic health promotion activities within the public health role that the government envisages for the profession. The specialist skills and unique knowledge of the local communities that the health visitors' serve offers them the most potential for health promotion amongst the wider community nursing groups. However, there are many barriers to overcome before the UK health visiting service can be fully capable of fulfilling its health promoting potential and for there to be a genuine synergistic relationship between health visiting and health promotion. The emergence of novel approaches to family centred support based on the expansion of positive child development activities offers new opportunities and potentially innovatory methods to enhance the health promoting role of the health visiting service, so that health promotion is seen as more than just an adjunct.

42 Health Promoting Practice

References

Acheson, D. (1998) *The Report of the Independent Inquiry into Inequalities in Health.* London: The Stationery Office.

Appleby, F. and Sayer, L. (2001) Public health nursing – health visiting. In Sines, D., Appleby, F. and Raymond, E. (eds) *Community Health Care Nursing*, second edition. Oxford: Blackwell Science.

Balbernie, R. (1999) Infant mental health: how events 'wire up' a baby's brain. *Young Minds Magazine* **39**: 17–18.

Bion, W. (1959) Attacks on linking. In *Second Thoughts* (1990). London: Karnac.

Brazelton, T., Koslowski, B. and Main, M. (1974) The origins of reciprocity: the early mother–infant interaction. In Lewis, M. and Rosenblum, L (eds) *The Effect of the Infant on its Caregiver.* London: Karnac.

Buchanan, A. and Hudson, B. (eds) (2000) *Promoting Children's Emotional Wellbeing: Messages from Research.* Oxford: Oxford University Press.

Community Practitioner and Health Visitor Association (1999) *Joined Up Working: Community Development In Primary Health Care.* London: CPHVA.

Coombes, R. (2003) Liberating the talents. *Community Practitioner* **76** (2): 46–7.

Council for the Education and Training of Health Visitors (1977) *An Investigation into the Principles of Health Visiting.* London: CETHV.

Cowley, S. (2002) What's in a name? Health Visiting is health visiting. *Community Practitioner* **75** (8): 304–7.

Cowley, S. (2003) A structured health needs assessment tool: acceptability and effectiveness for health visiting. *Journal of Advanced Nursing* **43** (1): 82–92.

Dalziel, Y. (2002) Community development as a public health function. In Cowley, S. (ed.) *Public Health in Policy and Practice.* London: Baillière Tindall.

Dalziel, Y. (2003) The role of nurses in public health. In Watterson, A. (ed.) *Public Health in Practice.* Basingstoke: Palgrave Macmillan.

Dalziel, Y. and McLachlan, S. (2000) *Preliminary Report of the CHART Project.* Edinburgh: Lothian Health.

Daniel, K. (1999) Working in partnership. *Community Practitioner* **72** (5): 117–18.

Deakin, A. (2002). Antenatal parent education – a new design for Stockport. *Association for Infant Mental Health (UK) Newsletter* **3** (2): 8–9.

Department for Education and Employment (1999) *Making a Difference for Children and Families: Sure Start.* London: DfEE.

Department for Education and Science (2003) *Every Child Matters.* London: The Stationery Office.

Department of Health (1999a) *Saving Lives: Our Healthier Nation.* London: HMSO.

Department of Health (1999b) *Making a Difference: Strengthening the Nursing, Midwifery and Health Visiting Contribution to Health and Healthcare.* London: HMSO.

Department of Health (1999c) *National Service Framework for Mental Health.* London: DoH.

Department of Health (2001) *Health Visitor Practice Development Resource Pack.* London: HMSO.

Department of Health (2002) *Liberating the Talents.* London: HMSO.

Department of Health (2003) *Liberating the Public Health Talents of Community Practitioners and Health Visitors.* London: HMSO.

Douglas, H. (1999) The Solihull Approach: helping health visitors help families with young children. *Young Minds* **40**: 19–20.

Douglas, H. (2001) *The Solihull Approach Resource Pack*. Birmingham: Solihull Primary Care Trust and the School of Primary Health Care, University of Central England.

Douglas, H. and Ginty, M. (2001) The Solihull Approach: changes in health visiting practice. *Community Practitioner* 74 (6): 222–4.

Eliot, L. (1999) *Early Intelligence: How the Brain and Mind Develop in the First Five Years of Life*. London. Penguin.

Elkan, R., Kendrick, D. and Hewitt, M. (2000) The effectiveness of domiciliary visiting: a systematic review of international studies and a selective review of the British literature. *Health Technology Assessment* 4 (13). ww.hta.nhsweb.nhs.uk/ htapubs.htm

Goleman, D. (1995) *Emotional Intelligence*. London: Bantam.

Gooding, L. (2003) Health promotion the 'natural way'. *Community Practitioner* 76 (6): 207.

Green, C. and Weeks, J. (2004) *My Time My Space: Arts Activities for Women with Postnatal Depression: an Initial Evaluation*. North East Somerset Arts (NESA) and Bath & North East Somerset Primary Care Trust, unpublished.

Hall, D. M. B. and Elliman, D. (eds) (2003) *Health for All Children*. Oxford: Oxford University Press.

Health Visitors Association (1985) *Health Visiting and School Nursing Reviewed*. London: HVA.

Henderson, C. (2000) Helping parents to help themselves and their children. *Community Practitioner* 73 (10): 801–3.

Home Office (1998) *Supporting Families*. London: The Stationery Office.

House of Commons Select Committee on Health (2001) *Report on Public Health, Second Report*. London: the Committee.

Houston, A. (2003a) Sure Start: a complex community initiative. *Community Practitioner* 76 (7): 257–60.

Houston, A. (2003b) Sure Start: the example of one approach to evaluation. *Community Practitioner* 76 (8): 294–7.

Huxley, P. (1997) *Arts On Prescription: an Evaluation*. Stockport: Stockport NHS Trust.

Kendall, S. (1993) Do health visitors promote client participation? An analysis of the health visitor–client interaction. *Journal of Clinical Nursing* 2: 103–9.

Labonte, R. (1998) *A Community Development Approach to Health Promotion*. Edinburgh: Health Education Board for Scotland.

Lowenhoff, C. (2004) Have talents: need liberating. *Community Practitioner* 77 (1): 23–5.

Macdonald, T. H. (1998) *Rethinking Health Promotion: a Global Approach*. London: Routledge.

Machen, I. (1996) The relevance of health visiting policy to contemporary mothers. *Journal Of Advanced Nursing* 24: 350–6.

McHugh, G. and Luker, K. (2002) Users' perceptions of the health visiting service. *Community Practitioner* 75 (2): 57–61.

Ministerial Group on the Family (1998) *Supporting Families: a Consultation Document*. London: The Stationery Office.

Murray, L. and Cooper, P. J. (1997) *Postpartum Depression and Child Development*. New York: Guildford Press.

Normandale, S. (2001) A study of mothers' perceptions of the health visiting role. *Community Practitioner* 74 (4): 146–50.

O'Hara, M. W. and Swain, A. M. (1996) Rates and risk of postpartum depression – a meta-analysis. *International Review of Psychiatry* **8**: 37–54.

Oliver, J. P. J., Huxley, P. J., Bridges, K. and Mohammed, H. (1996) *Quality of Life And Mental Health Services.* London: Routledge.

Pally, R. (1997) How brain development is shaped by genetic and environmental factors. *International Journal of Psychoanalysis* **78**: 587–93.

Perry, B. (1997) Incubated in terror: neurodevelopmental factors in the cycle of violence. In Osofsky, J. D. (ed.) *Children in a Violent Society.* New York: Guildford Press.

Poulton, B. (2003) Putting the 'public' back into public health. *Community Practitioner* **76** (3): 88–91.

St Aubyn, B. and Perkins, E. (2003) Health visitors listening to mothers' perspectives of self care. *Community Practitioner* **76** (2): 59–63.

Scriven, A. (2002) *Report of a Survey into the Impact of Recent National Health Policies on Specialist Health Promotion Services in England.* London: Brunel University.

Shaftoe, H. and Walker, P. (2000) Health and 'wicked issues'. *Community Practitioner* **73** (6): 632–3.

Shonkoff, J. P. and Phillips, D. A. (eds) (2000) *From Neurons to Neighbourhoods: the Science of Early Childhood.* Washington, DC: Institute of Medicine, National Research Council. www.nap.edu

Smith, M. (2004) Health Visiting: the public health role. *Journal of Advanced Nursing* **45** (1): 17–25.

Tones, K. (2001) Health promotion: the empowerment imperative. In Scriven, A. and Orme, J. (eds) *Health Promotion: Professional Perspectives*, second edition. Basingstoke: Palgrave Macmillan.

Twinn, S. and Cowley, S. (1992) *The Principles of Health Visiting: a Re-examination.* London: Health Visitors Association and United Kingdom Standing Conference on Health Visitor Education.

Tyldesley, R. and Rigby, T. (undated) *Arts on Prescription. Postnatal Depression Support Service: an Evaluation of a 12 week pilot.* Stockport: Stockport Primary Care Trust.

Wanless, D. (2004) *Securing Good Health for the Whole Population: Final Report.* London: HMSO.

Winkler, L. (1999) Neural pathways and the development of the brain. *Primary Practice* **20**: 30–5.

World Health Organisation (1986) *Ottawa Charter for Health Promotion.* Geneva: WHO.

Wright, C. (2001) Community nurses: crossing boundaries to promote health. In Scriven, A. and Orme, J. (eds) *Health Promotion: Professional Perspectives*, second edition. Basingstoke: Palgrave Macmillan.

CHAPTER 4

A Health Promoting Empowerment Approach to Diabetes Nursing

HELEN ASHTON AND JILL RODGERS

Living with a chronic disease such as diabetes mellitus demands lifestyle changes if short and long term complications are to be avoided. Short term complications of diabetes include low blood glucose levels (hypoglycaemia) potentially affecting a person's ability to work, drive a car and carry out many aspects of daily living that most take for granted. Long term complications can ultimately result in blindness, lower limb amputation, renal failure and in men, erectile dysfunction. There is a wealth of evidence that suggests that people with diabetes make their own decisions about whether or not to follow advice given by health professionals. These decisions are based on a number of factors not necessarily related to their health. So, the promotion of health in this vulnerable group is essential. If consultations are to be effective in facilitating this, a different approach is needed in chronic disease. A number of behaviour change models are available to give direction to practice. One that was developed and positively evaluated in the United States of America, and has also been found effective in Scandinavia and the United Kingdom, is that of facilitating self-care through empowerment (Funnell et al., 1991). This chapter will discuss a range of related issues including the need for change in nurses' health promotion practice, elements of the empowerment model, relevant government policy and the challenges facing nurses who care for people with diabetes and who wish to implement the empowerment philosophy in their healthcare practice.

The need for change in diabetes care

During an acute illness, the traditional medical model provides an appropriate framework of care. Elements of this model include the health professional being in overall charge of care, including diagnosis, treatment decisions, and ensuring treatment is carried out as prescribed (Anderson, 1995). It also expects the person receiving care to be passive, accept medical decisions, comply with instructions, and be dependent on the health professional.

There are a number of reasons why the medical model is inappropriate in chronic disease. Firstly, diabetes is a self-managed disease involving lifestyle changes and daily self-care routines. It carries no cure, but holds a threat of potential complications if not cared for adequately. Alongside this, people can feel relatively healthy with diabetes and therefore may consider there is no immediate benefit from taking their treatment or following a prescribed lifestyle regimen. Daily self-care can also be monotonous as it involves testing blood glucose, taking medication, eating healthily, caring for feet and balancing medication against food intake and physical activity. Type 2 diabetes is a progressive disease that can carry with it a sense of failure as, despite efforts to self-care, oral medication is required, doses are increased, and eventually insulin is introduced. Many people with diabetes become despondent or depressed if they fail to achieve the stringent targets set for them by health professionals, and motivation is lost (Polonsky, 1999).

There are a number of psychological factors contributing to how people view and care for their diabetes. One is their perception of the severity of their condition. If it is not viewed as serious, or they do not see themselves as vulnerable to complications, diabetes care is unlikely to be a priority (Weinstein, 1993). Another is their personal beliefs about their diabetes (Hampson et al., 1990). The work of Sutherland (1994) suggests that not only do people act in accordance with their beliefs, but they will also go to great lengths to avoid evidence that disproves their beliefs. Whether someone is ready or prepared to make changes will also influence their diabetes self-care, as will their self-efficacy or belief that they can achieve change (Anderson et al., 1995). Finally, perceived or actual barriers to self-management can prevent behaviour change (Glasgow, 1994).

There is also evidence that many people find it difficult to follow prescribed treatment regimens. For example, 28 per cent of young adults with Type 1 diabetes did not obtain enough insulin on prescription to meet their requirements (Morris et al., 1997) and only 20 per cent of people treated with insulin obtained enough blood glucose testing strips to test even once a day (Evans et al., 1999). Similarly, in Type 2 diabetes only a third of people taking a single type of tablet obtained enough of their medication on prescription to take it 90 per cent of the time (Donnan et al., 2002).

The difficulties of following advice are not confined only to taking medication. Some 10 per cent of young adults with Type 1 diabetes reported never following a healthy diet, with 58 per cent rarely following a healthy diet. Those with Type 2 diabetes reported following their dietary recommendations about 50 per cent of the time (Toobert et al., 2000). Also, people with Type 2 diabetes and young adults with Type 1 diabetes reported following their exercise recommendations only 33 per cent and 28 per cent of the time respectively (Toobert et al., 2000). Disposal of sharps is of particular concern, with approximately 50 per cent of diabetics failing to dispose of them safely, posing a potential hazard during waste collection (Reed et al., 2003).

Nurses provide much of the care for people with diabetes. The evidence discussed above, however, suggests that nurses are currently failing in their efforts to educate people to self-care and that they need to seek alternative health promotion and health education models to increase their success.

One approach that has been used successfully in the education of people with diabetes is that of empowerment, in which health practitioners aim to help individuals gain greater control over decisions and actions affecting their health (World Health Organisation (WHO), 1998a). As Whitehead points out in Chapter 2 of this book, this strategy relates to individual rather than community empowerment. The concept of empowerment is reflected in the Jakarta Declaration (WHO, 1997, 1998b) which reiterates the Ottawa Charter principles that highlighted the importance of empowering individuals as well as communities to improve health for all (WHO, 1986) (see Chapter 1 for further exploration of the Ottawa and Jakarta principles). Empowerment features in a number of the National Health Service (NHS) publications in England indicating, at least in the rhetoric, a commitment to the notion of empowerment. For example, *The NHS Plan* claims that far-reaching and fundamental reform, referred to as empowerment mechanisms, in the NHS will bring patients into decision making at every level (Department of Health (DoH), 2000).

The theme of empowerment of patients is reiterated in other United Kingdom (UK) government publications. These include *The Expert Patient* (DoH, 2001a), which considers the evidence for the efficacy of self-management programmes and sets out actions that need to be taken for successful implementation. Empowerment is a key feature of Standard 3 of the *National Service Framework for Diabetes: Standards* (DoH, 2001b: 21) in which the aim is to ensure that people with diabetes are empowered to enhance their personal control over the daily management of their diabetes in a way that enables them to experience the best possible quality of life.

The National Service Framework (NSF) also notes that the provision of information, education and psychological support that facilitates self-management is the cornerstone of diabetes care (DoH, 2001b: 22). Primary Care Trusts (PCTs) have been set the goal of reaching NSF Standards by 2013 (DoH, 2002).

The theme of empowerment can also be found in the government literature of other countries. For example, values identified by the Australian Capital Territory Government (2002: 13) include the pledge to ensure that consumers and carers are actively involved in making decisions about their own healthcare. Similarly, Health Canada Online (2003), presented by the Canadian federal department responsible for health, emphasises empowerment by reiterating the WHO's philosophy of helping people to increase control over and thus improve their health. These examples from the UK and other countries are advocating what is in essence a patient centred approach.

Benefits of a patient centred approach

Studies both in diabetes and in general psychology literature demonstrate the benefits of a patient centred approach (see also Chapters 8, 15 and 16 for further discussion on this methodology). Adult learning is concerned with making connections, and processing information, rather than simply being given information (Coles, 1989). A minimum level of knowledge is important for people with diabetes to self-care, but other factors, including motivation and attitudes, have a greater influence on behaviour (Lockington et al., 1988).

The more someone with diabetes is involved with decisions about their care and self-management, the more likely they are to be motivated to care for their diabetes. It was shown by Anderson and Funnell (2000) that behaviour changes to please the health professional or comply with advice are only sustained if the person is seen regularly. In contrast, if people set their own goals for treatment and behaviour changes, they develop problem solving skills and are better able to deal with their diabetes, taking a personal responsibility for their care and outcomes.

Studies involving adolescents identified that a health professional who listens, asks questions and is interested in their lifestyle increases their motivation, as opposed to one who does not listen to their views, but instead tells them what to do, who is seen as unhelpful (Kyngäs et al., 1998). This is also supported by some interesting evidence that suggests that when people with diabetes are able to interrupt and ask questions during a consultation they are not only more satisfied but also have lower blood glucose levels (Coles, 1990).

Autonomous motivation where people, for example, take medication because they believe it benefits their health rather than because they have been told to take it, is likely to result in long term behaviour change. Research has indicated that supporting autonomous motivation in a consultation increases the belief of the person with diabetes in their ability to deal with their disease and achieve targets, and also results in significant reductions in glycosylated haemoglobin values over a 12 month period (Williams et al., 1998). Self-determination theory also relates to this, with evidence to suggest that if people engage in an activity because it is important for them, they are more motivated to continue long term (Deci and Ryan, 1985).

Despite these compelling findings, diabetes nurses have not always achieved a patient centred approach in their consultations. In the Wikblad (1991) study, the experience of 55 people who had been diagnosed with Type 1 diabetes for at least five years identified that most consultations provided information that was not specific to their situation and that health professionals did not actively seek or welcome their input or opinion. The expectations of the participants were that they should be listened to, their fears discussed, and that they should be trusted to manage their own diabetes.

The current situation in diabetes nursing

The preceding discussion identified that empowerment is one of the fundamental principles of health promotion but it appears that some people with diabetes do not always feel empowered after consultations with health professionals, including nurses. Understandings of health promotion inevitably change according to the sociopolitical context of the times. The concept of health promotion is multifaceted and, even today, is used in different ways (Tones, 2001 and Chapter 1 of this text). It is this together with a number of other factors (outlined by Whitehead in Chapter 2 of this text) that have contributed to the lack of emphasis on health promotion in nursing. Of particular note is that traditionally, nurses have been trained in a biomedical model of care and the implications of this have been cogently analysed by Whitehead in Chapter 2. However, this is not just the case in the UK. Rafael (1999) highlights how the dominant biomedical model of health has influenced nursing in Canada. The problem with this model is that it ignores patients' subjective perceptions of their own health.

Current nursing literature shows evidence of greater understanding of the complexity of health promotion but Whitehead argues in Chapter 2 that nurses are continuing to use the terms health education and health promotion interchangeably. Until recently, nursing theories tended to focus on a reductionist, expert led approach to the health of the individual rather than any wider societal determinants of health (Robinson and Hill, 1998). Yet the promotion of health has been one of the nursing competencies necessary for registration since 1983 (Statutory Instrument, 1983, 1989) and more recently for entry to Parts 12–15 of the register held by the Nursing and Midwifery Council (NMC) (Statutory Instrument, 2000; NMC, 2002). Many authors have pointed to the challenges nurses face in meeting their health promotion role both in the UK and other countries such as Canada (Lindsey and Hartrick, 1996; Norton, 1998; Robinson and Hill, 1998; Whitehead, 2003).

Focussing on nursing practice, Whitehead (2001) points to how nurses tend to see health education in terms of giving information to individual patients, suggesting limited understanding of the impact of lifestyles and the major problems associated with attitude and behaviour change. Similarly, Roisin et al. (1999) were perplexed by the inability of some nurses to change their practice with patients with Type 2 diabetes from a biomedical model to a negotiated decision making framework. This framework was designed to increase people's involvement in their own care and the daily choices they made. Roisin et al. found that some nurses were torn between their professional responsibilities in terms of technical aspects of care such as biochemical measurements and encouraging patients with poorly controlled diabetes to decide what areas of their lifestyle they might be prepared to alter. Nurses often resorted to a directive model of health education where knowledge was imparted, suggesting that their socialisation into this way of working makes it extremely hard for them to take a more empowering approach to practice. It has been suggested that most health professionals experience a deep responsibility that shapes virtually every consultation they have and they feel effective when they find solutions for their patients and feel ineffective when they do not (Anderson et al., 2000).

Cooper et al. (2003) studied the effects of a theoretically constructed empowering education programme, delivered to people with diabetes by diabetes specialist nurses. The investigation focused on patients' perspectives of what they valued about the programme and it was found that nurses could educate patients to become more autonomous. However, when engaged in consultations with other health professionals, not all these practitioners were prepared to work in partnership with patients. In another study by Parkin and Skinner (2003) people with diabetes and the diabetes nurses and dietitians they saw were asked immediately after the consultation to report on what issues had been discussed, what decisions had been made and what goals had been set during the consultation. Both groups completely disagreed on issues almost 20 per cent of the time, with no common topic reported. There was complete disagreement on decisions made 20 per cent of the time and complete disagreement on goals set almost 45 per cent of the time. One conclusion that can be drawn from this evidence is that behaviour change is unlikely to result if patient and practitioner cannot reach a common understanding on what behaviour changes are needed.

Empowerment in practice

Reasons have already been iterated as to why people might find it hard to remain motivated to care for their diabetes. It has also been suggested that health professional training and the ethos of the NHS have generated an information giving approach to health education, without sufficient account taken of the psychosocial elements contributing to an individual's behaviour and other health promotion approaches. Notwithstanding, the NHS, in rhetoric at least, has shown a commitment to promoting health through an empowerment approach to patient care.

To adopt an empowerment approach to practice requires recognition that the education of people with diabetes needs to be substantially different from the traditional, compliance oriented approach. Funnell et al.'s (1991) model aims to increase patient autonomy and expand freedom of choice, rather than the compliance oriented methods of persuasion and encouragement to follow health professional recommendations. Patient consultations need to be based on a number of principles, detailed below.

Firstly the person with diabetes is equal to the health professional and a consultation is a meeting of two people who bring their own expertise to the situation. The health professional brings knowledge about diabetes, treatment options, preventative strategies and prognosis. The person with diabetes brings their existing knowledge plus their own experience of living with diabetes, their values and beliefs, social circumstances, habits and behaviour and attitudes to risk taking (Coulter, 1999).

Secondly, the beliefs, values, feelings and opinions of the person with diabetes are considered important and are actively sought out. They should be used in an exploratory manner, for example 'You said you believe it is inevitable that you will lose your sight, can you tell me what makes you think that?' rather than being judged as inaccurate or simply contradicted. Exploring why certain beliefs are held and providing information in a non-judgmental way about the facts of diabetes will help individuals identify when their beliefs are inconsistent with reality and help them adopt a more accurate view of their diabetes.

Diabetics should be encouraged to influence the content of the consultation, initially by being asked to identify any specific issues that impact on their self-care and then by mutual agreement as to what will be discussed. This helps to ensure that topics covered are directly relevant to their lives and experiences and decreases the chance of providing information that the health professional considers important but the person with diabetes does not.

Individuals living with diabetes should generate the solutions to the issues identified by them to ensure they fit within the context of their lifestyles, values, beliefs and support systems. This greatly increases the chances of behaviour change happening and being sustained. Suggestions from health professionals may not fit the individuals' lifestyle and although they may try and carry out suggestions made by health professionals, they are likely to revert to their former behaviour.

In an empowering consultation, the health professional adopts a facilitative role, asking open questions, helping individuals to look at alternatives, consider the consequences of different options and make their own decisions. Goal setting is also a vital part of the empowerment model. Identification of what specifically will happen as a result of a consultation, when it will happen, what barriers exist to implementing the plan and how these barriers can be overcome, all greatly increase the chances of a goal being achieved. Goals should be behavioural rather than based on results alone. For example, if the choice is to lose weight at a rate of one kilogram per week, the goal or goals should be elicited through questions that focus on what behaviour changes are needed to achieve it, for example 'What would you specifically need to change in order to achieve this weight loss?' The more specific and measurable goals are, the easier it is to see whether they are achievable and also whether they are likely to obtain the desired outcome.

The consultation should be a positive rather than a negative experience. Focussing on personal strengths and on successes in self-care, and discussing behaviour changes as experimental rather than as ultimate goals, reduces the feeling of failure experienced if they are not fully achieved and helps to maintain long term motivation.

In summary, empowering consultations should be seen as processes through which people with diabetes are guided, but the content should be steered by them. The health professional's role is to elicit individuals' issues and concerns, explore the feelings, beliefs and values around these issues, encourage them to identify options for change and help them commit to action they will take following the consultation. This process requires some counselling ability, with the nurse asking open questions, making direct eye contact, engaging in active listening and being interested in what people with diabetes have to say, reflecting back what they have said to check understanding and help with further exploration and summarising discussions, decisions made and goals agreed.

There are a number of other behaviour change models that can be used in consultations, for example motivational interviewing or assessment of willingness to change, which contain similar elements to the empowerment model. There is no single model that has been identified as more successful than another in achieving behaviour change, but using any patient centred model has been shown to increase motivation and self-care, increase self efficacy and improve glycaemic control (Williams et al., 1998).

Adopting an empowerment approach

For an empowerment approach to diabetes nursing to be widely adopted, the need for change has to be recognised. The fundamental basis of the empowerment approach is that it is not health professionals but people who have diabetes who make the most important choices about the management of their condition. They are the people in control of their self-management and they are the ones who will suffer the consequences of poor care, not the health professional (Anderson and Funnell, 2000). In accepting these basic principles, health professionals need to discard any judgmental and critical medical approach, such as blaming lack of self-care on the competence and motivation of people with diabetes and accept the part they play in this by moving towards using behavioural techniques to help people with diabetes to achieve and maintain better self-management (Dunn, 1990).

The need for a different approach has been recognised in the NSF for Diabetes Standards (DoH, 2001b) with recommendations for specialised training in counselling and behaviour change skills. A review of current workforce capabilities and the identification of local education needs are highlighted in the NSF for Diabetes Delivery Strategy (DoH, 2002). However, diabetes nursing is still driven by medical rather than behavioural and psychosocial targets and many nurses are reluctant to adjust their established practice (Rodgers and Walker, 2002), which must change if better self-care is to be embraced.

Recognition among health professionals of the need to access training in psychosocial aspects of diabetes and in behaviour change is slow to emerge, with many of the opinion that training in medical aspects of diabetes as more important (Gillibrand and Taylor, 2004). This is related in part to initial general training being focussed on the traditional medical model approach discussed earlier, and suggests that the concept of patient autonomy, equality and involvement in care decisions needs to be integrated into general health professional training from the outset, rather than being seen as an add-on when working in chronic disease.

Once the need for a different approach is accepted, there needs to be some consensus on how this should happen. Researched interventions aimed at behaviour change are often not described in enough detail to be able to replicate them (Rollnick et al., 2000). The outcomes measured vary greatly from one study to another, which makes them difficult to compare. Attempts are being made in the UK to provide standardised educational interventions for people with Type 1 diabetes through a programme named Dose Adjustment For Normal Eating (DAFNE) (DAFNE Study Group, 2002); and for people with Type 2 diabetes, an initiative referred to as Diabetes Education for Self-management: Ongoing and Newly Diagnosed (DESMOND) (Carey and Patel, 2004). Although the strengths of the DAFNE study include its randomised controlled design and 80 per cent follow up at six months, further study is needed to identify whether or not these results can be sustained over the longer term. The DESMOND initiative is currently being piloted in fifteen Primary Care Trust sites and formal evaluation took place during 2004 (Carey and Patel, 2004). More research is needed to establish and agree the main elements of educational approaches that will better facilitate behaviour change in people with diabetes.

Training courses are also required. Most diabetes courses focus on medical aspects of disease management, with a small amount of course time devoted to psychosocial aspects, with few courses with a primary focus on this aspect (Murray, 2001). This must change, so that high quality courses are available to nurses and other health professionals working in diabetes. It is important that training is not restricted to nurses alone, as individual nurses will find it hard to implement behaviour change strategies in a work environment dominated by the traditional medical model.

Even for those who are able to access specific skills training and then try to put this into practice, there are still a number of barriers to success. These include the discomfort that can arise when asking people about their feelings and beliefs. The uneasiness arises out of concern that the issues raised may need someone more competent to deal with them. The urge to give advice based on long practised behaviour, rather than eliciting options from the person with diabetes, can also cause anxiety and a feeling of not having held an effective consultation if advice is not given. There is also the perspective of the person with diabetes. Having been used to adopting a passive role in a consultation, many diabetes patients may be resistant to change and need time and encouragement to adopt a more interactive role.

Finally, it is important to recognise that nurses trained in the traditional medical model may find it equally as difficult to change behaviour as the people with diabetes. Accessing skills training can help, as can the building of peer review systems and developing opportunities to reflect on practice. It is only through investment in training and professional practice that the empowerment approaches described above will become the established methodology for promoting the health of people with diabetes.

References

Anderson, R. M. (1995) Patient empowerment and the Traditional Medical Model – a case of irreconcilable differences? *Diabetes Care* 18: 412–15.

Anderson, R. M. and Funnell, M. M. (2000) Compliance and adherence are dysfunctional concepts in diabetes care. *Diabetes Educator* 26: 597–604.

Anderson, R. M., Funnell, M. M., Butler, P. M., Arnold, M. S., Fitzgerald, J. T. and Feste, C. C. (1995) Patient empowerment: results of a randomised controlled trial. *Diabetes Care* 17: 943–9.

Anderson, R., Funnell, M., Carlson, A., Saleh-Stattin, N., Cradock, S. and Skinner, T. C. (2000) Facilitating self-care through empowerment. In Snoek, F. J. and Skinner, T. C. (eds) *Psychology in Diabetes Care*. Chichester: Wiley.

Australian Capital Territory Government (2002) *Health Action Plan*. Canberra: ACT Health. www.health.act.gov.au/c/health

Carey, M. and Patel, S. (2004) Welcome to DESMOND. *Keynotes* 1: 1. www.cgsupport. nhs.uk/downloads/NDST/DESMOND_newsletter.pdf (accessed 4 May 2004)

Coles, C. (1989) Diabetes education: theories of practice. *Practical Diabetes* 6: 199–202.

Coles, C. (1990) Diabetes education: letting the patient into the picture. *Practical Diabetes* 7: 110–12.

Cooper, H. C., Booth, K. and Gill, G. (2003) Patients' perspectives on diabetes health care education. *Health Education Research* 18: 191–206.

Coulter, A. (1999) Paternalism or partnership? *British Medical Journal* 319: 719–20.

DAFNE Study Group (2002) Training in flexible, intensive insulin management to enable dietary freedom in people with Type 1 diabetes: dose adjustment for normal eating (DAFNE) randomised controlled trial. *British Medical Journal* 325: 746–9.

Deci, E. and Ryan, R. (1985) *Intrinsic Motivation and Self-Determination in Human Behaviour*. New York: Plenum.

Department of Health (2000) *The NHS Plan: a Plan for Investment. A Plan for Reform*. Cm 4818-1. London: The Stationery Office.

Department of Health (2001a) *The Expert Patient: a New Approach to Chronic Disease Management for the 21st Century*. London: DoH.

Department of Health (2001b) *National Service Framework for Diabetes: Standards*. London: DoH.

Department of Health (2002) *National Service Framework for Diabetes: Delivery Strategy*. London: DoH.

Donnan, P. T., MacDonald, T. M. and Morris, A. D. (2002) Adherence to prescribed oral hypoglycaemic medication in a populations of patients with Type 2 diabetes: a retrospective cohort study. *Diabetic Medicine* 19: 279–84.

Dunn, S. M. (1990) Rethinking the models and modes of diabetes education. *Patient Education and Counselling* 16: 281–6.

Evans, J. M. M., Newton, R. W., Ruta, D. A., MacDonald, T. M., Stevenson, R. J. and Morris, A. D. (1999) Frequency of blood glucose monitoring in relation to glycaemic control: observational study with diabetes database. *British Medical Journal* 319: 83–6.

Funnell, M. M., Anderson, R. M., Arnold, M. S., Barr, P. A., Donnelly, M. B., Johnson, P. D., Taylor-Moon, D. and White, N. H. (1991) Empowerment: an idea whose time has come in diabetes education. *Diabetes Educator* 17: 37–41.

Gillibrand, W. and Taylor, J. (2004) Practice nurses' views of their diabetes care. *Practice Nursing* 15 (3): 144–9.

Glasgow, R. E. (1994) Social-environmental factors in diabetes: barriers to diabetes self-care. In Bradley, C. (ed.) *Handbook of Psychology and Diabetes.* Chur, Switzerland: Harwood Academic.

Hampson, S. E., Glasgow, R. and Toobert, D. J. (1990) Personal models of diabetes and their relations to self-care activities. *Health Psychology* 9: 632–46.

Health Canada Online (2003) *Achieving Health for All: a Framework for Health Promotion.* Health Canada. www.hc-sc.gc.ca/english/care/achieving_health.html

Kyngäs, H., Hentinen, M. and Barlow, J. H. (1998) Adolescents' perceptions of physicians, nurses, parents and friends: help or hindrance in compliance with diabetes self-care? *Journal of Advanced Nursing* 27: 760–9.

Lindsey, E. and Hartrick, G. (1996) Health-promoting nursing practice: the demise of the nursing process? *Journal of Advanced Nursing* 23: 106–12.

Lockington, T. J., Farrant, S., Meadows, K. A., Dowlatshahi, D. and Wise, P. H. (1988) Knowledge profile and control in diabetic patients. *Diabetic Medicine* 5: 381–6.

Morris, A. D., Boyle, D. I., McMahon, A. D., Greene, S. A., MacDonald, T. M. and Newton, R. W. (1997) Adherence to insulin treatment, glycaemic control and ketoacidosis in insulin-dependent diabetes mellitus. *The Lancet* 350: 1505–10.

Murray, J. (2001) *Importance of Psychosocial Aspects Of Diabetes Confirmed By Summit Meeting. Report of Oxford International Diabetes Summit, 2001.* Crawley: Novo Nordisk UK. www.novonordisk.co.uk/view.asp?ID = 1506

Norton, L. (1998) Health promotion and health education: what role should the nurse adopt in practice? *Journal of Advanced Nursing* 28: 1269–75.

Nursing and Midwifery Council (2002) *Requirements for Pre-registration Programmes.* London: NMC.

Parkin, T. and Skinner, T. C. (2003) Discrepancies between patient and professional recall and perception of an outpatient consultation. *Diabetic Medicine* 20: 909–14.

Polonsky, W. H. (1999) *Diabetes Burnout.* Alexandria, VA: American Diabetes Association.

Rafael, A. R. (1999) The politics of health promotion: influences on public health nursing practice in Ontario, Canada from Nightingale to the Nineties. *Advances in Nursing Science* 22 (1): 23–39.

Reed, J. A., Ashton, H., Lawrence, J., Hollinghurst, S. and Higgs, E. R. (2003) Diabetes self-management: how are we doing? *Practical Diabetes International* 20: 318–22.

Robinson, S. E. and Hill, Y. (1998) The health promoting nurse. *Journal of Clinical Nursing* 7: 232–8.

Rodgers, J. and Walker, R. (2002) Empowerment – not for all? *Journal of Diabetes Nursing* 6: 38–9.

Roisin, P., Rees, M. E., Stott, N. and Rollnick, S. R. (1999) Can nurses learn to let go? Issues arising from an intervention designed to improve patients' involvement in their own care. *Journal of Advanced Nursing* 29: 1492–9.

Rollnick, S., Mason, P. and Butler, C. (2000) *Health Behaviour Change.* Edinburgh: Churchill Livingstone.

Statutory Instrument (1983) *The Nurses, Midwives and Health Visitors Rules Approval Order.* SI no. 873. London: HMSO.

Statutory Instrument (1989) *The Nurses, Midwives and Health Visitors (Parts of the Register) Amendment (No.2) Order*. SI no. 1455. London: HMSO.

Statutory Instrument (2000) *The Nurses, Midwives and Health Visitors (Training) Amendment Rules Approval Order*. SI no. 2554. London: HMSO.

Sutherland, S. (1994) *Irrationality: the Enemy Within*. London: Penguin.

Tones, K. (2001) Health promotion: The empowerment imperative. In Scriven, A. and Orme, J. (eds) *Health Promotion: Professional Perspectives*. Basingstoke: Palgrave Macmillan.

Toobert, D. J., Hampson, S. E. and Glasgow, R. E. (2000) The Summary of diabetes self-care activities measure: results from seven studies and a revised scale. *Diabetes Care* 25: 943–50.

Weinstein, N. (1993) Testing four competing theories of health-protective behaviour. *Health Psychology* 12: 324–33.

Whitehead, D. (2001) Health education, behavioural change and social psychology: nursing's contribution to health promotion? *Journal of Advanced Nursing* 34: 822–32.

Whitehead, D. (2003) Evaluating health promotion: a model for nursing practice. *Journal of Advanced Nursing* 41 (5): 490–8.

Wikblad, K. F. (1991) Patient perspectives of diabetes care and education. *Journal of Advanced Nursing* 16: 837–44.

Williams, G., Freedman, Z. R. and Deci, E. L. (1998) Supporting autonomy to motivate patients with diabetes for glucose control. *Diabetes Care* 21: 1644–51.

World Health Organisation (1986) *Ottawa Charter for Health Promotion: an International Conference on Health Promotion, November 17–21*. Copenhagen: WHO.

World Health Organisation (1997) *The Jakarta Declaration on Leading Health into the 21st Century*. Geneva: WHO.

World Health Organisation (1998a) *Health Promotion Glossary*. Geneva: WHO.

World Health Organisation (1998b) *New Players for a New Era: Leading Health Promotion into the 21st Century. 4th International Conference on Health Promotion, Jakarta, Indonesia 21–25 July 1997*. Geneva: WHO.

CHAPTER 5

Health Promotion and the Role of the School Nurse

JANE THOMAS, PAUL WAINWRIGHT AND MELANIE JONES

Nursing as an occupation has its origins in the care and nurturing of children and nurses have always laid claim to the care of the person and the promotion of health and wellbeing, rather than the more narrow pursuit of diagnosis, prescription and the treatment of disease. The promotion of child health and the care of children in schools would therefore seem an obvious area for professional nursing to flourish. There is the added advantage that nurses tend to cost less and be more plentiful than doctors. The Audit Commission identified school nurses as key to school health functions (Audit Commission, 1994) and providing a context for their development in terms of interventions and health promotion. It is thus perhaps surprising that on the one hand there is so little evidence of the effectiveness of school nursing interventions (Wainwright et al., 1999) and that on the other school nurses are seldom mentioned in policy documents and reviews of child health policy. There is a tension between the two dynamics in school nursing: nursing care driven by bioscientific knowledge and medical models of health and care and the holistic, more person centred approach, the former exerting a reductionist effect and the latter being more eclectic. Historically the bioscientific model has dominated, as other authors in this part of the book testify, but as nursing matures as a profession more is expected and quality is viewed more widely. These two issues, the lack of evidence of effectiveness and the tension between disease oriented, biomedically driven interventions and holistic ones, do however reflect the general picture in nursing, as Whitehead so cogently argues in Chapter 2 of this text.

This chapter takes account of these tensions whilst exploring the nurse's contribution to the promotion of health from the school nursing perspective.

Historical background

School nursing grew from the extension of school medical services from 1912 onwards developing the surveillance and intervention aspects beyond

treatment and inspection functions. The specialism has experienced mixed for-
tunes since its establishment as a defined area of practice (Farrow, 2001). The
early years of school nursing saw the creation of substantive posts, funded by
health and education sectors in schools across the United Kingdom (UK) and
the integration of aspects of school health with areas of community nursing
practice and child health. The potential significance of school nursing as part
of child health should not be underestimated, given the extent to which events
in childhood impact on health throughout adult life. There can be no better
argument for investing efforts and resources in the health of children and the
role of the school nurse would seem to be a central part of that. So why is that
not the case? Why has school nursing experienced such difficult times in recent
years, to the point that the very survival of the service has been threatened in
many parts of the UK?

The Education Act of 1944 created an education system in which primary,
secondary and further education became a continuous process conducted in
three successive stages and became the responsibility of local government at
the county and county borough levels (Timmins, 1995: 93). The Act brought
in free school milk, meals, transport and medical inspections. There had been
some previous steps towards medical inspections through the Education Act of
1907 and free meals under the Liberal government of 1911 but Butler's 1944
Act, as part of the creation of the welfare state, set education firmly alongside
housing, employment, health and social security as the state's contribution to
the welfare of the people, whatever their class or economic status (Timmins,
1995). An effective, state provided education service, free at the point of delivery and compulsory up to the school leaving age, even if it had not included
direct health benefits such as medical inspections and free milk, arguably had
the potential to contribute to health and wellbeing as much as if not more than
any of the other aspects of the welfare state that Timmins (1995) critiques. It
is almost a cliché to argue that medical science and the National Health Service
(NHS) have contributed relatively little to the improvements in health and
increases in life expectancy that we have seen over the last century in the UK
(Baggott, 2000). Better housing and greater affluence have done more to
counter the threat of disease, and contemporary research still holds that the
most effective way to reduce inequalities in child health would be to eliminate
child poverty (see for example Acheson, 1998; Roberts, 2000). Poverty of
course undermines the ability of children to benefit from education but other
things being equal, education is regarded as one of the most important factors
in enabling individuals to improve their social and economic status (Marmot
and Wilkinson, 1999).

The development of the welfare state, and in particular the provision of
health and education services, can be seen as part of the humanistic project
that established both the academic disciplines of the child and childhood as we
know them today, including developmental psychology, paediatrics, child psychiatry, educational psychology, sociology, and the practices that intervene in
childcare, such as social work, and the institution of statutory protections in

the areas of health, work, and education (Rogers, 1993: 159). By this analysis, those responsible for the upbringing of children became increasingly responsible to the state and its agents, and children became a national asset (Rogers, 1993: 160).

If schools had no medical services, but simply delivered the curriculum, the benefits of education to the economy would still ensure that education led to improvements in the general health of society. The opportunity presented by bringing children together in a controlled, disciplined environment for significant periods of time resulted in an effective school medical service appearing a wise investment. This need was emphasised further by the health risks posed by the close proximity to each other of children from a variety of backgrounds, favouring the rapid transmission of infectious diseases such as measles, mumps, or more serious conditions such as diphtheria, polio and meningitis. Thus at the beginning of the twentieth century it was recognised that schoolchildren might spread infection between themselves through contact. Schools therefore deployed a regime of surveillance that stressed less the significance of sanitation and more the importance of personal hygiene (Armstrong, 1993: 58).

Development of school nursing

Historically school nursing has developed in diverse and uncoordinated ways across the UK (Bagnall and Dilloway, 1996). Nurses based in schools are either employed by the health service or by education departments in local authorities. Other school nurses are located in health service premises, providing a peripatetic service to a number of schools. Health visitors also assume school nursing duties in some geographical areas. Expenditure on school nursing varies widely, with Cotton et al. (2000) finding a range of spending from £5 to £9 per pupil per year. This diversity has not served to unify the school nursing service and one outcome has been that the professional profile of school nurses has been low (Wainwright et al., 1999). This in turn has resulted in little specific educational provision for the preparation and training of school nurses who are often characterised as predominantly female, part time, and lacking in ambition, working in education to take advantage of regular weekday working patterns and generous holidays to accommodate family responsibilities (Clarke et al., 2002). However unjust the stereotype, it has served to constrain school nursing and portray it as a less attractive area for ambitious and dynamic staff. But for the commitment and enthusiasm of nurses who work in the sector, policy change, funding constraints and recruitment problems might have consigned school nursing to history.

There is a distinct lack of any real or obvious interface between health services and the education system, despite their parallel development as part of the welfare state in the UK. This situation, characteristic of the division between health and social services, is not to the advantage of nurses working in schools in terms of funding, professional progression, working conditions and study leave. These structural problems, combined with the lack of a robust evidence base supporting the effectiveness of school nursing in the improvement of child health, results in school nursing being vulnerable to reduction and rationalisation. Even theoretical accounts of the contribution can explore the advantages of the educational setting and the potential contribution of teachers to health promotion with no mention of the place of school nursing (MacDonald, 2002). Not surprisingly, the calibre of the nurses who work in schools is variable (Clarke et al., 2002) but with support, training and encouragement most could improve their practice. Nurses in schools provide high level care for children, help for families, medical support for children with ongoing problems and health education and screening as part of child health services and their input may be particularly important in the provision of inclusive education (Sebba and Sachdev, 1997) and promoting wider community health (Dalziel, 2003). Given the clear strategic mandate for school nursing to play a fundamental part in improving of the health and wellbeing of children (Audit Commission, 1994; Department of Health (DoH), 1998, 1999; Welsh Office, 1998) it is time for school nursing to develop professionally to meet the challenge.

Professional development

Like many practitioners who move away from traditional, hospital based practice, school nurses have to sustain their clinical expertise through informal and professional networks, reading journals and attending courses. The specialist knowledge accrued in the educational setting has only comparatively recently been recognised and developed into formal, accredited programmes with parity of esteem alongside other nursing specialisms. The assessment skills, interpersonal skills tuned to the specific needs of children, awareness of legal, ethical and professional issues regarding children, autonomous decision making and responsibility required of school nurses exceed that of many colleagues working in mainstream healthcare. The ability to work interprofessionally, to prioritise and manage time effectively is taken for granted among nurses who work without direct supervision in school settings with children and young people. The school nurse is a professional with a particular contribution to make to the health of schoolchildren, and this specialist expertise has the potential to be fully exploited through health promotion and the range of activities it encompasses.

In spite of the increased statutory control of child rearing described by Rogers (1993), the lack of statutory requirements and national guidelines for specific school nursing services across the UK contributed to the problems of coordinating a proactive school nursing sector throughout the 1990s. A review of school nursing in Wales (Clarke et al., 2002) demonstrated the urgent need for the redefinition and redevelopment of school nursing. Political devolution in the UK, with responsibility for health services and education transferring to the National Assembly for Wales and to the Scottish Parliament, is likely to further influence the development of school nursing. The political and structural differences will undoubtedly increase over time unless the Nursing and Midwifery Council works through the devolved professional regulatory system and school nurses collaborate to provide standardisation and quality of provision across the UK. The current fragmentation of service undermines the coherent provision of health promotion as part of the fundamental education of children and young people, but the new public health agenda (Wanless, 2004: 69) provides opportunities to develop and evaluate the school nursing contribution to the health of children at school.

Educational context

The Health Promoting School movement (WHO, 1997) has developed education as a health promotion setting and provides the potential for extending school nursing interventions in this area. The establishment of health promotion as part of the Personal, Social and Health Education (PSHE) cross curricular theme following the Education Reform Act (Department for Education and Science [DfES], 1988) altered the status of health in the curriculum from a peripheral concern to stronger position as a theme across the statutory subjects. Bunton and MacDonald (2002) argue that the educational perspective challenges the assumptions of health promotion and this is particularly relevant to school nursing where issues of choice and autonomy are gaining momentum. The right to free choice, whether healthful or otherwise, is important in the context of adult health and presents complex issues in relation to children at school (Scriven and Stiddard, 2003).

The ethical aspects of health promotion for children at school are bound up with the whole debate about social control and the social construction of child rearing. However, if prevailing social attitudes are accepted and assumptions are made that the benefits of normative interventions outweigh any doubts about paternalism or loss of autonomy, and even if troubling questions about evidence of effectiveness are left aside, we must at the very least be convinced of the accuracy of any information disseminated in the name of health promotion and its benefits to health. There is also the responsibility to be truthful, to maintain confidentiality and respect privacy, to seek consent, to avoid harm and victim blaming and to promote freedom, justice, equity and choice. Such constraints are challenging and not infrequently contradictory, but nevertheless, partnerships between school nurses and teachers should foster shared approaches to promote healthy choice for children, their families and the wider community. The investment in every child as a national asset (Rogers, 1993) can be seen as an investment for future health, the health of the nation. However, such claims also carry overtones of the health of children as an instrumental rather than an intrinsic good and the danger of the health of children being seen more as a means than as an end.

The challenges in the current education system include testing, target setting and the competitive culture, fostering parental choice and providing public access to performance data. The local management of schools that involves decentralised budgets and the enhanced role of school governors complicates the situation, creating a climate in which academic achievement rather than empowerment is the objective (Scriven, 2001). Although attitudes to testing, target setting and league tables may be changing, with Wales taking a lead in discarding tests now seen to be unhelpful (National Literacy Trust, 2004), it is easy to see how areas such as health promotion can be sidelined if there is no support and enthusiasm from trained and experienced nurses. Indeed, one of the ironies of education policy over the last couple of decades is that the very activities that might be thought to contribute to health and wellbeing, such as sport and exercise, and non-academic activities such as clubs, hobbies and extracurricular music, have been driven out of the life of schools by the sale of playing fields (House of Commons Health Committee, 2004), a reluctance on the part of teaching staff to give time for extra curricular activities and the obsession with performance targets in core curriculum subjects (British Broadcasting Corporation [BBC], 2003).

The proportion of the day that children spend at school justifies substantial investment in creating health promoting environments and the promoting of health and wellbeing in a familiar learning environment (Scriven and Stiddard, 2003). The process of educating children and young people academically, physically, attitudinally, behaviourally and socially lends itself well to planned and opportunistic health promotion and the school nurse has the potential to play a direct role but also to contribute to strategic planning. Recognition of the school as a fundamental part of the welfare network for children is essential to the notion of the healthy school that takes account of the wider perspective on health and promotes the development of children and maximises their health potential (Beattie, 2001). Another perspective on contextual health promotion, developed in relation to relational fields is the Seedhouse (2002) concept of total health promotion. He cites the example of Healthy School development in relation to bullying and one can envisage the expansion of this way of working in school nursing.

Theoretical basis of practice

Wainwright et al. (1999) reviewed the school nursing literature with the intention of identifying factors influencing the success and effectiveness of school nurses in health promoting interventions. The difficulties of measuring effectiveness and of demonstrating impact from health promotion interventions make the production of evidence particularly problematic, as not all inputs are measurable or outcome related. Wainwright and his colleagues identified a lack of research and evidence to support the school nursing role and the effectiveness of interventions, issues also discussed by Bradley (1998). Their recommendations provide key areas for action in the development of school nurses nationwide and their contribution to the promotion of health among children and young people, as follows:

- prioritisation of health promotion skills, extending the role of the school nurse and resources available
- focussing of evaluative efforts on the effectiveness of particular school nurse led interventions
- development of flexible educational provision to support the development of research skills among school nurses
- involvement of academic institutions in the support of school nurse practice based research
- development of child health strategies that include school health strategies.

Wainwright et al. (1999) could not identify any concerted use of health promotion models in the health promoting practice of school nurses and there was no evidence to support the effectiveness or applicability of one model over another in any consistent manner. Although definitions, models and frameworks for health promotion may not have been widely used in school nursing practice several present themselves as appropriate and easily adapted for use in the sector. Tannahill's model (Downie et al., 1996) is familiar to many nurses and the applicability of the three domains to the school context would make it an appropriate and achievable framework for practice. Examples in use would include sex education in Tannahill's domain of health education, immunisation in the domain of prevention and citizenship relating to the domain of health protection issues, the three domains being drawn together through the national curriculum. Caraher (1994) proposed two models as useful to nursing, Becker's health belief model (1974) and Ewles and Simnett's taxonomy of approaches (revised in the fifth edition of Ewles and Simnett, 2003: 45). Caraher also recommended that nurses personally audit their health promotion practice. The proposition of questioning practice would enable nurses to easily encompass ethical, analytical and empowering in balanced interaction with adults and children.

Opportunities and barriers

Chapter 1 in this book provided a foundation from which to consider the contribution of school nurses to health promotion by appraising the context for health promoting practice. The policies, principles and perspectives that inform health and health promotion are examined and the potential for the movement to public health approaches explored. This chapter develops these issues now to consider the potential contribution of school nurses to the health of children in schools, their families and society at large. Examples of school nursing practice include:

- primary health promotion: immunisation or cardiac health (see also Jones and Hinton in Chapter 14 for further discussion of family approaches)
- secondary health promotion: anorexia (see also Harries in Chapter 10)
- tertiary health promotion: diabetes (see also Ashton and Rodgers in Chapter 4).

Harries' account of the occupational therapist's role in the management of anorexia in Chapter 10 of this text offers a connection with school nursing in the promotion of health, in terms of secondary health promotion. The issues around gender in relation to the condition and functional support for young people as they work to establish or re-establish patterns of eating conducive to their health and wellbeing are familiar to school nurses and there is the potential to develop innovative primary prevention by working collaboratively with colleagues outside the school system.

The previous chapter by Ashton and Rodgers on diabetes and health promotion explores the need for more empowering ways of working and this applies equally to diabetic children and adolescents. Behaviour change approaches, the lifestyle focus and secondary and tertiary health promotion have worked well in this area but there is scope for a more proactive approach. Concerns about diet, in school meals and tuck shops (House of Commons Health Committee, 2004) and the loss of sports facilities (Wanless, 2004) are particularly relevant in the context of the appearance of Type 2 diabetes in children. This development is particularly worrying, whether one is concerned with the welfare of the individual child or with the eventual consequences for society. It is a disturbing indication of the lack of coordination of services and the lack of recognition of this aspect of the role of school nurses that more work on snack food consumed in schools has been done by dental hygienists seeking to improve dental health than by school nurses worrying about obesity and its consequences. Media coverage suggests that there is also some scepticism in government as to the effectiveness of measures such as the removal of vending machines and the provision of more healthy options, particularly given the ease with which children can leave the school premises to purchase food and drink from local shops. This is not the place for a lengthy discussion of the broader social and cultural issues of junk food, advertising aimed at children and so on, but it does underline the difficulty of tackling problems of children's diets in schools in isolation from complex issues of social change (for further discussion of this issue see Caraher et al., 2005).

Whitehead, in Chapter 2 of this text, offers an appraisal of the culture, context and progress of health promotion in nursing from the original WHO assertion that nurses have the potential to be at the forefront of health promotion, through the professional sanction of that way of working, to ultimate recognition that nurses have, for a variety of reasons, failed to achieve this potential. One reason is the persistent attachment to health education and preventive practices which were effective in the 1980s but which have since been surpassed by methodological developments in health promotion practice. Nursing must regain its position within the mainstream of health promotion and find ways to adapt practice to suit diverse nursing contexts such as in the schools setting. The need for consistent and effective health promoting practice within nursing has been established more in some sectors of nursing than others and school nurses can learn from examples in these areas.

The dominance of disease reduction approaches and nurses' alliance with the medical model of health and treatment (see also Whitehead's discussion in Chapter 2) has held school nursing back in health promoting terms. The study by Cotton et al. (2000) also found that a substantial amount of time was spent on routine screening and health surveillance. Although health appears as one of the so called metaparadigm concepts for nursing (Fawcett, 1995) the nursing literature is surprisingly short of clear, well developed accounts of the concept of health as it might be understood in nursing terms. The preoccupation of school nursing with traditional expectations of first aid provision, the treatment of head lice, and sex education has served only to marginalise the specialism and to reinforce the view of it as a peripheral area of practice rather than a central aspect of child health. Health promotion has been established as a fundamental activity in health visiting (see Weeks et al., Chapter 3 in this text) but the same emphasis has not been achieved in school nursing. The lack of evidence of effectiveness (Wainwright et al., 1999) has compounded the situation and school nursing has paid the price.

The future for health promotion in school nursing

Health service reform has brought the need for a more responsive service to the forefront (DoH, 1997) and school nursing is now building a future perspective with health promotion as a central feature of the role, extending beyond the school and into the community (Dalziel, 2003), in keeping with the developing public health agenda and in collaboration with the multidisciplinary workforce in health, education and social care contexts (see for example Law et al. in Chapter 18 of this text on speech therapy or Verne and Scott in Chapter 9 on dietetics). The opportunity for role development in school nursing is clear but it needs support at strategic and operational levels if the change to an integrated and proactive school nursing service is to be achieved and if school nursing is to assert itself alongside other health promoting professions.

The role of the school nurse has long been publicly valued and has reemerged in recent years with child health issues prominent in our national health agenda. Farrow (2001) has identified the diversity of the role as key to school nursing. The impact of the role on children and their families is relatively constant but so are the problems of combating the lack of an effective health and education interface, the need for investment and resources and the need to demonstrate effectiveness. Role extension is a significant challenge for school nursing but development and prioritisation of the health promotion work of school nurses provides one way forward. The time is right for practice development in school nursing but there is a need to sustain the prominence of areas of strength such as health promotion. That is not to argue in favour of either specialism or generalism, but to add another dimension, embracing educational innovation and a research base. School nursing has done well to survive the shift of focus from care provision and first aid to a more integrated approach, working across boundaries with other disciplines in a more preventive and health promoting way. Skill mix has not been an issue for school nurses in the UK until recently but in America support workers are involved to a much greater extent in the care of children at school while France has no standard school nursing provision. The work force definitions used by planners in the National Assembly for Wales recognise both the school nurse with the specialist qualification and the school nurse, unqualified (Richards, 2004), which suggests that the value of the qualification is not widely acknowledged. School nurses need to defend their role in the health of school age children in terms of quality of input with regard to skill mix and workload, as caseloads also vary widely across the UK, influencing the type and range of potential interventions available to the school nurse.

The presence of a nurse in a health promoting capacity within schools has the potential to develop health and wellbeing in children beyond the physical and psychological aspects of health. Middleton (1997) identified education as a form of health promotion in itself, exploring its role in preventing crime. The extended role of education provides particular opportunities for school nursing to expand its contribution to health promotion. Weare (2002) has championed the educational context for health promotion proposing a breadth of strategy and approach to empowerment and the promotion of autonomy in schools.

An interesting example of an area where school nurses might develop health promoting practice, but one that also demonstrates the difficulties inherent in such an approach, is the concept of resilience. Resilience has been defined as the maintenance of competent functioning despite an interfering emotionality (Newman and Blackburn, 2002: 3). Newman and Blackburn argue that children have become less able to cope with obstacles and stress compared with earlier generations and recent trends in health and social care have tended to highlight risk factors, a development that can be seen also in schools. They argue that risk factors can be seen as opportunities for growth and adaptation and that, while our increased awareness of such risks has led to improvements in the physical health of children there has also been an increase in psychological and conduct disorders in most developed countries in the last 50 years and children have themselves reported an increase in long term illnesses. Thus if there were agreement about the kind of activities and interventions that might increase resilience in children there might be substantial gains to be had in terms of physical and psychosocial health, in the short as well as the longer term. The notion of risk raises issues around risk reduction and the potential for overreaction that is more detrimental than the original risk. The fear of litigation has resulted in identified risks being excluded or controlled in schools (see, for example, Hinsliff, 2004), innately risky activities such as sport and play can be curtailed and this in turn impairs child health and wellbeing.

As with many attempts to pursue more holistic ideas of health and wellness, resilience turns out to be a complex and multifaceted concept, and one that emerges as a result of a multitude of factors. There are no specific health promoting interventions which primarily focus on resilience. Unfortunately for the school nurse, interventions in health, education and social care may do harm as well as good and resilience may be weakened by unnecessary or harmful interventions (Newman and Blackburn, 2002: 10). Excessive preoccupation with identifying and eliminating risk factors may also undermine resilience, and thus by this account many traditional school nursing activities may be counterproductive.

Wainwright et al. (1999) identified a lack of research into school nursing health promotion practice and a resultant lack of evidence to support the role and contribution of the school nurse. This was supported by the review by Clarke et al. (2002) and their recommendation that research be commissioned to improve the evidence base on school nursing and effective school health provision. School nursing is at a critical point where the pressure is not only to promote the health of children, but also to do so thoroughly, appropriately and with regard to the available evidence. Where there is a lack of evidence to support school based practice, nurses should engage as users of and participants in research to demonstrate effectiveness, efficiency and reliable relationships. Not all school nurses want to undertake research but they need to be users of research, as a means of enhancing practice and sustaining currency.

The development of clearer theoretical perspectives on school nursing, utilising a strong evidence base, will demand a much greater clarity of what it is that health promotion in schools can realistically provide. The valuable contribution of school nurses to specific healthcare activities has been alluded to, such as the support of children with chronic illnesses, the organisation and conduct of medical examinations and surveillance programmes, immunisation and so on. However, these activities reflect a highly reductive, bioscience approach and a biostatistical rather than a holistic view of health (Nordenfeldt, 1993). Even initiatives to improve eating habits or encourage exercise, while less obviously disease specific, can reflect the medical approach. However, if school nurses are to function to their full potential it would seem important that they address the nursing function of nurturing and promoting wellbeing. This is arguably more likely to produce lasting benefit but much more difficult to justify in terms of evidence based practice, at least as this is narrowly conceived by those who subscribe to the systematic review of randomised controlled trials as the gold standard of evidence (Rolls, 1999).

There can be no doubt that the years of compulsory education provide an excellent opportunity to shape the future health and wellbeing of those who pass through it (Moon, 1999). Nurses, historically, have the motivation and the skills required to support the healthy development of children in schools and there might be more opportunities in future for nurses to develop their role in relation to the National Curriculum Personal, Social and Health Education input. However, if they are to succeed, they must develop a clear philosophical and theoretical basis for their practice, balancing the important and necessary bioscience based interventions with more holistic strategies to promote health and wellbeing and finding the means to justify these. This will present a considerable challenge. The centrality of health promotion as a health investment strategy has been emphasised by Levin and Ziglio (2003) but with a clearer emphasis on a critical approach. School nurses are in a unique position to develop theoretically, strategically, operationally and critically in terms of their health promotion function. National occupational standards devised for use in public health practice (Faculty of Public Health, 2004) provide a context within which school nursing can make a strong, specific and substantial impact on the health and wellbeing of children across the UK. Over time and with commitment, school nursing will emerge with a body of evidence to support its practice and become recognised as a valued constant in the health of all school age children.

References

Acheson, D. (1998) *The Report of the Independent Inquiry into Inequalities in Health.* London: The Stationery Office.

Armstrong, A. (1993) From clinical gaze to regime of total health. In Beattie, A., Gott, M., Jones, L. and Sidell, M. (eds) (1993) *Health and Wellbeing: a Reader.* Basingstoke: Palgrave Macmillan.

Audit Commission (1994) *Seen but not Heard: Co ordinating Community Child Health and Social Services for Children in Need.* London, HMSO.

Baggott, R. (2000) *Public Health, Policy and Politics.* Basingstoke: Palgrave Macmillan.

Bagnall, P. and Dilloway, M. (1996) *In Search of a Blue Print: a Survey of School Health Services.* London: DoH/Queen's Nursing Institute.

Beattie, A. (2001) Health Promoting Schools as Learning Organisations. In Scriven, A. and Orme, J. *Promoting Health: Professional Perspectives.* Basingstoke: Palgrave Macmillan.

Becker, M. H. (1974) The health belief model and personal health behaviour. *Health Education Monographs 2 4.*

Bradley, B. J. (1998) Establishing a research agenda for school nursing. *Journal of School Nursing* 14 (1, February): 4–13.

British Broadcasting Corporation (2003) Teachers denounce national tests. http://news.bbc.co.uk/1/hi/education/3209245.stm (accessed 7 July 2004)

Bunton, R. and MacDonald, G. (eds) (2002) *Health Promotion: Disciplines, Diversity and Development.* London: Routledge.

Caraher, M. (1994) Health promotion: time for an audit. *Nursing Standard* 8 (2, 9 February).

Caraher, M., Coveney, J. and Lang, T. (2005) Food health and globalisation: is health promotion still relevant? In Scriven, A. and Garman, S. (eds) *Promoting Health: Global Perspectives*. Basingstoke: Palgrave Macmillan.

Clarke, J., Buttigieg, M., Bodycombe-James, M., Eaton, N., Kelly, A., Merrell, J., Thomas, J., Parke, S. and Symonds, A. (2002) *Recognising the Potential: the Review of Health Visiting and School Health Services in Wales*. Cardiff: National Assembly for Wales.

Cotton, L., Brazier, J., Hall, D., Lindsay, G., Marsh, P., Polnay, L. and Williams, S. (2000) School nursing: costs and potential benefits. *Journal of Advanced Nursing* **31** (5): 1063.

Dalziel, Y. (2003) The role of nurses in public health. In Watterson, A. (ed.) *Public Health in Practice*. Basingstoke: Palgrave Macmillan.

Department for Education and Science (1988) *Education Reform Act*. London: HMSO.

Department of Health (1997) *The New NHS: Modern, Dependable*. London: The Stationery Office.

Department of Health (1998) *The Health of the Nation: a Policy Assessment*. London: The Stationery Office.

Department of Health (1999) *Reducing Health Inequalities: an Action Report*. London: The Stationery Office.

Department of Health (1999) *Saving Lives: Our Healthier Nation*. London: The Stationery Office.

Downie, R. S., Tannahill, C. and Tannahill, A. (1996) *Health Promotion: Models and Values*, second edition. Oxford: Oxford University Press.

Ewles, L. and Simnett, I. (2003) *Promoting Health: a Practical Guide*, fifth edition. London: Baillière Tindall.

Faculty of Public Health (2004) *The National Occupational Standards for the Practice of Public Health*. London: FPH.

Farrow, S. (2001) The Role of the school nurse in promoting health. In: Scriven, A. and Orme, J. (eds) (2001) *Promoting Health: Professional Practice*, second edition. Basingstoke: Palgrave Macmillan.

Fawcett, J. (1995) *Analysis and Evaluation of Conceptual Models of Nursing*. Philadelphia, PA: F. A. Davis.

Hinsliff, G. (2004) New blitz on compensation culture. *Education Guardian* http://education.guardian.co.uk/schooltrips/story/0,10621,1228482,00.html (accessed 7 July 2004)

House of Commons Health Committee (2004) *Obesity: Third Report of Session 2003–2004, Volume 1*. London: The Stationery Office.

Marmot , M. and Wilkinson, R. G. (1999) *Social Determinants of Health*. Oxford: Oxford University Press.

Middleton, J. (1997) Crime is a public health problem. In Siddell, M., Jones, L., Katz, J., Peberdy, A. and Douglas, J. *Debates and Dilemmas in Promoting Health*. Basingstoke: Palgrave Macmillan/Open University.

Moon, A. (1999) Rationale of work in school settings. In Perkins, E. R., Simnett, I. and Wright, L. (1999) *Evidence-based Health Promotion*. Chichester: Wiley.

National Literacy Trust (2004) www.literacytrust.org.uk/Database/tables.html#14-year-old (accessed 7 July 2004)

Newman, T. and Blackburn, S. (2002) *Transitions in the Lives of Children and Young People: Resilience Factors*. Edinburgh: Scottish Education Development Department.

Nordenfeldt, L. (1993) Concepts of health and their consequences for health care. *Theoretical Medicine* **14**: 277–85.

Richards, D. (2004) Personal communication, 16 January.

Roberts, H. (2000) *What Works in Reducing Health Inequalities in Child Health?* Basildon: Barnardos.

Rogers, R. S. (1993) The social construction of child rearing. In: Beattie, A., Gott, M., Jones, L. and Sidell, M. (eds) (1993) *Health and Wellbeing: a Reader.* Basingstoke: Macmillan (now Palgrave Macmillan).

Rolls, E. (1999) The challenge of evidence-based practice. In Perkins, E. R., Simnett, I. and Wright, L. (1999) *Evidence-based Health Promotion.* Chichester: Wiley.

Scriven, A. (2001) The influence of government policy on the provision of health education in schools. In Scriven, A. and Orme, J. (eds) *Promoting Health: Professional Perspectives.* Basingstoke: Palgrave Macmillan.

Scriven, A. and Stiddard, L. (2003) Empowering schools: translating principles into practice. *Health Education* **103** (2): 110–18.

Sebba, J. and Sachdev, D. (1997) *What Works in Inclusive Education?* Basildon: Barnardos.

Seedhouse, D. (2002) *Total Health Promotion: Mental Health, Rational Fields and the Quest For Autonomy.* Chichester: Wiley.

Timmins, N. (1995) *The Five Giants: a Biography of the Welfare State.* London: Fontana.

Wainwright, P., Thomas, J. and Jones, M. (1999) *School Nursing: A Review of the Literature.* Cardiff: Health Promotion Wales.

Wanless, D. (2004) *Securing Good Health for the Whole Population: Final Report.* London: HMSO.

Weare, K. (2000) *Promoting Mental, Emotional and Social Health: A Whole School Approach.* London: Routledge.

Weare, K. (2002) *The Contribution of Education to Health Promotion.* In Bunton, R. and MacDonald, G. (eds) (2002) *Health Promotion: Disciplines, Diversity and Development.* London: Routledge.

Welsh Office (1998) *Better Health, Better Wales.* Cardiff: Welsh Office.

World Health Organisation (1997) *The Health Promoting School: An Investment in Education, Health and Democracy.* Conference report on the first conference of the European Network of Health Promoting Schools, Thessaloniki, Greece. Copenhagen: WHO.

CHAPTER 6

A Hospital Nursing Based Osteoporosis Prevention Study: Action Research in Action

DEAN WHITEHEAD

The focus of this chapter is an innovative and comprehensive hospital nurse initiated and led preventative health education strategy. Its relevance to this book is twofold in that it firstly relates to a health promotion challenge facing health services, that of preventative osteoporosis service provision, and secondly mirrors a number of current health policy trends, such as multiprofessional, multiagency collaboration, service reform and the employment of organisational action change strategies.

The National Health Service (NHS) South West Regional Executive/Office (NHSE-SW, NHS-SWRO) in the United Kingdom (UK) originally commissioned the research on which the chapter is based, as part of its project *Our Healthier Nation: Improving the Competence of the Workforce in Health Promotion*. The overarching aim of the project was to work with educationalists and healthcare practitioners to explore ways of improving the knowledge, skills and competencies of healthcare professionals in taking forward health promotion within clinical settings in a way that was timely, appropriate and sensitive to patient needs. Several regional reports from this NHS project have already been published (NHSE-SW, 1999a, 1999b; NHS-SWRO, 2002). Whitehead et al. (2003) elaborate on the process and outcomes of the overall project as well as offering a detailed description of the research design used in this particular study.

As mentioned previously, from the overall NHS project, this localised osteoporosis research study was conceived as the collaboration between a hospital Trust and its neighbouring university, hence the differing agencies involved. The research team was composed of senior practitioners from both agencies and differing health professional disciplines, combining the role of academic researchers with that of the clinical interventionist. Although an equal partnership approach was adopted, the study was nevertheless deemed to be both nurse initiated and nurse led. After general agreement amongst the research team, the programme design of choice was a participatory action research (PAR) approach, through which the existing hospital based osteoporosis service was explored.

The intention of this study was to affect and implement organisation based service delivery and reform. In action research (AR) studies, change is not imposed or even knowable, but is discovered as it happens and as part of an ongoing learning process (Bate, 2000). Nevertheless, the study participants wanted to avoid the situation faced by Waller et al. (2002), whereby their preventative osteoporosis programme produced no significant effect. The PAR design helped to facilitate this process by allowing the participants to initially assess the existing preventative osteoporosis service, determine the issues and problems and decide on an appropriate service reform programme. Over the two year life span of this study, the osteoporosis service in question expanded its health education and health promotion activities to include a wider range of preventative services. This chapter chronicles the change process and details the programme outcomes.

The extent of the osteoporosis problem

Osteoporosis is a preventable disease that is known to place both a huge economic and a social burden on societies worldwide. Despite this, evidence suggests that preventative osteoporosis activity is afforded a low priority within health services. Far less emphasis is placed upon supporting clients through preventative health promotion activities than on reactive screening and pharmacological interventions.

The true extent of the global osteoporosis problem should not be underestimated and cannot be overstated. The evidence clearly indicates that the osteoporosis situation is already a major public health burden for many if not most health services throughout the world. Osteoporosis places a huge economic and social burden on societies throughout the world in terms of human suffering, loss of productivity and dramatically increased healthcare costs (Epstein and Goodman, 1999; Ribeiro and Blakeley, 2001). Each year it costs the UK's health service an estimated £942 million, Canada's CN$1.3 billion and the USA's over US$10 billion (Dolan and Torgerson, 1998; Scheiber and Torregrosa, 1999). These figures are set to spiral in the near future. It is predicted that the burden to the US economy alone will increase to more than US$60 billion by the year 2020 (National Osteoporosis Foundation, 1997). What is particularly surprising in this fact is that osteoporosis and its predecessor, osteopenia, are almost entirely preventable. This situation is set to further escalate over the next decade or so until, if left unchecked, osteoporosis has the potential to become the biggest global disease epidemic. The failure of many health services to address the preventative determinants of osteoporosis provision has exacerbated the situation.

The dilemmas faced by nurses in dealing with osteoporosis

Many health professionals, including hospital nurses, are either unaware of the extent of the osteoporosis problems that health services face and of the growing evidence surrounding its progression or remain unmoved by the necessity to actively engage in preventative, rather than reactive, health promotion or health education programmes. Fleming and Patrick (2002) state that most physicians, even if they appreciate the value of osteoporosis prevention, still fail to preventatively counsel their clients. In essence, medically focussed and reactive management represents the mainstay of most osteoporosis services. This is despite the fact that Freedman et al. (2000) claim that current physician led treatments for osteoporosis in postmenopausal women are often inadequate or inappropriate, while Westesson et al. (2002) argue that most osteoporosis sufferers remain underdiagnosed and undertreated. Torgerson (1998) states that half of all women sustaining a hip fracture do not receive any osteoporosis related treatment as follow up.

Many nurses are in a better position than doctors to support and advise clients about the treatment and prevention of osteoporosis, as well as make a significant contribution to research in this area (Cavalieri, 1998; Leslie, 2000; Schmitt, 2000; Wilson, 2001). In reality, however, this is rarely the case. Limited evidence is available to indicate that existing osteoporosis services have been initiated, developed or evaluated by nurses, apart from a few notable exceptions that have been conducted mostly in North America (Sutcliffe, 1999; Sedlak et al., 2000; Ribeiro and Blakeley, 2001; Curry et al., 2002). Sutcliffe (1999) states that client interventions for osteoporosis remain medically dominated with limited support provided by nursing staff, even within a reactive medical role. The osteoporosis knowledge base of both nurses and clients is seriously lacking and represents an acute need for nurses to be further educated in this field (Hunt and Repa-Eschen, 1998; Allanach, 2000).

Health education programmes in institutional settings

As part of recently emerging reform programmes throughout the world, many hospitals are required to pursue a notable shift from their focus on a medical and curative service function, towards the delivery of wider health services across the whole health and social care continuum. Underpinning this reform, the Health Promoting Hospital (HPH) movement has singled out the hospital setting for particular attention, advocating broad health promotion and health education activities as the mainstay of such reform. The progress and reform of the Health Promoting Hospital movement continue to be well documented and have resulted in a series of influential reports, which include

The Budapest Declaration on Health Promoting Hospitals and *The Vienna Recommendations on Health Promoting Hospitals* (World Health Organisation (WHO), 1990, 1991, 1997). The WHO subsequently devotes an extensive website to the European HPH movement's international progress (WHO, 2003a 2003b). In essence, hospitals, as institutions with the potential to actively promote the health and wellbeing of their users and workforce, have been concertedly targeted, in an attempt to bring about radical health promotion expansion and reform.

Healthcare resources and priority have shifted from institutional and curative based service delivery, towards community driven preventative social action, cohesion and capital. Subsequently, hospitals are compelled to demonstrate notable shifts in practice, as are the health professionals employed within them. It is argued here that the best vehicles for such shifts and reform lie with the concerted health education and health promotion strategies and programmes that incorporate the principles of capacity building and organisational change, as part of a concerted reorientation of service delivery that promotes health within and outside physical health service boundaries. The challenge here, however, lies in convincing hospital organisations as a whole that sustained health education and health promotion initiatives ease rather than add to any organisational reform burden and improve chances for overall effectiveness, while also providing fresh ways to tackle existing problems (Pelikan et al., 1997).

It is known that many hospitals are still hesitant about incorporating broader health promotion initiatives into their structure, organisation and culture (Bakx et al., 2001). Similarly, Guilmette et al. (2001) state that the hospital demands of reducing inpatient stay periods and other functional outcomes mean that health promotion and health education issues do not receive the attention that they deserve. Specific health related projects in hospitals could be used as a vehicle towards a broader aim of wider development within the organisational setting (Whitelaw et al., 2001). This said, the majority of hospital based, nursing related health promotion programmes almost exclusively involve health education activities that focus on behavioural and individualistic aspects, at the expense of organisational and structural reform (Haddock and Burrows, 1997; Preston, 1997; Galvin et al., 2000; Bolman et al., 2002; Kim et al., 2003). Some nursing examples, however, do exist that demonstrate some degree of organisational transition towards broader health promotion initiatives (Glasper, 1995; Bensberg et al., 2003).

Action research as a method for organisational change

The participants in the osteoporosis prevention study were from the outset motivated to see through a programme of reform and hence action research was the preferred choice for all involved. It is known that organisational and service change strategies are often ineffective, but AR has been successfully used to facilitate effective change processes in health service organisations (Hampshire, 2000). The changes emerge from the creation of knowledge constructed by a process of consensus building through observing and reflecting on immediate experiences, forming abstract generalisations and concepts, and testing and applying these experiences in new situations. Figure 6.1 demonstrates the typical cyclical process of an organisational Participatory Action Research approach. Action research is particularly relevant when applied to health service organisations and represents a best practice approach for investigating and achieving service and organisational change in these settings (Thassri et al., 2000; Earl-Slater, 2002). A number of authors state that AR methods are also particularly appropriate when applied to health related programmes (Green et al., 1996; Tones, 2000; Whitehead et al., 2003). Some have highlighted the fact that action research closely fulfils the goals and principles of the participatory learning processes that underpin health education programmes (WHO, 1998; Tones, 2000).

The study process

A more detailed account of this study's methodological and findings based processes can be found in Whitehead et al. (2004). The study began with the research participants defining their roles within the programme and agreeing the nature and determinants of an ongoing equal and shared power and decision making capacity. This happened once the study participants had been voluntarily selected from initial forums of interested clinicians and academics. The initial forums included senior medical staff, nursing managers, physiotherapists and occupational therapists working in a range of settings, including women's health, orthopaedics, elderly care, health information services and the osteoporosis service. Each potential participant was directly involved in some way in the management of osteoporosis in their own discipline and clinical setting. From the initial forums, appropriate and willing participant co-researchers were coopted into the study. Once the study participants were assembled the aim was to gather their knowledge of current osteoporosis prevention activity and then work collaboratively to further observe, understand and eventually bring about any agreed programme reform.

In collecting data, action research studies generally adopt a wide variety of data collection techniques within the frameworks of differing designs. The data was mainly gathered from PAR group interviews involving all the research participants. The group sessions took place every one to two months over a period of two years, with each session lasting between 60 to 90 minutes. During each session, detailed real time notes with the aid of a laptop computer were taken throughout. Written notes were also collected that highlighted key points and significant non-verbal cues. Key open ended questions were formulated for each session in order to maintain focus and direction. The sessions

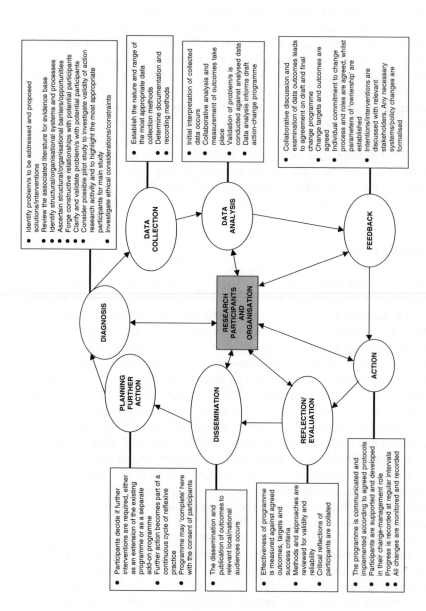

Figure 6.1 An organisational change action research cycle

Source: Adapted from Whitehead et al. (2003), with kind permission from *Health Education Journal*

enabled the group to review progress, identify emerging issues and agree and implement plans of action. Each session finished with a debriefing, while each new group session started with a re-review of the previous session notes. To supplement the group session data, further data were collected via the use of ongoing personal reflective diary accounts. Each of the participants maintained an up to date reflective account that they brought to each focus group session. Action research is seen to be more effective if the participants are actively self-reflecting and critically reflecting on the objective problem (Dickens and Watkins, 1999).

In terms of analysing the collected data after each group session, the transcribed notes were compared and contrasted against the reflective diary notes for similarities and emerging themes. The contextual detail of each session transcript was read in full by all the participants for familiarisation purposes and for extracting significant statements, then accompanied by a line by line analysis of the full transcripts, then unitised as a basis for defining categories later on. A systematic analysis of all the data involved the processes of immersion, open coding, development of broad categories, the coding of data into identified categories using content analysis, individual analysis involving thematic analysis and organising and writing up the results (Vaughn et al., 1996; Krueger, 1998). Meanings were composed and statements organised into clusters of themes and compared with initial ideas. The data were then combined and treated as a whole for analysis purposes. Once the initial analysis was conducted, the interpretation was discussed between all of the participants and negotiated as a valid interpretation of the data.

What results showed in terms of hospital nurses' health promoting approaches

Initial observations of the osteoporosis service informed the study participants that it was mostly confined to a biomedically defined and reactive role. Furthermore it left the participants with the impression that only limited preventative health education activity existed within the service. While the medical treatment of osteoporosis may have improved over recent years, a similar improvement is needed in preventative health promotion work (Epstein and Goodman, 1999). Those involved in this study mirrored this sentiment. It was agreed by all of the participants, even those that were already working in the osteoporosis service setting, that a preventative reform programme package was required to bridge the preventative deficit. Osteoporosis is a preventable disease and therefore preventative interventions should be offered long before the onset of disease (Ihrke, 1997; McClung, 1999; Healy, 2000). It is noted, however, that preventative information strategies are best integrated into the total health care package of osteoporosis sufferers (MacLennan, 1997), as was the intention in this particular programme. All clients and staff who responded to the aims and intentions of this study unanimously supported the need for a preventative osteoporosis programme and reported that they had already benefited from the information and services that it provided. The research participants were encouraged and motivated by the positive response that, in turn, prompted further programme reform and progress.

The level of information uptake in this study was encouraging throughout most of the previously mentioned clinical areas, women's health, orthopaedics and elderly care. In both the elderly and orthopaedic clinical settings all of the produced information packs were utilised. The most surprising finding of this study, however, was the level of uptake of information from the women's health setting. Only about half the number of packs taken up in the orthopaedic and elderly settings were taken up and used here. This echoes the concerns of the European Osteoporosis Study (1995), emphasising a reputed lack of understanding surrounding the disease on the part of women clients at risk of osteoporosis. The European study found that half of the women interviewed regarded osteoporosis as an inevitable consequence of an ageing process rather than a disease process, with little that they could do to prevent or alter this.

Upon further investigation it was found that organisational factors had significantly contributed to the fact that the osteoporosis service had existed mainly as a medically governed and reactive service. Alongside this, it was also concluded that such factors had ensured that further resources were unavailable for any planned preventative programme activity. Despite the fact that the Department of Health (DoH) (1995) stated its commitment to offer a seamless service by which osteoporosis would be prioritised and dealt with effectively, this appears not to have been the case in practice. Certainly, as this study suggests at its local level, this commitment had been lacking in terms of prioritisation and resourcing. The initial findings reflected the National Osteoporosis Society (NOS, 1995) study that suggested that half of the local health commissions and their purchasing authorities were still failing to comply with government guidelines.

One of the main findings of this study did not directly relate to the issue of osteoporosis prevention itself, but the collaborative nature of the study. It highlighted the usefulness of adopting participatory styles of clinical research activity and proved to be a liberating and helpful process for the participants when evaluating their experiences. The empowering action research framework that was adopted meant that the research team were able to explore their power relationships with each other, in line with a health promotion ideology (Sturt, 1999). Issues such as organisational political tension, lack of managerial authority, unequal power relationships and disempowered participants had the potential to influence the findings of this study but, where they existed, were overcome due to the nature of the chosen design. Each participant had the ability and authority to challenge existing structures without real threat and already had the advantage of being in a position to implement effective service reform within the parameters of professional autonomy. The closeness that was generated between the participants is the strength of action research in generating change and new knowledge in nursing (Williamson and Prosser, 2002).

Action cycle

Eventually, the participants were able to put into effect a long term preventative osteoporosis programme that spanned a two year period, with its effects continuing to be evident today. It targeted four different hospital based areas, the three clinical areas mentioned previously as well as the hospital public concourse area, as part of its ongoing programme. By the time the programme was fully implemented a range of health promoting activities were in place which included:

1. Designing and developing comprehensive *healthy bones* client health information packs. The information contained focused primarily on lifestyle related issues such as diet, exercise and falls prevention. The packs included contact and self-referral information for the hospital based health information centre and the Trust osteoporosis service. Negotiated contact details were contained for the local National Osteoporosis Society (NOS) sponsored osteoporosis support group
2. Designing and developing specific awareness raising osteoporosis prevention information packs for the clinical staff in the three designated clinical areas
3. Setting up osteoporosis awareness raising display boards in prominent area of each of the chosen clinical areas
4. Setting up formal health information referral processes for at risk clients and their relatives between the osteoporosis service and the health information centre
5. Developing in house posters for placing around the hospital with contact details of the osteoporosis service and health information centre
6. Developing several osteoporosis awareness campaign days for the general public in the main concourse area of the hospital
7. Revising several postqualifying clinical modules, including orthopaedic, health promotion and evidence based practice, delivered at the local university, to include osteoporosis related content.

As part of a concerted reform of the existing osteoporosis service, running alongside the preventative programme of this study other related activity was taking place. One of the participants in this study was an active member of another team set up to implement further review activities. They were subsequently able to report between the teams on the progress of both activities. This ongoing dialogue meant that the preventative programme activities were able to complement the overall service reform process. Further osteoporosis service reform activities included:

1. Approaching a major drugs company, which had provided short term funding for the employment of an osteoporosis nurse specialist. A business case had been put to the Trust for long term funding of this post. Funding had also been secured to send a physiotherapist and physician to visit an innovative fracture intervention service in Scotland

2. The participant in question became an active member of a regional multia-gency task group for a falls reduction pathway programme. A report came out of the findings of this task group (Devon County Implementation Group, 2002)
3. Setting up a formal fundraising group for a new osteoporosis scanner, involving members of this research study and the local osteoporosis support group. A senior representative of the National Osteoporosis Society was also involved
4. Establishing, in conjunction with the local NOS support group, an osteo-porosis community road show programme, running four times a year
5. Developing a formal osteoporosis service referral guideline for local general practitioners (GPs) based on the Royal College of Physicians guidelines
6. Initiating a rolling programme of osteoporosis awareness education days with local physiotherapists
7. Creating an ongoing and increasing level of preventative exercise classes linked to osteoporosis service referred clients. These include both *fit and flexi* and *weak and wobbly* programmes and involve a recently appointed Tai Chi instructor. These classes are run by one of the study participants.

Over the two year cycle of this study, a preventative and awareness raising hospital nurse led health promotion programme has been set up, achieving a significant number of outcomes. Its impact is ongoing, specifically because one of the study participants is still actively involved in the day to day running and activities of the osteoporosis service and is continuing to extend the range of preventative services on offer. Final reflections of the group participants uncovered a number of positive outcomes, particularly related to the level of organisational change that had been achieved and the clinical benefits accrued over the lifetime of the study and beyond. The successes of the study have prompted the impetus to develop the service further. Another potential study has been discussed that would measure and evaluate the direct impact of the osteoporosis service changes as it has continued to expand, although it would be principally aimed at the clinical staff and client interface. It would probably also adopt a PAR design in line with the previous programme.

As nurses seek to challenge and change their hospital based health promot-ing practices, they are reminded of the methods and approaches used in this study. Action Research methods are recommended to any health practitioner who is interested in a mutual learning process within which people work together to discover what the issues are, why they exist and how they might be addressed (Bate, 2000). This chapter particularly calls on hospital nurses, con-sidering their collective size and scope in institutional health service arenas, to make themselves instrumental in developing broad and wide reaching health education and health promotion strategies. This study is presented as an example of what can be achieved through adopting health promotion principles of participation, collaboration and multiprofessional partnership approaches to health promoting practice, in hospital nursing settings that traditionally have been less receptive to promoting health in a more holistic manner.

References

Allanach, V. (2000) Call for osteoporosis campaign. *Nursing Standard* 14 (44): 7.

Bate, P. (2000) Synthesising research and practice: using the action research approach in health care settings. *Social Policy and Administration* 34: 478–93.

Bakx, J., Dietscher, C. and Visser, A. (2001) Editorial – Health promoting hospitals. *Patient Education and Counselling* 45: 237–8.

Bensberg, M., Kennedy, M. and Bennetts, S. (2003) Identifying the opportunities for health promoting emergency departments. *Accident and Emergency Nursing* 11: 173–81.

Bolman, C., de Vries, H. and van Breukelen, G. (2002) Evaluation of a nurse managed minimal contact smoking cessation intervention for cardiac patients. *Health Education Research* 17: 99–116.

Cavalieri, R. J. (1998) Nursing presence in osteoporosis research. *American Journal of Nursing* 98: 60–3.

Curry, L. C., Hogstel, M. O., Davis, G. C. and Frable, P. J. (2002) Population based osteoporosis education for older women. *Public Health Nursing* 19: 460–9.

Department of Health (1995) *Advisory Group on Osteoporosis Report.* London: HMSO.

Devon County Implementation Group (2002) *The Health Forum: Tackling Inequalities in Health Through Partnership. Reducing Falls Among Older People, Task Group Report,* November. Devon: DCIG.

Dickens, L. and Watkins, K. (1999) Action research: rethinking Lewin. *Management Learning* 30: 127–40.

Dolan, P. and Torgerson, D. J. (1998) The cost of treating osteoporotic fractures in the United Kingdom female population. *Osteoporosis International* 8: 611–17.

Earl-Slater, A. (2002) The superiority of action research? *British Journal of Clinical Governance* 7: 132–5.

Epstein, S. and Goodman, G. R. (1999) Improved strategies for diagnosis and treatment of osteoporosis. *Menopause* 6: 242–50.

European Osteoporosis Study (1995) *European Osteoporosis Study.* London: Gordon Simmons Research Group.

Fleming, R. and Patrick, K. (2002) Osteoporosis prevention: paediatricians' knowledge, attitudes and counselling practices. *Preventative Medicine* 34: 411–21.

Freedman, K. B., Kaplan, F. S., Bilker, W. B., Strom, B. L. and Lowe, R. A. (2000) Treatment of osteoporosis: are physicians missing an opportunity? *Journal of Bone and Joint Surgery* 82A: 1063–70.

Galvin, K., Webb, C. and Hillier, V. (2000) The outcome of a nurse led health education programme for patients with peripheral vascular disease who smoke: assessment using attitudinal variables. *Clinical Effectiveness in Nursing* 4: 54–66.

Glasper, E. A., Lowson, S., Manger, R. and Phillips, L. (1995) Developing a centre for health information and promotion. *British Journal of Nursing* 4: 693–7.

Green, L. W., O'Neill, M., Westphal, M. and Morisky, D. (1996) The challenges of participatory action research for health promotion. *Promotion et Education* 3: 3–5.

Guilmette, T. J., Motta, S. I., Shadel, W. G., Mukand, J. and Niaura, R. (2001) Promoting smoking cessation in the rehabilitation setting. *American Journal of Physical Medicine & Rehabilitation* 80: 560–2.

Haddock, J. and Burrows, C. (1997) The role of the nurse in health promotion: an evaluation of a smoking-cessation programme in surgical pre-admission clinics. *Journal of Advanced Nursing* **26**: 1098–1110.

Hampshire, A. J. (2000) What is action research and can it promote change in primary care? *Journal of Evaluation in Clinical Practice* **6** (4): 337–43.

Healy, P. (2000) Bone of contention. *Nursing Standard* **14** (48): 11.

Hunt, A. H. and Repa-Eschen, L. (1998) Assessment of learning needs of registered nurses for osteoporosis education. *Orthopaedic Nursing* **17**: 55–60.

Ihrke, K. (1997) Osteoporosis: risk factors, diagnostic measures and treatment options. *Internet Journal of Academic Physician Assistants* **1** (1): 5.

Kim, C.-G., June, K.-J. and Song, R. (2003) Effects of a health promotion program on cardiovascular risk factors, health behaviours, and life satisfaction in institutionalized elderly women. *International Journal of Nursing Studies* **40**: 375–81.

Krueger, R. A. (1998) *Analyzing and Reporting Focus Group Results*. Thousand Oaks, CA: Sage.

Leslie, M. (2000) Issues in the management of osteoporosis. *Nursing Clinics of North America* **35**: 189–97.

MacLennan, A. (1997) Osteoporosis: menopause and beyond. *Australian Family Physician* **26**: 123–31.

McClung, B. L. (1999) Using osteoporosis management to reduce fractures in elderly women. *Nurse Practitioner* **24** (3): 26–36.

National Osteoporosis Foundation (1997) *Boning up on Osteoporosis: a Guide to Prevention and Treatment*. Washington, DC: NOF.

National Osteoporosis Society (1995) *Local Provision for Osteoporosis: Essential Requirements for a Hospital-based Clinical Service in the Health District*. Bath: NOS.

NHS Executive – South West (1999a) *Our Healthier Nation: Improving the Competence of the Workforce in Health Promotion*. Bristol: NHSE-SW.

NHS Executive – South West (1999b) *Our Healthier Nation: an Evaluation of Clinical Placements – Health Promotion Audit Tool*. Bristol: NHSE-SW.

NHS South West Regional Office (2002) *Our Healthier Nation: Improving the Competence of the Workforce – Practice Placements as Learning Environments*. Bristol: NHS-SWRO.

Pelikan, J., Lobnig, H. and Krajic, K. (1997) Health-promoting hospitals. *World Health* **3**: 24–5.

Preston, R. M. (1997) Ethnography: studying the fate of health promotion in coronary families. *Journal of Advanced Nursing* **25**: 554–61.

Ribeiro, V. and Blakeley, J. A. (2001) Evaluation of an osteoporosis workshop for women. *Public Health Nursing* **18**: 186–93.

Scheiber, L. B. and Torregrosa, L. (1999) Early intervention for postmenopausal osteoporosis: part 1: risk factors, prevalence, diagnosis. *Journal of Musculoskeletal Medicine* **16**: 153–7.

Schmitt, M. (2000) Osteoporosis: focus on fractures. *Patient Care Nurse Practitioner* **3**: 61–71.

Sedlak, C. A., Doheny, M. O. and Jones, S. L. (2000) Osteoporosis education programs: changing knowledge and health behaviours. *Public Health Nursing* **17**: 398–402.

Sturt, J. (1999) Placing empowerment research within an action research typology. *Journal of Advanced Nursing* **30**: 1057–63.

Sutcliffe, A. M. (1999) A regional nurse-led osteoporosis clinic. *Nursing Standard* **13** (37): 46–7.

Thassri, J., Kala, N., Chusington, L., Phongthanasarn, J., Boonsrirat, S. and Jirojwong, S. (2000) The development of a health education programme for pregnant women in a regional hospital, southern Thailand. *Journal of Advanced Nursing* 32: 1450–8.

Tones, K. (2000) Evaluating health promotion: a tale of three errors. *Patient Education and Counselling* 39: 227–36.

Torgerson, D. J. (1998) Prescribing by general practitioners after an osteoporotic fracture. *Annals of Rheumatic Disease* 57: 378–9.

Vaughn, S., Schumm, J. S. and Sinagub, J. (1996) *Focus Group Interviews in Education and Psychology.* London: Sage.

Waller, J., Eriksson, O., Foldevi, M., Grahn-Kronhed, A. C., Larsson, L., Lofman, O., Toss, G. and Moller, M. (2002) Knowledge of osteoporosis in a Swedish municipality – a prospective study. *Preventative Medicine* 34: 485–91.

Westesson, P. L., Lee, R. K., Ketkar, M. A. and Lin, E. P. (2002) Underdiagnosis and undertreatment of osteoporosis. *The Lancet* 360 (9348): 1891.

Whitehead, D., Taket, A. and Smith, P. (2003) Action research in health promotion. *Health Education Journal* 62: 5–22.

Whitehead, D., Keast, J., Montgomery, V. and Hayman, S. (2004) A preventative health education programme for osteoporosis. *Journal of Advanced Nursing* 47 (1): 15–24.

Whitelaw, S., Baxendale, A., Bryce, C., MacHardy, L., Young, I. and Witney, E. (2001) 'Settings' based health promotion: a review. *Health Promotion International* 16: 339–53.

Williamson, G. R. and Prosser, S. (2002) Action research: politics, ethics and participation. *Journal of Advanced Nursing* 40: 587–93.

Wilson, A. (2001) Diagnosis and treatment of osteoporosis. *British Journal of Community Nursing* 6: 535–41.

World Health Organisation (1990) *Initiation of International Network of Health Promoting Hospitals at WHO-EURO Workshop.* Vienna: WHO.

World Health Organisation (1991) *The Budapest Declaration of Health Promoting Hospitals.* Copenhagen: WHO.

World Health Organisation (1997) *The Vienna Recommendations on Health Promoting Hospitals.* Copenhagen: WHO.

World Health Organisation (1998) *Health Promotion Evaluation: Recommendations to Policy-Makers. Report of the WHO European Group on Health Promotion Evaluation.* Copenhagen: WHO.

World Health Organisation (2003a) www.who.dk/healthpromohosp (accessed 25 November 2003)

World Health Organisation (2003b) www.who.dk/eprise.main/WHO/progs/INC/About/20020726_1 (accessed 25 November 2003)

PART II

PROMOTING HEALTH THROUGH OCCUPATIONAL THERAPY

CHAPTER 7

The Culture and Context for Promoting Health through Occupational Therapy

ANN WILCOCK

This chapter will critically assess the culture and context of occupational therapy with regard to its current and potential contribution to health promotion. The basic rationale for the profession is the close association between what people do and their health, so there is substantial justification for occupational therapists to aim practice towards positive health and wellbeing for their clients. This applies to those clients with physical or mental dysfunctions who are the more usual recipients of occupational therapy, and can be extended to the population at large.

To begin, an historical examination of the place of occupational therapy within healthcare will be outlined, including the profession's philosophical stance, changing practice and research directions followed by discussion concerning the relationship between occupation and health. Within these discussions, the effect of occupational therapy's association with medicine will be suggested as a factor that has inhibited its participation in health promotion initiatives. This is despite the findings of recent research that supports the potential contribution that occupational therapists could make to the promotion of health. The compatibility between the actual and potential role of occupational therapy and the World Health Organisation's (WHO) Ottawa Charter for Health Promotion will then be discussed with regard to the Charter's call for action to build healthy public policy, create supportive environments, strengthen community action, develop personal skills, and reorient health services towards the promotion of health.

The place of occupational therapy within healthcare

There is limited understanding of the role of occupational therapy in healthcare from both within the healthcare fraternity and in the population at large

(Scriven and Atwal, 2004). This ties in with a limited understanding of the relationship between health and occupation within the population generally. In high income countries this is due, in part, to the materialist and economic focus given to how people spend their time. Within population healthcare this manifests as a focus on work place occupational health and safety, and in occupational therapy on encouraging independence and reducing risk and litigation in domestic situations usually for people with medically defined dysfunction. Whilst both these emphases are valuable in themselves it is also important that other difficulties caused by limited understanding about occupation and health are addressed and overcome. With respect to health promotion, although ideas about health and wellbeing do differ between individuals, communities, professions, societies and cultures, actual experiences of health, ill health and engagement in occupation are often affected by underlying occupational determinants such as the type of economy, national policies and priorities, and cultural values. So it is of use to trace the effects of those and to address concerns at the underlying levels when considering health from an occupational perspective.

Philosophical stance, changing practice and research directions

Occupational therapy is a profession that emerged in the twentieth century. It is founded upon a basic understanding that what people do can affect their health status (Wilcock, 1998). This understanding has been acted upon, to some extent, throughout time, and indeed, was integral within the six rules for health known as the Regimen Sanitatis that form the basis of modern medicine. The Regimen was an assembly of sensible regimes concerned with people's physical, mental, social and rest activity, their eating and drinking patterns, and the environments in which they lived and worked. Based on Hippocratic medicine these health rules were reintroduced into Europe via Arabia during the early Middle Ages (Daremberg, 1870; Risse, 1993). The Regimen message was in ascendance until well into the nineteenth century slowly becoming disregarded as advances in knowledge of physiology, pharmaceutics and surgical techniques led to different directions for medicine in the twentieth century. It is somewhat ironic that occupational therapy as a separate profession should be born as the influence of the Regimen declined, but it accounts for the medicalisation of occupation as therapy that typified practice in the twentieth century.

The 1987–89 Blom-Cooper Commission of Inquiry into occupational therapy in the United Kingdom (UK) described one reason why occupational therapy might have developed at that time, and that marked its difference from many of the other allied health professions. They suggested that it did not develop primarily to enable medicine to exploit new technologies but developed when it became possible to save the lives of those who would in earlier times have died. With this increased ability there was a growing awareness that the job of restoring individuals to health and maximising their functional capacity was not completed by the clinical or medical skills (Blom-Cooper, 1990: 13).

Formally named and framed in the United States of America (USA) in 1917, the profession's first objectives were the advancement of occupation as a therapeutic measure; the study of the effect of occupation upon the human being; and the scientific dispensation of this knowledge (American Occupational Therapy Association, 1967: 4–5).

Psychiatrist Adolf Meyer is widely recognised as providing the philosophical foundation of occupational therapy in a seminal paper given in 1922 (Meyer, 1922). He based much of his philosophy on broad concepts of instincts, habits, interests and specific experiences and capacities, and advocated that the wholesome pluralism of practical life should not be surrendered to medical ideology (Henderson, 1951: xiii). He believed occupation used therapeutically could maintain and enhance healthful living particularly if staff and patients shared in occupations in a homelike environment (Gelder, 1991: 422).

One of the earliest definitions of occupation therapy in the United Kingdom includes remedial and preventive roles as well as health maintenance through the creation of new habits. It stated that occupational therapy was:

... treatment, under medical direction, of physical or mental disorders by the application of occupation and recreation with the object of promoting recovery, of creating new habits, and of preventing deterioration. (Board of Control, 1933: 2)

In the same decade, an occupational therapist explained in newspaper reports that occupational therapy involved the patient's whole day, so that work, leisure, recreation, eating and sleeping formed a balanced whole, varied and directed in accordance with his or her individual needs (Clarke, 1938). Early concepts and definitions were soon narrowed and simplified to something along the lines of any activity, mental or physical, prescribed and guided for the definite purposes of contributing to, and hastening recovery from disease or injury (Casson, 1955: 98–100). These acknowledged a medical rather than a holistic health giving value to occupation.

According to the 1966 report *Occupational Therapy, Present and Future* (Dunkin, 1966) the major aim of the profession in the 60s was forwarding the recovery of patients from mental or physical illness according to the demands of home and job and fostering wellbeing, independence, initiative, responsibility, judgement and resettlement. Aimed at maximum social and vocational adjustment, intervention strategies included advice on equipment, home alterations, leisure and social needs, and training for returning function or residual abilities. In the following decade ideas about social or developmental problems, and fulfilling people's needs for optimum function in social environments gained ground (Grove, 1977). That continued to the present day along with other contemporary ideas like partnership, personal, social, cultural and

economic needs, lifestyle, problem solving, and sensitivity to social, techno-
logical and demographic influences and changes. Most important in terms of
health promotion, has been the growth of conceptual recognition over the last
decade of occupational therapists' potential to promote people's health and
wellbeing by enabling meaningful occupation (Wilcock, 2002).

The earlier reference to prescription is testament to occupational therapy's
alliance with medicine since the earliest days. It can even be suggested that the
profession would not have evolved at all had it not been for the interest and
involvement of physicians, psychiatrists and surgeons, some of whom made
great contributions in order to meet the holistic health needs of their patients.
One such explained that the prescribing of suitable occupations for patients is
as important as the prescribing of drugs (Eager, 1936: 6). For many decades
occupational therapists were totally committed to the idea of medical prescription that provided them with a place in the complex scheme of healthcare
(Wilcock, 2002). Today, the issue of prescription is a somewhat murky issue to
both occupational therapists and medical personnel. A recent factor in that
issue for occupational therapists has been a more mature appreciation of the
depth and potential of occupation as an agent of health in its own right and
different views of treatment or purpose from reductionist medical thought.

As medical interest and practice became more pharmaceutically and techni-
cally driven its practitioners declined as close and influential allies of occupational therapy. So, from the 60s on, occupational therapists began to seek
alliances with others who held different kinds of expertise such as research or
business skills or government influence. By the end of the 1980s occupational
therapy embraced many areas of specialisation but even then in the UK the
Blom-Cooper Commission of Inquiry (1990) was still able to legitimately
describe it as a submerged profession. Indeed, an apparent loss of direction
had been evident for a decade or more. This led to a search for a more
contemporary image, by, for example, reducing interest in creativity, sidelining
diversion as unscientific, and even putting aside, for some 30 years, the word
occupation in favour of the term activity (Wilcock, 2002). Occupation has
re-entered the professional vocabulary of a great majority of occupational therapists worldwide over the last decade, to the extent that it forms the lynchpin
of the World Federation of Occupational Therapists' 2002 minimum standards
for professional education (Hocking and Ness, 2002).

The contribution occupational therapy can undoubtedly make towards
improvement of health generally has been largely ignored both within and
outside its ranks as individual members of the profession have sought to meet
the requirements imposed upon their work by those in charge of healthcare
services. There are notable exceptions. From the 1960s the voices of occupational therapists such as West (1969), Cromwell (1970) and Finn (1977) tell
of the need for members of the profession to subject the basic relationship
between occupation and health to in-depth research in order to advance
programmes to promote health and to prevent ill health. From outside the
profession, Bockoven, a psychiatrist, writing about community mental health

in the 1970s recognised the critical moral importance of occupation in human life, arguing that occupational therapists have acquired a body of moral perspectives and occupational lore of unique value to society that can be more effectively utilised if it is not limited to being a service solely for sick people, whilst recognising that their contribution was prevented from realising either the depth or breadth of their role as a moral and scientific force (Bockoven, 1972: 219).

More recent works by occupational therapists have echoed those calls with texts beginning to address these issues as the way forward (Wilcock, 1998; Crepeau et al., 2003; Christiansen and Baum, 2004).

Even early in the twentieth century when occupation based programmes were largely used as a remedy to assist people with medically recognised illness or dysfunction, such as tuberculosis, mental handicap, blindness, or orthopaedic problems, within them were the seeds of health promoting practice. Indeed, although, initially, treatment was prescribed for particular medical purposes, secondary advantages were apparent in many cases. Individuals gained in economic and social terms as well as experiencing improvements in function and wellbeing generally. With hindsight such benefits are not surprising, as recent population based research has demonstrated connections, for older people at least, between social and productive activities and mortality (Glass et al., 1999) and between occupation and wellbeing (Clark et al., 1997).

In the latter of those studies, occupational therapists from the University of Southern California researched the connection between occupational therapy preventive programmes and health risks of older people (Clark et al., 1997). Their randomised controlled study of three groups living independently in community housing in Los Angeles showed benefits across health, function, and quality of life domains for subjects who were engaged in a purpose designed occupational therapy programme. The programme enabled subjects to gain appreciation of and to consciously articulate how occupations affect health. It also enabled them to employ successfully occupationally based principles of healthy living. The control groups, a social activity group and a non-treatment group, in contrast, tended to decline over the study interval. The other study, though by researchers outside the profession, is worthy of promulgating by occupational therapists. It was also a randomised controlled trial. In a study over 13 years involving 2761 male and female older Americans, Glass and colleagues found that social and productive activities, occupations, that involve little or no enhancement of fitness lower the risk of all causes of mortality to the same level as fitness activities. The data suggest that in addition to increased cardiopulmonary fitness, activity may confer survival benefits through psychosocial pathways (Glass et al., 1999: 478–83).

Other randomised controlled studies such as these need to be undertaken by occupational therapy researchers, as well as there being a continuance of qualitative studies that question, in more depth, the what, whys and hows of experiences of occupation and health. This might lead to more interest in the potential of occupation as a health agent that has received little encouragement from the ranks of public health authorities, or health promotion experts. Notwithstanding lack of interest from outside the profession, exploring the culture, context, actual and potential role of occupational therapists to promote health and wellbeing for all people is in line with the direction advocated by the World Health Organisation (WHO).

Over the last two decades the WHO has made calls for all health professionals to aim their practice towards people's attainment of complete physical, mental, and social wellbeing as well as the remediation of illness. It is timely, therefore, that the College of Occupational Therapists in the United Kingdom has recently adopted a new definition. This states that occupational therapy enables people to achieve health, wellbeing and life satisfaction through participation in occupation (College of Occupational Therapists, 2004: 7).

For occupational therapists to do this it is necessary for them first to understand occupation as an agent of physical, mental and social health.

The relationship between occupation and health

The word occupation is used in this chapter and in other chapters in this part of the book to comprise all that people do in order to fulfil basic needs essential for survival. This includes occupation to meet their innate needs and learned potential; to be and become according to individual talent and societal opportunities; and to enable adaptation to biological, social and environmental challenges. It is central to the human experience. Indeed, occupation calls upon and allows expression of the particular mix of complex human characteristics and capacities that have enabled humans to survive healthily and successfully as a species throughout time. For humans the particular mix of an upright posture that allows hands to be free to engage in multiple tasks aided by their dexterity and ability to oppose the thumb were major factors supporting different ways of meeting survival needs. So, too, has been the expansion of the brain and subsequent cognitive capacity, language, creativity and conscious awareness of self. All support the premise of archaeological and anthropological opinion that, throughout their existence, humans have engaged in occupation in a more complex manner than other animals. That has often been in response to sociocultural as well as ecological factors (Bronowski, 1973; Campbell, 1988; Jones et al., 1992).

In *An Occupational Perspective of Health* (Wilcock, 1998) an occupational theory of human nature was set out based on Stevenson's analysis of theories of human nature (Stevenson, 1987). Stevenson proposed that such theories needed to be based on a background theory of the universe and a basic theory of the nature of people. Set against a background of evolutionary sciences as they are presently understood, more than sufficient evidence was found to argue that all people are occupational beings who, unless prevented by acquired or congenital dysfunction, engage, daily, in complex, self- or socially initiated behaviour. The unconscious purpose of such behaviour is survival and health maintenance. The theory about the occupational nature of people holds true, too, if set against creationists' beliefs about the theory of the universe. In Genesis, Adam was set to tend the garden before the fall from grace, and the links to survival and health are manifest in the requirement to toil after he and Eve were expelled from Eden. This biblical explanation formed part of the recognition of the links between occupation and health that were central within monastic doctrine for centuries. The Benedictine Rule, organised around alternating periods of prayer, labour and rest, provides an example of a long period of time when disease was often attributed to sin, idleness seen as the enemy of the soul (Bettenson, 1963), and occupation seen as integral to spiritual health as well as meeting physical, mental and social health needs.

Stevenson considered that theories of human nature require a diagnosis of what is wrong with humans and a prescription of how to right those wrongs (Stevenson, 1987: 9). From an individual perspective, the general lack of appreciation of people as occupational beings and in particular of the complex and multidimensional connections between occupation and health forms the diagnosis of what is wrong. The prescription to right that wrong requires sustained and serious attention to promulgating the connections between occupation and positive or negative health across populations generally. That is a health promoting role that occupational therapists might well undertake in a similar way to the strategies used over recent decades to increase understanding of the links between nutrition and health.

In the theory, the term occupation encompasses all the activities that people engage in across the sleeping/waking continuum, including those that are economically, socially or politically driven, obligatory or self-chosen, and meet individual physical, social, mental or spiritual needs, pleasures and purposes. Individual potential for and engagement in different occupations results from genetically inherited capacities coupled with what individuals learn, particularly early in life, from the familial, sociocultural and natural environments in which they live. All people unless prevented by congenital or acquired dysfunction engage in many different occupations each day. These reflect integrated functioning of mind and body not as separate entities but simply one and the same (Lorenze, 1987: 93), and may be self-initiated or a requirement of others.

The integrated functioning of mind and body as people engage in occupation is part of the process of minding the body and maintaining health. Ornstein and Sobel (1988) claim, in *The Healing Brain*, that in daily life and daily pursuits the brain makes countless adjustments which enable health by preserving stability between social worlds, mental and emotional lives, and internal physiology. In considering how much that is reflected in people's understanding of health Blaxter's (1990) survey of 9000 adults across the United Kingdom is useful. Her findings revealed many different ways that people described health, and perhaps, surprisingly, that these included ideas that had occupational links. Indeed, over 30 per cent of all respondents defined health for themselves in functional terms and many described health for others in that way, particularly when talking about men or about older people. They incorporated ideas about the ability to perform physically demanding work, to work despite an advanced age, and to engage in social, family and community activity. Some saw health as being able to do what you want to when you want to (Blaxter, 1990: 28–9). Some respondents said that health is being function-ally able, having energy, being physically or psychosocially fit, or engaging in healthy behaviour. They sometimes used words such as being alert, lively, and full of get up and go, and women of any age and many older men used energy and vitality to describe enthusiasm about work. Women also defined health as being keen and interested, doing everything easily, and feeling like conquering the world (Blaxter, 1990: 25–7).

Some health experts have also linked health with occupation. Sigerist, the medical historian, for example, maintained that work is essential to the main-tenance of health because not only does it determine the chief rhythm of our life, balance it, and give meaning and significance, but also without occupation the body and mind are likely to atrophy (Sigerist, 1955: 254–5). Writers in health promotion texts have observed similar links. Kass (1981), a case in point, defined health as the well working of the whole organism and as a state of being revealed in activity. More recently, Greiner, Fain and Edelman (2002) see it as a state of functioning that realises a person's potential. Included within what the authors describe as functional health patterns are those concerned with activity, exercise, sleep, rest, cognition, perception, self-perception, self-concept, roles, relationships, and coping and stress tolerance. They propose that functioning is integral to health. Their thesis is that there are physical, mental and social levels of function reflected in terms of performance and social expectations. Loss of function may be a sign or symptom of a disease, a state of ill health.

Despite some links having been made between health and occupation by people in the field and in the population generally there remains substantial difficulty in the application of occupational issues to health promotion policy and action. In part this is due to people's limited understanding of themselves as occupational beings and to the fact that health maintaining needs and func-tions, rather like the autonomic nervous system, are built into the organism to just go on working. It is also due to little being written in mainstream health-care about the benefits of a natural lifestyle, or of the need for a balance of ongoing physical, mental, and social occupations as integral aspects of health, because it is based on the Western medical model.

Occupational therapists and the Ottawa Charter for Health Promotion

The Ottawa Charter for Health Promotion (WHO, 1986) despite being some 20 years old, is recognised as a classic document that has not been superseded

in terms of providing fundamental definitions, descriptions and recommendations for the way forward in the new millennium (see Chapter 1 of this text for
a full discussion of the Charter). Throughout, the Charter calls for action to
build health public policy, create supportive environments, strengthen community action, develop personal skills, and reorient health services towards the
promotion of health. Whilst written in a terminology different to that which
occupational therapists have used traditionally much of the Charter addresses
issues occupational therapists might pick up on in terms of health promoting
personal, communal, environmental and sociopolitical initiatives. For example
in describing health promotion the Charter recognises the fundamental relationship between what people do or are unable to do and their health status in
the explanation that:

> To reach a state of complete physical, mental and social wellbeing, an individual or
> group must be able to identify and realise aspirations, to satisfy needs, and to change
> or cope with the environment. Health is, therefore, seen as a resource for everyday
> life not the objective of living. (WHO, 1986: 2)

Recognition of links with the Charter has already occurred at occupational
therapy national association levels, and the 2002 strategy developed by the
British College of Occupational Therapists (COT) (COT, 2002) has been
chosen, here, as an example to illustrate such links. The strategy argues for an
occupational therapy client centred health focus that answers the WHO call for
the reorientation of all health professionals towards the pursuit of health as
well as the remediation of illness. It combines the population health promoting vision of the Charter with the more recent *International Classification of
Functioning, Disability and Health* (ICF) (WHO, 2001). The mix of ICF and
Charter are put forward as the legitimate domain of occupational therapists.
The diagram illustrating the strategy is shown as Figure 7.1.

The strategic actions as put forward by the Charter and required of occupational therapists are those of enablers, advocates and mediators for disadvantaged communities and population groups as well as for individuals with
dysfunction. The expression enabling occupation has been widely used since
the publication of the Canadian Occupational Performance Model that
adopted it as its catch cry (Townsend, 1997). However, although occupational
therapists have traditionally taken an enabling role and are comfortable
with that concept, they have been more hesitant to act as mediators and advocates. This entails a more active role in social planning at political levels than
has been part of normal practice.

The health promoting foci of the COT strategy is fourfold. Aimed at individuals and communities they target increased levels of participation and
decreased levels of handicap. They focus on advocating for and enabling occupationally just environments and promoting physical, mental and social wellbeing. The COT strategy recognises occupational ill health or dysfunction is
not confined to people with medically defined illness or disability, highlighting

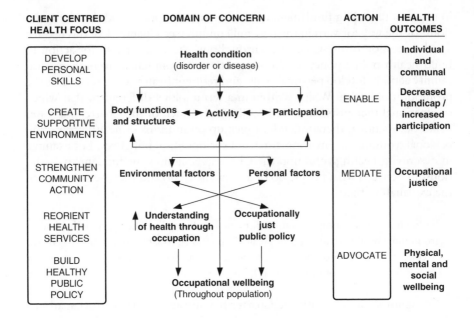

Figure 7.1 COT Strategy 2002: a mix of Ottawa Charter for Health Promotion and ICF

Source: Reprinted with permission from The British Association and College of Occupational Therapists (2002)

the need for occupational therapists to understand how health is maintained and increased through occupation. The strategy also recognises that occupational health and wellbeing is a right of all people and that therefore a population health promotion approach is an appropriate responsibility for occupational therapists. Occupational therapists can bring to population based health promotion programmes their distinct view of people as occupational beings, analysing, challenging and advocating research and practice policies, initiatives, and interventions from that viewpoint. That involves a commitment to advocate and mediate for the provision of occupationally just policies.

The central place of the ICF within the strategy is indicative of the wide acceptance by occupational therapists of this new way of considering what had previously been a disability descriptor. On the issue of health promotion it provides a strong link between it and the former disability focus of occupational therapy in that it applies to everybody, not just people with medically based dysfunction. The ICF also has potential use as a research, a social policy or an educational tool.

In conclusion, it is important to highlight some directions that occupational therapists need to attend to if they are to offer a distinct and valuable contribution in the field of health promotion. Firstly, they need to advance understanding of the relationship between health and occupation in public and political forums. Secondly, they need to extend their enabling role, and become better advocates and mediators. Thirdly, they need to explore socio-cultural and political factors that determine underlying occupational determinants of health such as those that create situations that might be described as occupationally unjust or imbalanced, and finally, they need to address cultural and environmental contexts as well as individual problems in occupation based personal, communal or sociopolitical initiatives.

References

American Occupational Therapy Association (1967) *Then and Now: 1917–1976.* Rockville, MD: AOTA.

Bettenson, H. S. (ed.) (1963) *Documents of the Christian Church.* New York: Springer.

Blaxter, M. (1990) *Health and Lifestyles.* London/New York: Tavistock/Routledge.

Blom-Cooper, L. (1990) *Occupational Therapy: an Emerging Profession in Healthcare.* Report of a Commission of Inquiry. London: Duckworth.

Board of Control (1933) *Memorandum on Occupation Therapy for Mental Patients.* London: His Majesty's Stationery Office.

Bockoven, J. S. (1972) *Moral Treatment in Community Mental Health.* New York: Springer.

Bronowski, J. (1973) *The Ascent of Man.* London: British Broadcasting Corporation.

Campbell, B. G. (1988) *Humankind Emerging*, fifth edition. New York: HarperCollins.

Casson, E. (1955) Occupational therapy. Reprinted from a report of conference on 'Welfare of Cripples and Invalid Children' held at the Drapers' Hall, London, 7 and 8 November 1935. *Occupational Therapy* 18 (3): 98–100.

Christiansen, C. H. and Baum, C. M. (eds) (2004) *Occupational Therapy: Enabling Function and Wellbeing*, third edition. Thorofare, NJ: Slack.

Clark, F., Azen, S. P., Zemke, R., Jackson, J., Carlson, M., Mandel, D., Hay, J., Josephson, K., Cherry, B., Hessel, C., Palmer, J. and Lipson, L. (1997) Occupational therapy for independent-living older adults: a randomised controlled trial. *Journal of the American Medical Association* 278 (16): 1321–6.

Clarke, N. I. R. (1938) Work as a stimulant: value of occupational therapy. *Birkenhead News* 27 August. Also reported in *Birkenhead Advertiser* 27 August.

College of Occupational Therapists (2002) *COT Strategy: From Interface to Integration.* London: COT.

College of Occupational Therapists (2004) OT definition agreed. *Occupational Therapy News* 12 (2): 7.

Crepeau, E. B., Cohn, E. S. and Schell, B. A. B. (eds) (2003) *Willard and Spackman's Occupational Therapy*, tenth edition. Philadelphia, PA: Lippincott, Williams and Wilkins.

Cromwell, F. S. (1970) Our challenges in the seventies: occupational therapy today – tomorrow. In *Proceedings of the 5th International Congress.* Zurich: World Federation of Occupational Therapists.

Daremberg, C. (1870) On the Glosses of the Four Salernitan Masters. In Ordronaux, J. (ed.) *Regimen Sanitatis Salernitatum: Code of Health of the School of Salernum.* Philadelphia, PA: J. B. Lippincott.

Dunkin, E. N. (1966) Summary of the report *Occupational Therapy, Present and Future* to the Council of the Association of Occupational Therapists from the Advisory Board of the Sub-Committee. *Occupational Therapy* 29 (8): 6–13.

Eager, R. (1936) *Aids to Mental Health: the Benefits of Occupation, Recreation and Amusement*. Exeter: W. V. Cole.

Finn, G. L. (1977) Update of Eleanor Clarke Slagle Lecture: the occupational therapist in prevention programs. *American Journal of Occupational Therapy* 31 (10): 658–9.

Gelder, M. (1991) Adolf Meyer and his influence on British psychiatry. In Berrios, G. E. and Freeman, H. (eds) *150 Years of British Psychiatry, 1841–1991*. London: Gaskell.

Glass, T. A., de Leon, C. M., Marottoli, R. A. and Berkman, L. F. (1999) Population based study of social and productive activities as predictors of survival among elderly Americans. *British Medical Journal* 319 (21 August): 478–83.

Greiner, P. A., Fain, J. A. and Edelman, C. L. (2002) Health defined: objectives for promotion and prevention. In Edelman, C. L. and Mandle, C. L. (eds) *Health Promotion Throughout the Lifespan*, fifth edition. St Louis, MO: Mosby.

Grove, E. (1977) Occupational therapy in the United Kingdom. Paper given at the first European Occupational Therapy Congress, Edinburgh, UK.

Henderson, D. K. (1951) Introduction. In Winters, E. E. (ed.) *The Collected Papers of Adolf Meyer, Volume II: Psychiatry*. Baltimore, MD: Johns Hopkins University Press.

Hocking, C. and Ness, N. E. (2002) *The 2002 Revised Minimum Standards for the Education of Occupational Therapists*. Zurich: World Federation of Occupational Therapists.

Jones, S., Martin, R. and Pilbeam, D. (eds) (1992) *The Cambridge Encyclopaedia of Human Evolution*. Cambridge: Cambridge University Press.

Kass, L. R. (1981) Regarding the end of medicine and the pursuit of health. In Caplan, A. L., Englehart, H. T. and McCartney, J. J. (eds) *Concepts of Health and Disease: Interdisciplinary Perspectives*. Boston, MA: Addison-Wesley.

Lorenze, K. (1987) *The Waning of Humaneness*. Boston, MA: Little, Brown.

Meyer, A. (1922) The philosophy of occupational therapy. *Archives of Occupational Therapy* 1: 1–10. Reprinted (1977) in *American Journal of Occupational Therapy* 31 (10): 639–42.

Ornstein, R. and Sobel, D. (1988) *The Healing Brain: a Radical New Approach to Healthcare*. London: Macmillan (now Palgrave Macmillan).

Risse, G. B. (1993) History of Western medicine from Hippocrates to germ theory. In Kipple, K. F. (ed.) *The Cambridge World History of Human Disease*. Cambridge: Cambridge University Press.

Scriven, A. and Atwal, A. (2004) Occupational therapists as primary health promoters: opportunities and barriers. *British Journal of Occupational Therapy* 67 (10): 424–9.

Sigerist, H. E. (1955) *A History of Medicine , Volume 1: Primitive and Archaic Medicine*. New York: Oxford University Press.

Stevenson, L. (1987) *Seven Theories of Human Nature*, second edition. New York: Oxford University Press.

Townsend, E. (ed.) (1997). *Enabling Occupation: an Occupational Therapy Perspective*. Ottawa: Canadian Association of Occupational Therapists.

West, W. (1969) The growing importance of prevention. *American Journal of Occupational Therapy* 23: 223–31.

Wilcock, A. A. (1998) *An Occupational Perspective of Health*. Thorofare, NJ: Slack.

Wilcock, A. A. (2002) *Occupation for Health, Volume 2: a Journey from Prescription to Self Health*. London: COT.

World Health Organisation (1986) *Ottawa Charter for Health Promotion*. Geneva: WHO.

World Health Organisation (2001). *International Classification of Functioning, Disability and Health*. Geneva: WHO.

CHAPTER 8

Promoting Health through Client Centred Occupational Therapy Practice

THELMA SUMSION

Client centred practice has formed the foundation of occupational therapy in Canada since the early 1980s. The Canadian Model of Occupational Performance guides this approach and has undergone several revisions since its inception. The current version, and principles that underlie this approach, are clearly outlined in the text *Enabling Occupation* (Townsend, 2002). The inherent concepts are also featured in the codes of ethics of occupational therapy organisations in both Canada and the United Kingdom (UK) (Canadian Association of Occupational Therapists (CAOT), 2002; College of Occupational Therapists (COT), 2000).

Likewise, health promotion has been a focus of practice for Canadian therapists since 1919 as shown by the original slogan presenting the philosophy of 'through mind and hands to health' (Robinson, 1981: 2). More recently the publication *For the Health of It: Occupational therapy within a Health Promotion Framework* (Letts et al., 1996) has refocussed the profession on this issue. The occupational therapy literature clearly demonstrates this shift in focus with many articles on health promotion programmes including wellness programmes in seniors' apartment complexes (Jackson et al., 1998; Matuska et al., 2003), encouragement to focus on building healthy communities (Baum and Law, 1998), discussion of roles in community practice, the work place and in education (Madill, Townsend and Schultz, 1989), and day treatment programmes for persons with AIDS (Gutterman, 1990).

The links between client centred practice and health promotion therefore warrant investigation, as both are integral components of occupational therapy practice. This chapter will discuss definitions of both client centred practice and health promotion, reviewing key components of a client centred process and a barrier to the implementation of this approach. The discussion will conclude with a brief consideration of strategies for linking client centred practice and health promotion. The possibility that the link only exists theoretically or that it has not been realised in practice will be critically examined throughout.

Occupational therapy definitions of client centred practice

There are now several definitions of client centred practice in occupational therapy and the following are examples of those that have originated in North America.

Law et al. (1995: 253) describe the approach as one that embraces a philosophy of respect for, and partnership with, people receiving services. It recognises the autonomy of individuals, the need for client choice in making decisions about occupational needs, the strengths clients bring to an occupational therapy encounter and the benefits of client–therapist partnership and the need to ensure that services are accessible and fit the context in which a client lives. Client centred occupational therapy practice is therefore seen as an alliance formed between client and therapist and is designed to combine their skills and strengths to work toward client goals related to occupational performance (Fearing et al., 1997: 8).

The Canadian Association of Occupational Therapists (1997: 5) also believes that to be client centred is to understand and develop particular types of collaborative working with clients, rather than doing things for or deciding what is best for clients. It also means advocating with and for clients so they are empowered to share in decision making to create fair opportunities for living despite disability, development, ageing, social or other circumstances (Townsend, 1998a: 2).

In the UK client centred occupational therapy is a partnership between the client and the therapist that empowers the client to engage in functional performance and fulfil their occupational roles in a variety of environments. The client participates actively in negotiating goals that are given priority and are at the centre of assessment, intervention and evaluation. Throughout the process the therapist listens to and respects the client's values, adapts the interventions to meet the client's needs and enables the client to make informed decisions (Sumsion, 2000: 308).

The ideas of partnership, alliances and collaboration dominate these explanations of a client centred approach. Respect and the importance of considering the client's context, the achievement of client goals concerning occupational performance, the therapist's role as an advocate and involving the client in decision making are also featured. The notion of autonomy, client's strengths, accessible services, focus on client's needs, defining the client, recognising client opinions and knowledge, the client engaging the support and assistance of the therapist and empowerment are also important elements.

Definitions of health promotion

Health promotion has been explored fully in Chapter 1 of this book, so it is not the intention to discuss it in any depth here. There are, however, three specific definitions that show clear links to client centred practice. Edwards (1990: 5) draws explicitly on the World Health Organisation (WHO) in describing health promotion as the process of enabling people to increase control over and improve their own health. This definition arose from the Ottawa Charter of Health Promotion (WHO, 1986: 1) where it was claimed that to achieve health an individual or group must be able to identify and to realise aspirations, to satisfy needs and to change or cope with the environment. Bowen (1999: 14) took a slightly different approach by defining health promotion as the process of furthering the condition of being sound in body, mind and spirit. There is a clear objective of working with people to realise their goals or aspirations as they define the health issues to be improved.

These definitions demonstrate a strong link between client centred practice with a focus on positive alliances that consider the client's context or environment while working toward the achievement of the client's goals, and health promotion, that also emphasises the identification and development of aspirations in order to change relevant environments with a focus on improving health.

Components of client centred practice

There are numerous components of client centred practice. However, further investigation of some key components should strengthen the link between client centred practice and health promotion. These components are partnership, communication, choice and power.

Partnership

Health professionals are being challenged to change the way they have traditionally related to clients and to make the shift from a focus on authoritarianism to one of partnership (Rosenbaum et al., 1998). An effective professional and client partnership is required to ensure that the best care is being provided as it adds to the strength and effectiveness of that care (Roberts and Magrab, 1991; Kalmanson and Seligman, 1992; Ellers, 1993; Gatterman, 1995; Edgman-Levitan, 1997). However, Jadad (1999) expressed caution as he found little evidence that professionals were actually implementing this concept. Additional characteristics of a partnership presented by Banks et al. (1997) include flexibility or the recognition that the relationship can change, and egalitarianism shown through a sense of similar status for both the client and therapist.

Hall, Roter and Katz (1988) undertook a meta-analysis of the literature from 1966 to 1985 regarding medical visits to healthcare providers. They concluded that a partnership was built only when the clinician went beyond providing the clients with information and actually elevated their position to full partnership. These same authors also found a clear positive association between partnership building and client satisfaction with the interaction. The two parties should be seen as equals and each has specific roles within this partnership (Brewer et al., 1989; Skelton, 1997). However, the client has a more active role in defining goals and outcomes and the therapist is the technical expert with knowledge about the condition and its treatment and the facilitator who provides the required information (Law et al., 1995; Rosenbaum et al., 1998). Overall, this needs to be an active partnership (Corring, 1996) that moves beyond token representation to true partnership (Wertlieb, 1993; Dressler and MacRae, 1998).

Thibeault and Hebert (1997) link the concepts of partnership in client centred practice and health promotion by reminding us that in any community that is attempting to implement change there are degrees of control, the decision making must be given to the group, and that the plans created by the partnership must be true to the goals set by the client. Planning, which is a crucial ingredient of both health promotion and client centred practice, can only be done in partnership with the client (Letts et al., 1996).

Communication

Effective communication, through the use of appropriate language, is an important element in ensuring the success of the therapist–client partnership (Boumbulian et al., 1991; Delbanco, 1992; Corring, 1996; Edgman-Levitan, 1997; Ellis, 1997; Townsend, 1998c). This communication should occur between all members of the treatment team, the client and where relevant their family (Matheis-Kraft et al., 1990). Communication skills are essential to enable all those involved to discuss issues openly in an atmosphere of mutual decision making (Pesznecker, Zerwekh and Horn, 1989; Logan, 1997). However, professionals need to be trained how to use information with clients to promote informed decision making (College of Health, 1999).

Hall et al. (1988) found that client satisfaction was directly related to the amount of information provided by clinicians. This view is further supported by the results of a survey of clients in four countries regarding their satisfaction with primary care, which reported that they received insufficient information (Calnan et al., 1994). Therefore, communication of appropriate and relevant information is an important component of client centred practice. Law and Mills (1998), following a review of six client centred frameworks, also concluded that the provision of information and an emphasis on person centred communication were common to all models.

Communication is also a vital component of health promotion that involves providing information so people can address their identified health needs

(Letts et al., 1996). Health professionals can assist client competence through understanding the clients' position and ensuring their wishes and voices are heard (Reutter and Ford, 1997). Clients are empowered through the provision of information and careful listening also enhances the process of development (Finlayson and Edwards, 1995). The Ottawa Charter for Health Promotion (WHO, 1986) emphasises the importance of access to information to enable clients to take control of the issues that for them will determine their health. Hotz et al. (1997) provide an example of this control through their discussion of the importance of parents having information about lead and the effects it can have on child development.

Choice

Clients can only make informed choices if they are given full information about relevant outcomes (Law et al., 1995). England and Evans (1992: 1223), for example, studied clients in a cardiovascular risk management clinic and found that relevant information had a major impact on the treatment clients chose. Other authors have expressed the opinion that clients also have a right to receive information that is understandable in order to make decisions (Hostler, 1991; Law et al., 1995) and the education that comes with information increases the individual's opportunities for making meaningful choices (Capitman and Sciegaj, 1995).

Several authors have identified choice as an important component of client centred practice (Fraser, 1995; Sweeney, 1997; Allen and Petr, 1998). Choice is essential in meeting client centred occupational needs and the lack of choice can lead to unnecessary reliance on the hospital system (Rebeiro, 2000). Others have stated that a sense of choice should be created by outlining available options whenever possible, even if in small amounts, as everyone is capable of some level of choice (Abramson, 1990; Baum and Law, 1997). It is important, therefore, to acknowledge that control and choice are related to each person's healthcare programme and to his or her quality of life (Matheis-Kraft et al., 1990; Raeburn and Rootman, 1998). In reality, clients' choice is important, as they are the only ones who truly understand their daily experiences and the impact on their lives of the choices to be made (Law et al., 1995).

A further group of authors have expressed the view that clients have the right to make choices about personal things in their environment (Happ et al., 1996), the role and degree of involvement with professionals (Leviton et al., 1992) and ultimately who will be involved and the nature and level of that involvement (Allen and Petr, 1998). Therefore, it appears to be important for occupational therapists to respect the choices made by clients even if they think a wrong choice has been made, as competent clients have the right to make decisions even if they appear to be unsafe (Speechley, 1992; Clemens et al., 1994; Law, 1998). The choices made by clients preserve their autonomy and their right to take risks (Happ et al., 1996).

Overall, allowing the client to exercise choice indicates the occupational therapist is willing to look at the meaning of the problem from the client's perspective and recognises that the client's values, interests and goals are at the foundation of a client centred approach (Pesznecker et al., 1989; Grol et al., 1990; Smith, 1995). Supporters of client centred practice have expressed the view that clients should be allowed to set their own goals (Happ et al., 1996) and therapists should enable clients to implement the strategies to achieve the goals they have set (Leviton et al., 1992; Krupa and Clark, 1995; Law et al., 1995). From a health promotion perspective, clients can make choices and assume control when their actions are based on internal, self-motivated goals (Phillips, 1994). They are more likely to be able to work toward independence when health professionals support their choices (Reutter and Ford, 1997) and they can only achieve their chosen levels of health if they have access to information (WHO, 1986).

Power

The impact of power must be clearly understood, as it is a central element in client centred practice. Henderson (1994), in a discussion of the power of knowledge, describes day-to-day relations that place one person in a position of power over another. The concept of power over another person also influences behaviour and decisions of others to obey or conform (Raatikainen, 1994). Power over clients is attributed to a sense of strength and creativity rather than weakness and inferiority (Hokanson Hawks, 1991). These authors place the emphasis on strength, control and competitiveness, which supports the idea that health professionals do have power over clients, that power influences goal attainment and that clients are disempowered by the system (Hugman, 1991; Corring, 1996). Avis (1994, cited in Law, 1998) found that this power differential was an important factor in lessening people's ability to participate in their healthcare. Language is the medium of power and a medical vocabulary can be very confusing to clients and hence places the therapist in a position of power over the client (Gerhardt, 1989). This power even enables professionals to determine what a client is or should be (Hugman, 1991). To solve this problem, simple language should be used in the provision of information to clients and the time taken to ensure that all components of any discussion or written material have been understood (Law, 2000). Therapists do have power over clients and may use their ability and knowledge to get clients to do something they would not otherwise have done (Hokanson Hawks, 1991). Therefore, power cannot be ignored and warrants careful consideration in any intervention but particularly in those that are meant to be client centred. Rather than exerting power over clients, occupational therapists should be attending to the balance of power where the shift in that balance is toward the client (Epstein et al., 1993; Corring, 1996; Honey, 1999).

Law et al. (1995) outline the core concepts of power, and link power to partnership, by defining power as a process by which the client and therapist achieve together what neither could achieve alone. Giving power to people relates to effectiveness and the ability to set goals, achieve objectives and effect outcomes, which gives control to individuals (Swaffield, 1990; Raatikainen, 1994). This power should be both informal and formal. Informal power provides access to decision makers and formal power encompasses the responsibility for making decisions (Honey, 1999).

Townsend (1998b) proposes a profile of empowerment that enables client participation in both client centred practice and health promotion. She suggests that people should be invited to participate in programmes by being treated as persons rather than patients. Individual and social action should be facilitated and collaborative decision making encouraged. Therapists need to facilitate experiential learning and recognise that clients become empowered through taking risks to learn and determine a future course for themselves. The final component of her profile is promoting inclusiveness rather than the segregation that comes with being different. Honey (1999) referred to this as objective power where structures exist to ensure consumers' views do make a difference. Ellis (1997) also supported these elements through a discussion of empowerment that includes facilitation, encouragement and the provision of information.

It has been argued that the therapist should no longer lead the client centred process and therefore the power is no longer assigned to the therapist (Crepeau, 1991). Rather, it is the client who directs the process and therefore has the power. Once this power is understood and accepted, clients become equal partners in healthcare and can foster their own health rather than always seeking professional help (Sumsion, 1999). Enabling clients to accept power is an important concept within health promotion and this is how people can control the impact of external factors on their lives (Thibeault and Hebert, 1997).

Barrier to health promoting client centred practice

The above components will facilitate the link between client centred practice and health promotion but a barrier to this implementation arises when occupational therapists face the challenge of assigning power and choice. Power may be a factor that interferes with the therapist's ability to truly listen to the client, which is an integral component of both client centred practice and health promotion. Meeson (1998) interviewed 12 community occupational therapists and found that very few made direct reference to embedding client empowerment in their approach to practice. Townsend (1998b) also found that empowerment was a problem that formed the basis of her institutional ethnographic study and she proposed a profile of empowerment that would enable client participation. The components of this profile are inviting clients to participate in all levels of planning, facilitating individual and social action, encouraging collaborative decision making, guiding critical reflection and experiential learning, supporting risk taking and promoting inclusiveness. This profile would also enhance client participation in all levels of health promotion. It may be uncomfortable for therapists to give more power to clients and in fact they may not be willing to share the power of decision making (Glenister, 1994; Law et al., 1995). However, the challenge is to learn how to incorporate the shared expertise and power of both the provider and the client into the therapeutic relationship (Chewning and Sleath, 1996).

Occupational therapists must relinquish power and control if they are to work in partnership with clients (Corring and Cook, 1999; Honey, 1999). Therapists who are truly client centred and advocates of health promotion work as collaborators and facilitative teachers who give up control, recognise the client is the one directing the decisions and accepts those decisions (Sumsion, 1993). Adopting client centred approaches requires changing the balance of power so that those who are directly affected are driving the process (Raeburn and Rootman, 1998). This will be difficult for some occupational therapists that fear they may be giving control to clients who have neither the knowledge nor the will to accept this challenge (Laine and Davidoff, 1996). Others may fear liability if they do not maintain complete control (Johns and Harvey, 1993).

This control also relates to the professionals' need to direct the process, which negates their ability to be client centred (Allen and Petr, 1998). Ellis (1997) found that nurses needed to do for clients, which undermined the client's autonomy and empowerment. They were also paternalistic and therefore felt they knew what was best for the client as well as being compulsive helpers. All of these behaviours led to burnout and placed nurses in a position of not being able to care for themselves and subsequently not being able to care for others. Therefore, services became nurse driven rather than client led where clients are given time and opportunity to express their views about their care (Goodall, 1992).

Perhaps this reluctance to share power is based on working within the traditional medical model. Grol et al. (1990) studied doctors in Belgium, Britain and the Netherlands, and found that a considerable number maintained a disease or doctor centred attitude. Specialisation within teams is also a problem that can create territories and hinder communication (Lawlor and Mattingly, 1998). Occupational therapists do want to be more client centred but often the teams they work with do not have a clear structure for applying this approach (Meyer, 1996).

Clients also present many barriers that will inhibit their involvement in client centred practice and their assuming responsibility for their own health. The largest issue appears to be their reluctance to become involved in the process (Ersser, 1996; Fiveash, 1998). There will be clients who want little or no information or involvement, who do not want to participate in decision making or who are unwilling or unable to take responsibility for their own healthcare (Speechley, 1992). Deber (1994) reviewed several studies and concluded that all clients want information but not all want to participate in decision making. Ende et al. (1989) concurred with this conclusion as they found support for situations where the doctor kept the client informed and engaged in decision making rather than the client being the main decision maker. Pendleton and House (1984) administered the Health Opinion Survey to clients with diabetes in a low income neighbourhood. They found a low score in this group for individuals wanting involvement either in obtaining information or carrying out health related functions. They concluded that the variables affecting this preference were socioeconomic status and affliction with a chronic disease.

Overall, it is the optimistic clients with a positive attitude who will be able to maintain their independence (Ende et al., 1989; McWilliam et al., 1994). Growing awareness has encouraged clients to become more informed consumers of healthcare and to participate in that care. Clients will obtain the best outcome when the treatment they receive fits their expectations and their usual coping style (Krantz et al., 1980).

Strategies for linking client centred practice and health promotion

The above discussion has presented many strategies for implementing both client centred practice and health promotion, particularly in relation to partnership working. Finlayson and Edwards (1997) remind us that the clients's role in active or primary prevention is to do something for themselves. Chandra et al. (2003) also stress that the accepted model of practice within health promotion is now one that considers the client to be an active participant in an environment that will support each person's potential (Phillips, 1994). Overall, individuals should be regarded as active participants in the process of maintaining and achieving health and encouraged to engage in partnerships to reach these goals (Madill et al., 1989; Letts et al., 1996).

There is a clear and positive link between client centred practice and health promotion. The concepts of partnership, communication, choice and power are foundational to both client centred practice and health promotion and must be implemented by occupational therapists committed to ensuring that clients have every chance of obtaining their health goals. The links between the two are strong, and when these two approaches are supported and clearly connected, the clients will be empowered to assume responsibility for their health, which is a unifying goal in both health promotion and client centred practice.

References

Abramson, J. S. (1990) Enhancing patient participation: clinical strategies in the discharge planning process. *Social Work in Health Care* **14** (4): 53–71.

Allen, R. I. and Petr, C. G. (1998) Rethinking family centred practice. *American Journal of Orthopsychiatry* **68** (1): 4–15.

Avis, M. (1994) Choice cuts: an exploratory study of patients' views about participation in decision-making in a day surgery unit. *International Journal of Nursing Studies* **31** (3): 289–98.

Banks, S., Crossman, D., Poel, D. and Stewart, M. (1997) Partnerships among health professionals and self-help group members. *Canadian Journal of Occupational Therapy* **64** (3): 259–69.

Baum, C. M. and Law, M. (1997) Occupational therapy practice: focusing on occupational performance. *American Journal of Occupational Therapy* **51** (4): 277–88.

Baum, C. and Law, M. (1998) Community health: a responsibility, an opportunity, and a fit for occupational therapy. *American Journal of Occupational Therapy* **52** (1): 7–10.

Bowen, J. E. (1999) Health promotion – opening the lens. *OT Practice* **20** (December): 14–18.

Boumbulian, P. J., Day, M. W., Delbanco, T. L., Edgman-Levitan, S., Smith, D. R. and Anderson, R. J. (1991) Patient-centred patient-valued care. *Journal of Health Care for the Poor and Underserved* **2** (3): 338–46.

Brewer, E. J., McPherson, M., Magrab, P. R. and Hutchins, V. L. (1989) Family-centred, community based, co-ordinated care for children with special health care needs. *Paediatrics* **83** (6): 1055–60.

Calnan, M., Katsouyiannopoulos, V., Ovcharov, V. K., Prokhorskas, R., Ramic, H. and Williams, S. (1994) Major determinants of consumer satisfaction with primary care in different health systems. *Family Practice* **11** (4): 468–78.

Canadian Association of Occupational Therapists (2002) *Enabling Occupation: an Occupational Therapy Perspective*. Ottawa: CAOT Publications.

Capitman, J. and Sciegaj, M. (1995) A contextual approach for understanding individual autonomy in managed community long term care. *The Gerontologist* **35** (4): 533–40.

Chandra, A., Malcolm, N. and Fetters, M. (2003) Practising health promotion through pharmacy counselling activities. *Health Promotion Practice* **4** (1): 64–71.

Chewning, B. and Sleath, B. (1996) Medication decision-making and management: a client-centred model. *Social Science Medicine* **42** (3): 389–98.

Clemens, E., Wetle, T., Feltes, M., Crabtree, B. and Dubitzky, D. (1994) Contradictions in case management: client-centred theory and directive practice with frail elderly. *Journal of Ageing and Health* **6** (1): 70–88.

College of Health (1999) *Patient-Defined Outcomes*. London: College of Health.

College of Occupational Therapists (2000) *Code of Ethics and Professional Conduct*. London: COT.

Corring, D. (1996) *Client-centred care means I am a valued human being*. Unpublished Masters thesis, University of Western Ontario.

Corring, D. and Cook, J. (1999) Client-centred care means that I am a valued human being. *Canadian Journal of Occupational Therapy* **66** (2): 71–82.

Crepeau, E. B. (1991) Achieving intersubjective understanding: examples from an occupational therapy treatment session. *American Journal of Occupational Therapy* **45** (11): 1016–25.

Deber, R. B. (1994) Physicians in health care management: 8. The patient–physician partnership: decision-making, problem solving and the desire to participate. *Canadian Medical Association Journal* **151** (4): 423–7.

Delbanco, T. L. (1992) Enriching the doctor–patient relationship by inviting the patient's perspective. *Annals of Internal Medicine* **116** (5): 414–18.

Dressler, J. and MacRae, A. (1998) Advocacy, partnerships and client-centred practice in California. *Occupational Therapy in Mental Health* **14** (1/2): 35–43.

Edgman-Levitan, S. (1997) On the value of patient centred care. *Journal of American Academy of Physician Assistants* **10** (3): 9–21.

Edwards, J. (1990) Health promotion – an opportunity for occupational therapy. *Canadian Journal of Occupational Therapy* **57** (1): 5–7.

Ellers, B. (1993) Innovations in patient centred education. In Gerteis, M., Edgman-Levitan, S., Daley, J. and Delbanco, T. L. (eds).*Through the Patient's Eyes*. San Francisco: Jossey-Bass.

Ellis, S. (1997) Patient and professional centred care in the hospice. *International Journal of Palliative Nursing* **3** (4): 197–202.

Ende, J., Kazis, L., Ash, A. and Moskowitz, M. A. (1989) Measuring patients' desire for autonomy. *Journal of General Internal Medicine* **4**: 23–30.

England, S. L. and Evans, J. (1992) Patients' choices and perceptions after an invitation to participate in treatment decisions. *Social Science Medicine* **34** (11): 1217–25.

Epstein, R. M., Campbell, T. L., Cohen-Cole, S. A., McWhinney, I. R. and Smilkstein, G. (1993) Perspectives on patient–doctor communication. *Journal of Family Practice* **37** (4): 377–88.

Ersser, S. (1996) Ethnography and the development of patient-centred nursing. In Fulford, K. W. M., Ersser, S. and Hope, T. (eds) *Essential Practice in Patient-Centred Care*. Oxford: Blackwell Science.

Fearing, V. G., Law, M. and Clark, J. (1997) An occupational performance process model: fostering client and therapist alliances. *Canadian Journal of Occupational Therapy* **64** (1): 7–15.

Finlayson, M. and Edwards, J. (1995) Integrating the concepts of health promotion and community into occupational therapy practice. *Canadian Journal of Occupational Therapy* **62** (2): 70–5.

Finlayson, M. and Edwards, J. (1997) Evolving health environments and occupational therapy: definitions, descriptions and opportunities. *British Journal of Occupational Therapy* **60** (10): 456–60.

Fiveash, B. (1998) Client-managed care. *European Nurse* **3** (3): 186–93.

Fraser, D. M. (1995) Client-centred care: fact or fiction? *Midwives* June: 174–7.

Gatterman, M. I. (1995) A patient-centred paradigm: a model for chiropractic education and research. *Journal of Alternative and Complementary Medicine* **1** (4): 371–86.

Gerhardt, U. (1989) *Ideas about Illness: an Intellectual and Political History of Medical Sociology*. Basingstoke: Macmillan (now Palgrave Macmillan).

Glenister, D. (1994) Patient participation in psychiatric services: a literature review and proposal for a research strategy. *Journal of Advanced Nursing* **19**: 802–11.

Goodall, C. (1992) Preserving dignity for disabled people. *Nursing Standard* **6** (35): 25–8.

Grol, R., De Maeseneer, J., Whitfield, M. and Mokkink, H. (1990) Disease-centred versus patient-centred attitudes: comparison of general practitioners in Belgium, Britain and the Netherlands. *Family Practice* **7** (2): 100–3.

Gutterman, L. (1990) A day treatment program for persons with AIDS. *American Journal of Occupational Therapy* **44** (3): 234–7.

Hall, J. A., Roter, D. L. and Katz, N. R. (1988) Meta-analysis of correlates of provider behaviour in medical encounters. *Medical Care* **26** (7): 657–75.

Happ, M. B., Williams, C. C., Strumpf, N. E. and Burger, S. G. (1996) Individualised care for frail elders: theory and practice. *Journal of Gerontological Nursing* March: 7–14.

Henderson, A. (1994) Power and knowledge in nursing practice: the contribution of Foucault. *Journal of Advanced Nursing* 20: 935–9.

Hokanson Hawks, J. (1991) Power: a concept analysis. *Journal of Advanced Nursing* 16: 754–62.

Honey, A. (1999) Empowerment versus power: consumer participation in mental health services. *Occupational Therapy International* 6 (4): 257–76.

Hostler, S. L. (1991) Family centred care. *Paediatric Clinics of North America* 38 (6): 1545–60.

Hotz, M., Knieomann, K. and Kohn, L. (1997) Occupational therapy in paediatric lead exposure prevention. *American Journal of Occupational Therapy* 52 (1): 53–9.

Hugman, R. (1991) *Power in Caring Professions*. London: Macmillan (now Palgrave Macmillan).

Jackson, J., Carlson, M., Mandel, D., Zemke, R. and Clark, F. (1998) Occupation in lifestyle redesign: the well elderly study occupational therapy program. *American Journal of Occupational Therapy* 52 (5): 326–36.

Jadad, A. R. (1999) Promoting partnerships: challenges for the internet age. *British Medical Journal* 319: 761–4.

Johns, N. and Harvey, C. (1993) Training for work with parents: strategies for engaging practitioners who are uninterested or resistant. *Infants and Young Children* 5 (4): 52–7.

Kalmanson, B. and Seligman, S. (1992) Family–provider relationships: the basis of all interventions. *Infants and Young Children* 4 (4): 46–52.

Krantz, D. S., Baum, A. and Wideman, M. (1980) Assessment of preferences for self-treatment and information in health care. *Journal of Personality and Social Psychology* 39 (5): 977–90.

Krupa, T. and Clark, C. C. (1995) Occupational therapists as case managers: responding to current approaches to community mental health service delivery. *Canadian Journal of Occupational Therapy* 62 (1): 16–22.

Laine, C. and Davidoff, F. (1996) Patient-centred medicine. *Journal of the American Medical Association* 275 (2): 152–6.

Law, M. (1998) Does client-centred practice make a difference? In Law, M. (ed). *Client-centred Occupational Therapy*. Thorofare, NJ: Slack.

Law, M. (2000) Identifying occupational performance issues. In Fearing V. G. and Clark, J. (eds) *Individuals in Context: a Practical Guide to Client-centred Practice*. Thorofare, NJ: Slack.

Law, M., Baptiste, S. and Mills, J. (1995) Client-centred practice: what does it mean and does it make a difference? *Canadian Journal of Occupational Therapy* 62 (5): 250–7.

Law, M. and Mills, J. (1998) Client-centred occupational therapy. In Law, M. (ed). *Client-centred Occupational Therapy*. Thorofare, NJ: Slack.

Lawlor, M. C. and Mattingly, C. F. (1998) The complexities embedded in family-centred care. *American Journal of Occupational Therapy* 52 (4): 259–67.

Letts, L., Fraser, B., Finlayson, M. and Walls, J. (1996) *For the Health of It! Occupational Therapy within a Health Promotion Framework*. Toronto, Ontario: CAOT Publications.

Leviton, A., Mueller, M. and Kauffman, C. (1992) The family-centred consultation model: practical applications for professionals. *Infants and Young Children* 4 (3): 1–8.

Logan, H. L. (1997) The patient and the shifting health-care paradigm. *Journal of the American College of Dentists* 64 (1): 16–18.

Madill, H., Townsend, E. and Schultz, P. (1989) Implementing a health promotion strategy in occupational therapy education and practice. *Canadian Journal of Occupational Therapy* 56 (2): 67–72.

Matheis-Kraft, C., George, S., Olinger, M. J. and York, L. (1990) Patient driven healthcare works. *Nursing Management* **21** (9): 124–8.

Matuska, K., Giles-Heinz, A., Flinn, N., Neighbor, M. and Bass-Haugen, J. (2003) Outcomes of a pilot occupational therapy wellness program for older adults. *American Journal of Occupational Therapy* **57** (2): 220–4.

McWilliam, C. L., Brown, J. B., Carmichael, J. L. and Lehman, J. M. (1994) A new perspective on threatened autonomy in elderly persons: the disempowering process. *Social Science Medicine* **38** (2): 327–38.

Meeson, B. (1998) Occupational therapy in community mental health, Part 2: Factors influencing intervention choice. *British Journal of Occupational Therapy* **61** (2): 57–62.

Meyer, C. (1996) *The Development of a Client-centred Approach for Community Occupational Therapy Practice: a National Survey.* Unpublished doctoral thesis, University of Leeds.

Pendleton, L. and House, W. C. (1984) Preferences for treatment approaches in medical care. *Medical Care* **22** (7): 644–6.

Pesznecker, B. L., Zerwekh, J. V. and Horn, B. J. (1989) The mutual-participation relationship: key to facilitating self care practices in clients and families. *Public Health Nursing* **6** (4): 197–203.

Phillips, D. E. (1994) Health promotion – framework and application for the long-term care setting. *Canadian Nursing Home* **5** (2): 4–10.

Raatikainen, R. (1994) Power or lack of it in nursing care. *Journal of Advanced Nursing* **19**: 424–32.

Raeburn, J. and Rootman, I., (1998) *People-centred Health Promotion.* New York: Wiley.

Rebeiro, K. L. (2000) Client perspectives on occupational therapy practice: are we truly client-centred? *Canadian Journal of Occupational Therapy* **67** (1): 7–14.

Reutter, L. and Ford, J. S. (1997) Enhancing client competence: melding professional and client knowledge in public health nursing practice. *Public Health Nursing* **14** (3): 143–50.

Roberts, R. N. and Magrab, P. R. (1991) Psychologists' role in a family-centred approach to practice, training, and research with young children. *American Psychologist* **46** (2): 144–8.

Robinson, I. M. (1981) Muriel Driver Memorial Lecture 1981: The mists of time. *Canadian Journal of Occupational Therapy* **48** (4): 145–52.

Rosenbaum, P., King, S., Law, M., King, G. and Evans, J. (1998) Family-centred service: a conceptual framework and research review. *Physical and Occupational Therapy in Paediatrics* **18** (1): 1–20.

Skelton, A. M. (1997) Patient education for the millennium: beyond control and emancipation. *Patient Education and Counselling* **31**: 151–8.

Smith, R. (1995) A client-centred model for equipment prescription (client's values and roles, effective use of adaptive equipment). *Occupational Therapy in Health Care* **9** (4): 39–52.

Speechley, V. (1992) Patients as partners. *European Journal of Cancer Care* **1** (3): 22–6.

Sumsion, T. (1993) Client-centred practice: the true impact. *Canadian Journal of Occupational Therapy* **60** (1): 6–8.

Sumsion, T. (1999) A study to determine a British occupational therapy definition of client-centred practice. *British Journal of Occupational Therapy*, **62** (2): 52–8.

Sumsion, T. (2000) A revised occupational therapy definition of client-centred practice. *British Journal of Occupational Therapy* **63** (7): 304–9.

Swaffield, L. (1990) Patient power. *Nursing Times* **86** (48): 26–8.

Sweeney, M. M. (1997) The value of a family-centred approach in the NICU and PICU: one family's perspective. *Paediatric Nursing* 23 (1): 64–6.

Thibeault, R. and Hebert, M. (1997) A congruent model for health promotion in occupational therapy. *Occupational Therapy International* 4 (4): 271–93.

Townsend, E. (1998a) Using Canada's 1997 guidelines for enabling occupation. *Australian Occupational Therapy Journal* 45: 1–6.

Townsend, E. (1998b) *Good Intentions Overruled*. Toronto: University of Toronto Press.

Townsend, E. (1998c) Occupational therapy language: matters of respect, accountability and leadership. *Canadian Journal of Occupational Therapy* 65 (1): 45–50.

Townsend, E. (2002) *Enabling Occupation: an Occupational Therapy Perspective*. Ottawa: CAOT Publications.

Wertlieb, D. (1993) Special section editorial: Toward a family-centred paediatric psychology – challenge and opportunity in the international year of the family. *Journal of Paediatric Psychology* 18 (5): 541–7.

World Health Organisation (1986) *Ottawa Charter for Health Promotion*. Geneva: WHO.

CHAPTER 9

Healthy Discharges for Older Persons: a Health Promotion Role for Occupational Therapists in Acute Healthcare

ANITA ATWAL

Discharge planning is a process that can enable resources to be used more effectively and efficiently and entails bridging the gap between hospital and home. The discharge process is complicated by an absence of a consensus on its purpose and aims (Evans and Hendricks, 1992; Mamon et al., 1992). When discussing the discharge process it is essential to take into account it is not a single isolated event. It involves the admission procedure and the documentation of the expected problems and outcomes, the referral process, multidisciplinary assessment, the setting of goals, the planning of interventions, the implementation of the plan and the evaluation of the discharge. The multifaceted nature of discharge planning makes it a difficult process to manage for both occupational therapists and health and social care professionals. The emphasis has to be on ensuring healthy discharges, as poor discharge planning can impact upon the quality of life and wellbeing of older persons, their carers and the community.

This chapter explores, from an occupational therapy perspective, the factors that promote and inhibit healthy discharges for older people, drawing on issues from a research study that explored the discharge process within the acute healthcare setting (Atwal, 1999). The six objectives for health promotion for older persons outlined in Table 9.1 and published by the World Health Organisation (WHO) (1983) will be used to discuss discharge planning in relation to primary, secondary and tertiary health promotion practices. The current challenges that occupational therapy faces in relation to promoting healthy discharges for older people will then be explored.

Table 9.1   Health promotion goals for older people

- To prevent unnecessary loss or functional capacity
- To maintain quality of life by preventing distressing symptoms
- To assist older persons to live in their own homes and to prevent
- Unnecessary admissions too residential care
- To prevent unnecessary decline in functional capacity and quality of life if admission to long-stay care is essential
- To prevent the breakdown of informal networks of care.

Source: World Health Organisation (1983)

Discharge planning and health promotion

Ageing is a process that occupational therapists take seriously, as the proportion of people aged 60 and over in the general population is growing faster than any other age group (WHO, 2002). Increasing life expectancy is, however, often viewed as a problem by governments, communities and health and social care professionals because it is anticipated that an ageing population will lead to unmanageable health and social care costs (Tonks, 1999; Lothian and Philp, 2001; WHO, 2002). Jones (1993) argues that such attitudes are reinforced by the negative images of older people that are sometimes presented in the mass media. Demographic problems are less likely to occur if policy makers examine strategies to deliver a more efficient healthcare service and reduce the cost of long term care through the implementation of health promotion and informal care (WHO, 2002). If used effectively, discharge planning might have an impact on the economics of population ageing being managed in a successful way, although currently there is no clear evidence that discharge planning actually reduces healthcare costs or has an impact on mortality or length of hospital stay (Parker et al., 2002, Parkes and Shepperd, 2003). Occupational therapists therefore must demonstrate the effectiveness of discharge planning and associated health promotion initiatives for healthcare providers as well as for older people.

Using the United Nations Standard of over 60 years of age to describe older people, there is evidence that this population group have not always been at the forefront of occupational therapy and health promotion professional agendas (Killoran et al., 1997; Atwal et al., 2003). This is surprising as occupational therapists work predominantly with older people and health promotion has much to contribute to the enhancement of levels of health and wellbeing, reduction of incidence of illness, disease and accidents in this population group (National Council for Ageing and Older People, 1998; WHO, 2002).

Currently in the United Kingdom (UK), Australia and the United States of America (US) there are more positive moves toward promoting quality of life of older persons through broad national health promotion standards (see Table 9.2).

These health promotion standards offer wide ranging opportunities. Occupational therapists can enhance older persons' quality of life in numerous

Table 9.2 Comparison of active ageing, health promotion and occupational therapy core values

Active ageing (WHO, 2002: 12)	Health promotion (WHO, 1986)	Occupational therapy core values (College of Occupational Therapists, 2000)
'Active ageing' refers to continued participation in society, to realise potential for physical, social, and mental wellbeing whilst ensuring adequate protection, security and care when assistance is needed. This includes continued participation in social, economical, cultural, spiritual and civic affairs	• Equity • Empowerment • The reorientation of the health service	• OT practice is culturally sensitive and culturally relevant. • OTs promote personal identity by giving information and choices to their clients • The client's goals take precedence in the treatment programme • Each OT has a responsibility to ensure that's they provide a high quality service that meets the client's needs and does no harm. • OT is part of the total care of the client and OTs are members of the multidisciplinary team

ways through meaningful occupation, the promotion of safe environment and health behaviours and through the prevention of disease and disorders. Whilst health policy changes have resulted in opinion papers being published (see Wilcock, 1998a, 1998b, 2002; VanderPloeg, 2001) they contain little discussion of the health promoting role of occupational therapist in discharge planning for older persons.

This lack of discourse might be a result of occupational therapists' lack of association with health promotion in general (see Chapter 7 in this text for further discussion) or with a health promotion role within discharge planning. It might also be a reflection of occupational therapists' reluctance to become experts within discharge planning or their failure to recognise its importance. The College of Occupational Therapists (COT) (2002) and the Audit Commission (Audit Commission, 2000) have expressed concern that the role of the occupational therapist in the acute setting is limited and there is a move by the occupational therapy profession to adopt a stronger health promotion role (Wilcock, 1998a, 2002; COT, 2002). It is therefore an opportune time for a radical shift in the way occupational therapists perceive their discharge planning functions. This shift might have other positive repercussions, as the profession is frequently misunderstood and has a limited evidence and theoretical base (Marriott, 1997; Atwal and Reeves, 2003; Lillywhite and Atwal, 2003).

Occupational therapists' failure to value discharge planning must be examined within the political and historical context. Discharge planning is a powerful political tool that has been used to highlight failures within health and social care. The media has highlighted the numerous problems that older persons can experience accessing acute medical care and it has also been responsible for promoting the belief that some of these problems could have been avoided if older persons awaiting social care input had not occupied beds, rather than presenting the alternative argument, that the health and social care system cannot meet the needs of older persons (Victor et al., 2000; Atwal, 2002).

Active ageing and discharge planning

Active ageing is a concept that aims to optimise opportunities for health, participation and security in order to enhance quality of life as people age (WHO, 2002: 2) and has much in common with the goals of health promotion and occupational therapy. It signifies an important paradigm shift away from a needs based approach to a rights based approach which promotes the participation of older people both in the community and the political process. See Table 9.3 for a comparison of active aging, health promotion and occupational therapy core values.

Table 9.3   Health promotion standards outlined in key policy documents in the United States of America, the United Kingdom and Australia

Country and documents	Standards
United States of America *Healthy People 2010* (US Department of Health and Human Services, 2000): a revision of *Healthy People 2000*, where specific targets were given for older people	Two key goals: ● Increase quality and years of healthy life ● Eliminate health disparities Priority areas: ● promoting healthy behaviours ● promoting healthy and safe communities ● improving systems for personal and public health ● preventing and reducing diseases and disorder
United Kingdom *National Service Framework for Older People* (DoH, 2001a)	Standard 5: Stroke: prevent strokes Standard 6: Falls: prevent falls Standard 7: Mental health in older people: provide access to integrated mental health services Standard 8: Promote health and active life in older age
Australia *Goals and Targets for Australia's Health in the Year 2000 and Beyond* (Nutbeam et al., 1993): a revision of the 1989 strategy 'A Better Health Program'	Two important targets that have importance relevance to older people and discharge planning are the inclusion of objectives for: ● healthy environment, such as home, housing, transport, health care settings ● health literacy

The active ageing concept should be used throughout the discharge process as a philosophical guide to occupational therapists in promoting healthy discharge planning for older people.

Health promoting objectives relating to discharge planning

To prevent unnecessary loss or functional capacity

Occupational therapists aim to optimise health and wellbeing through meaningful occupation (Wilcock, 1998a). Currently, occupational therapists predominantly practice at a secondary health promotion level, restoring, maintaining and enhancing functional wellbeing both within inpatient settings and in the community. Restoring function is an essential component of enabling an older person to sustain their role within the community and consequently is an essential component of a healthy discharge.

Within discharge planning there is evidence that an older person may not always have reached their optimum level or received appropriate rehabilitation prior to their discharge (Audit Commission, 2000). The College of Occupational Therapists (2002) suggests that the dominance of the medical model rather than the salutogenic model of health (Antonovsky, 1996) has resulted in occupational therapists being powerless partners in assessing people to return home with preventable levels of dysfunction. Consequently the goals of an organisation and of the government can impact upon how, when and whether an older person is discharged (McKenna et al., 2000; Lester-Boutlin and Gibson, 2002; Atwal and Caldwell, 2003). Indeed the emphasis on releasing acute beds can mean that the total health needs of the older persons are not assessed or not resolved (Mistiaen et al., 1997; Waters et al., 2001; Atwal, 2002).

To ensure effective partnership

Discharge planning is a process that is dependent upon teamwork and interagency working (Bull and Roberts, 2001; Atwal, 2002). Occupational therapists must work in partnership with members of the multidisciplinary team and the older person and their carers in order to ensure healthy discharges. In doing so, they must possess excellent team working skills and ensure that the autonomy of the older person and their carer is respected even if it conflicts with professional opinion.

The locus of control, however, often lies with the medical establishment and not with the occupational therapist and the interprofessional team. These inequalities in power can constrain effective teamwork, which in turn can impact upon communication and the outcome of the discharge process

(Caldwell and Atwal, 2003). In order to facilitate partnership working current health and special care policy in the UK has highlighted the need for integrated and person centred care (Department of Health (DoH), 2000, 2001a). Whilst there is currently an opportunity to improve partnership and participatory working, new health and social care policy contradicts this ethos. The Delayed Discharge Bill (DoH, 2003) will impose financial penalties on social services for delayed discharges for non-medical reasons. Consequently this could result in older persons being discharged from hospital before they are ready in order that financial penalties are avoided.

To prevent unnecessary decline in functional capacity and quality of life

Whilst the role of the occupational therapist is well established with older people in a wide range of health and social care settings, there is a noticeable absence of input in care homes in the UK (Green and Cooper, 2000). A rationale given for the lack of participation by occupational therapists in care homes is the limited evidence to demonstrate the effectiveness of occupational therapy in such settings (Duncan-Myers and Huebner, 1999; Green and Cooper, 2000; Mayers, 2000). It is also suggested that the reluctance to employ occupational therapists could be associated with the perception that older persons have reached their final discharge destination, and that resources could be targeted more effectively to older persons awaiting discharge. There is, however, evidence that older persons in care homes would benefit from rehabilitation to maintain function and wellbeing, which could result in significant saving in terms of nursing staff costs (Przybylski et al., 1996; Atwal et al., 2003) and that older persons in care homes valued continued engagement in meaningful occupations (Raynes, 2000; Atwal and Caldwell, 2003). The introduction of national minimum standards for care homes (DoH, 2001b) will enable occupational therapists to demonstrate that they have an important health promotion role in enhancing quality of life in activities of daily living, leisure and social activities, cultural interests and personal and social relationships.

To respect the autonomy of the individual

Within the ethos of client centred practice occupational therapists must uphold the autonomy of the client even if it conflicts with professional opinion. Whilst respecting the autonomy of the client, occupational therapists must also avoid harm to the older person (Atwal and Caldwell, 2003). An important distinction is between those risks that are taken voluntarily and those that are involuntary, as the excessive concerns of professionals about safety may override the wishes of an older person (Clemens, 1995).

Occupational therapists must discuss the findings of any assessment they undertake and ensure that the older person's opinions are documented, acknowledged and not dismissed (Caldwell and Atwal, 2003). An older patient can be frustrated by the discharge procedure and their perception of not being involved within the discharge decision making process can increase their anxiety about returning home. To ensure that the autonomy of the patient is respected it is essential that occupational therapists are able to explain clearly the aims of their interventions and of the discharge process.

To enable independent living

Maintaining and enhancing independence in order that older persons can continue to live in their own homes is a primary goal of occupational therapists working both within the acute hospital setting and the community. Occupational therapists within the community are more likely to engage in primary and secondary health promotion with regard to the discharge process, involving rehabilitation or accident prevention in the home. An older person may have been discharged but still might not be able to undertake some everyday tasks such as going shopping. The older person can be supported in achieving these goals by an occupational therapist working within intermediate care and in community teams. The aim of intermediate care is to prevent unnecessary hospital admission, provide effective rehabilitation services to enable early discharge from hospital and to prevent premature or unnecessary admission to long term residential care (DoH, 2001b). For occupational therapists this is the ideal opportunity to participate within primary, secondary and tertiary health promotion. Whether occupational therapists will be able to utilise this opportunity is doubtful for a couple of reasons, one being a national shortage of occupational therapists in the UK (Audit Commission, 2000) and the other being that occupational therapists are too preoccupied with equipment and housing adaptation assessment. This final point might be why Glasman (1996: 7) challenges occupational therapist to consider what they want to achieve for their older clients, arguing that they have lost their sense of purpose.

Discharge planning can lead to the wrong outcome for the client and their carers in terms of the final discharge destination and with regard to readmission, the latter being a quality indicator of a successful discharge. Methods of assessments used by health and social care professionals could impact upon the discharge process. One such example is the use of predischarge visits by occupational therapists to predict whether older persons have the capacity to return home (Clark et al., 1997; Mountain and Pighills, 2003). Whilst this is an integral part of occupational therapy practice and discharge planning there is a lack of evidence to demonstrate that they are effective (Patterson and Mulley, 1999). Mountain and Pighills (2003) suggest that predischarge visits can only provide a snapshot in time judgement to be made at the point of discharge.

Occupational therapists and health and social care professionals now have the opportunity to utilise intermediate care services that can give older persons the opportunity to focus on rehabilitation and ensure that the right decision is made at the appropriate time for the client.

In order for the older person to make an informed decision about their discharge it is essential that they be given accurate information from occupational therapists and other professionals. Honest, continuous and timely communication is considered an essential component of the discharge process (Driscoll, 2000; Bull and Roberts, 2001). Occupational therapists must ensure that the information that is given is presented in the most appropriate way to the older person and their carer, taking into account physical aspects of ageing as well as cultural, social and educational factors. Furthermore they must be mindful of older persons' literacy and must become critical consumers of educational materials in order to ensure their effectiveness and quality (Griffin et al., 2003). There is however little evidence about the role of health education interventions in improving the healthy discharge of older persons from hospital, although there is some evidence that readmission to hospital is less frequent in patients who received complex educational interventions (Parker et al., 2002). However older persons no longer have to rely on professionals for health education materials since many other media are available through information technology such as the Internet. Within discharge planning this can enable older persons and their carers to be able to direct professionals to request types of services that could enhance their quality if life once discharged from hospital.

To maintain quality of life

Quality of life is defined by the WHO Quality of Life Group [WHOQOL Group], (1995: 405) as a person's perception of their position in life in the context of the culture and value systems in which they live and in relation to their goals, expectations, standards and concerns. It is a broad ranging concept influenced in a complex way by the person's physical health, psychological state, level of independence, social relationships, and their relationships to salient features of their environment.

Occupational therapists are involved in promoting quality of life through various interventions such as rehabilitation, helping older people remain socially active, improve the quality of their homes, and maintain independence. Within discharge planning it is suggested that the care management process appears not to be valued since occupational therapists do not associate it with quality of life and health promotion. A systematic review of the effectiveness of home care (Godfrey et al., 2000) demonstrated that such services can delay admission to long term institutional care for those who are physically frail and are assessed at being at risk of admission. What occupational therapists must ensure is that older persons are able to continue to perform occupations that they value and regard as important. Wenger (1992) found that many older people placed high value on shopping and cooking as it gave them an opportunity for social contact. The continued participation in these activities was perceived as an important component of maintaining their independence. Similarly Godfrey (1995) found that older people placed higher value on certain activities of daily living and preferred to struggle with self-care tasks as these were perceived as central to their sense of autonomy.

To facilitate informal care

The importance of informal carers within health and social care has been addressed under health and social care legislation (United Kingdom Parliament, 1995, 2000). Informal carers are family members, neighbours or friends who provide physical, social and psychological or spiritual support that enable older persons to be maintained within the community and without whom additional statutory provision would be needed. A study by Victor et al. (2000) found that older patients who did not have a family carer experienced discharge delays. Research into the experiences of carers has highlighted issues in relation to caring and discharge planning, identifying a lack of awareness of the important role that carers play within the discharge process. This perhaps accounts for carers' complaints about the lack of consultation about the discharge plans to return home, lack of appropriate notice prior to discharge, slow or complete lack of information exchange between professionals, services not delivered and delays in providing essential equipment (Princess Royal Trust for Carers, 1998; Holzhausen, 2001).

This failure to take the carer's opinions into account has consequences not only for the client and the carer but also for health and social care Trusts. Research by Carers UK (Holzhausen, 2001) into carers' perceptions of discharge planning found that the proportion of people who had been readmitted within two months of being discharged doubled from 19 per cent in 1999 to 43 per cent in 2001. Some older persons are also caring for another older person, with a survey by the Princess Royal Trust for Carers (1998) showing that 9 per cent of their sample consisted of people over 75 years of age who were caring for another person over 75. In the same study, eight out of ten carers said that caring had a negative impact on their own health, and only 3 per cent of carers who responded to the survey claimed to have been taught moving and handling skills.

Discharge planning and primary, secondary and tertiary health promotion

Primary health promotion

Currently most occupational therapists are not overtly involved with primary health promotion, even though there is evidence demonstrating the relationship between occupation, health and wellbeing (Clark et al., 1997; Iwarsson et al., 1998; Glas et al., 1999; Lennarysson and Silverstein, 2001 and see also Wilcock, Chapter 7 in this text). There is evidence that social and productive activities are effective in promoting fitness (Glass et al., 1999; Lennarysson and Silverstein, 2001), ensuring quality of life (Clark et al., 1997; Glass et al., 1999), decreasing the risk of dementia (Wang et al., 2002) and preventing disability (de Leon et al., 2003). Occupation based interventions can contribute to the discharge process by preventing ill health, decline in function and the need for readmission into hospital and/or a care home. Specific occupational therapy based programmes need to enhance social support and social networks for older people. Hence any occupational therapy based programme needs to take place in facilities that are designed to offer opportunities for social contact, such as bingo halls or church halls. Moreover, occupations need to be evaluated to demonstrate that they can prevent ill health and are of interest to an older person and their carer and must be utilised in a way that will ensure an older person can achieve individual goals.

Primary prevention includes targeting the macro and micro environments in which an older person lives, which may need modification as the ageing process occurs or as they relocate. The challenge for occupational therapists is to work with the local community and housing and environmental officers to build healthy environments in order that older people may maintain functional independence and their role in and links with the community.

Secondary health promotion

Secondary health promotion strategies relating to older people could include programmes that optimise residual abilities, support and enable management of losses such as bereavement, and support informal care relationships and networks (Grams and Albee, 1995). By optimising residual abilities occupational therapists can contribute to the discharge process by preventing readmissions and reducing the levels of support that statutory agencies need to provide.

Occupational therapists have an important role in implementing coping strategies to avoid the harmful effect of stressful situations. In particular the challenge for occupational therapists is to promote the wellbeing of informal carers. Such interventions could include manual handling or stress management advice that might ensure that the carer does not experience unnecessary physical or psychological ill health.

Tertiary health promotion

Occupational therapists have a significant tertiary health promotion role within the discharge process, through the provision of equipment, home visits, discharge education, rehabilitation and packages of care. The challenge for occupational therapists is to value their contribution within tertiary health promotion and to ensure that the full needs of an older person are met. This can be particularly challenging when working within organisations that demand older persons be discharged quickly from acute medical beds. Occupational therapists need to ensure that other professionals value their current health promotion role within discharge planning. Most importantly occupational therapists need to value their unique role within the care management process.

Health and social care policies now offer occupational therapists and the professions with which they work new and innovative health promoting ways of discharging older persons. Within a health promotion approach to discharge planning there is a tension between individual autonomy, client participation and organisational efficiency. Efficiency need not be viewed in negative terms but should correspond with the requirment to ensure that interventions and discharge planning are based on best evidence. More research is needed on discharge procedures (Vetter, 2003) and on how best to develop models of discharge planning that integrates primary, secondary and tertiary health promotion. In order to promote healthy discharge planning the occupational therapy profession needs to ensure that educational establishments provide appropriate training on the ageing process, health promotion and discharge procedures. Whilst the discharge materials published by the Department of Health (1994, 2003) provide a guide to the discharge process, occupational therapists are not always equipped with the complex skills that are needed to plan a health promoting discharge.

Occupational therapists need to collaborate with government departments, experts on ageing and health promoters so that they can expand their role within health promotion. Furthermore, promoting healthy discharges will require occupational therapists to become confident in their vision of the future direction of the profession. It is important to emphasise that discharge planning is an interprofessional activity that is dependent upon a team approach. If discharge planning is to enhance quality of life for older persons, occupational therapists must be aware of the importance of primary, secondary and tertiary health promotion in enabling a healthy discharge.

References

Antonovsky, A. (1996) The salutogenic model as a theory to guide health promotion. *Health Promotion International* **11** (1): 11–18.

Atwal, A. (1999) *The Battlefield: Discharge Planning and Multidisciplinary Teamwork.* Unpublished doctoral thesis, Middlesex University.

Atwal, A. (2002) Nurses' perceptions of discharge planning in acute healthcare: a case study in one British teaching hospital. *Journal of Advanced Nursing* **39** (5): 450–9.

Atwal, A. and Caldwell, K. (2003) Ethics, occupational therapy and discharge planning: four broken principles. *Australian Journal of Occupational Therapy* **50** (4): 245–51.

Atwal, A., Owen, S. and Davies, R. (2003) Struggling for occupational satisfaction: older people in care homes. *British Journal of Occupational Therapy* **66** (3): 118–24.

Audit Commission (2000) *The Way to Go Home: Rehabilitation and Remedial Services for Older People*. London: Audit Commission.

Bull, M. J. and Roberts, J. (2001) Components of a proper hospital discharge for elders. *Journal of Advanced Nursing* **35** (4): 571–81.

Caldwell, K. and Atwal, A. (2003) The problems of interprofessional practice in hospitals. *British Journal of Nursing* **12** (20): 1169–1236.

Clark, C., Azen, S. P., Jackson, J., Carison, M., Mandel, D., Hay, J., Josephson, K., Cherry, B., Hessel, C., Palmer, J. and Lipson, J. (1997) Occupational therapy for independent-living older adults. *Journal of the American Occupational Therapy Association* **278** (16): 1321–26.

Clemens, E. L. (1995) Multiple perceptions of discharge planning in one urban hospital. *Health and Social Work* **20**: 254–62.

College of Occupational Therapists (2000) *Code of Ethics and Professional Conduct for Occupational Therapists*. London: COT.

College of Occupational Therapists (2002) *From Interface to Integration: a Consultation Document*. London: COT.

de Leon, C. M., Glas, T. A. and Berkman, L. F. (2003) Social engagement and disability in a community population of older adults. *American Journal of Epidemiology* **157**: 633–42.

Department of Health (1994) *Hospital Discharge Workbook*. London: HMSO.

Department of Health (2000) *The NHS Plan: a Plan for Investment. A Plan for Reform*. London: HMSO.

Department of Health (2001a) *National Service Framework for Older People*. London: HMSO.

Department of Health (2001b) *Care Homes for Older People: National Minimum Standards*. London: HMSO.

Department of Health (2003) *Discharge from Hospital: Pathway, Process and Practice*. London: HMSO.

Driscoll, A. (2000) Managing post-discharge care at home: an analysis of patients' and their carers' perceptions of information received during their stay in hospital. *Journal of Advanced Nursing* **31** (5), 1165–73.

Duncan-Myers, A. M. and Huebner, R. A. (1999) Relationship between choice and quality of life among residents in long term-care facilities. *American Journal of Occupational Therapy* **54** (5): 504–8.

Evans, R. and Hendricks, R. (1992) Evaluating hospital discharge planning: a randomised clinical trial. *Medical Care* **31**: 357–9.

Glass, T. A., de Leon, C. M., Marottoli, R. A. and Berkman, L. F. (1999) Population based study of social and productive activities as predictors of survival among elderly Americans. *British Medical Journal* **319**: 478–83.

Glasman, D. (1996) Circles of support. *Therapy Weekly* **22** (29 February): 7.

Godfrey, M. (1995) *Casualties of Change: from Home Help to Home Care*. London: London Borough of Hounslow Social Services Department.

Godfrey, M., Randall, T., Long, A. and Grant, M. (2000) *Home Care: a Review of Effectiveness and Outcomes*. Exeter: Centre for Evidence-based Social Work, University of Exeter.

Grams, A. and Albee, G. W. (1995) Primary prevention in the service of ageing in LA. In Bond, L. A., Cutler, S. J. and Grams, A. (eds) *Promoting Successful and Productive Ageing*. Thousand Oaks, CA: Sage.

Green, S. and Cooper, B. A. (2000) Occupation as a quality of life constituent: a nursing home perspective. *British Journal of Occupational Therapy* **63** (1): 17–24.

Griffin, J., McKenna, K. and Tooth, L. (2003) Written health education materials: making them more effective. *Australian Occupational Therapy Journal* **50** (3), 170–7.

Holzhausen, E. (2001) *You Can Take Him Home Now; Carers' Experience of Hospital Discharge.* London: Carers National Association.

Iwarsson, S., Isacesson, A., Persson, D. and Schersten, B. (1998) Occupation and survival: a 25 year follow-up study of an ageing population. *American Journal of Occupational Therapy* **52** (1): 65–70.

Jones, H. (1993) Altered images. *Nursing Times* **89** (5): 58–60.

Killoran, A., Howse, K. and Dalley, D. (1997) *Promoting the Health of Older People: a Compendium.* London: Health Education Authority.

Lennarysson, C. and Silverstein, M. (2001) Does engagement with life enhance survival of elderly people in Sweden? The role of social and leisure activities *The Journal of Gerontology Series B: Psychological Sciences and Social Sciences* **56**: 335–42.

Lester-Boutlin, P. and Gibson, R. W. (2002) Patients' perceptions of home health occupational therapy. *Australian Occupational Therapy Journal* **49** (3): 146–54.

Lillywhite, A. and Atwal, A. (2003) Occupational therapists' perceptions of the role of community learning disability teams. *British Journal of Learning Disabilities* **31** (3): 130–5.

Lothian, K. and Philp, I. (2001) Care of older people: maintaining the dignity and autonomy of older people in the healthcare setting. *British Medical Journal* **322**: 668–70.

Mamon, J., Steinwarks, D., Fahey, D., Bone, M., Oktay, J. and Klein, L. (1992) Impact of hospital discharge planning in meeting patients needs after returning home. *Health Service Research* **2** (2): 155–75.

Marriott, A. A. (1997) Using the core values and skills of occupational therapy in management. *British Journal of Occupational Therapy* **60** (4): 169–73.

Mayers, C. (2000) The Casson Memorial Lecture 2000: Reflect on the past to shape the future. *British Journal of Occupational Therapy* **63** (8): 358–66.

McKenna, H., Keeney, S., Glenn, A. and Gordon, P. (2000) Discharge planning: an exploratory study. *Journal of Clinical Nursing* **9** (4): 594.

Mistiaen, P., Duijnhouwer, E., Wijkel, D., Bont, de M. and Veeger, M. (1997) The problems of elderly people at home one week after discharge from an acute care setting. *Journal of Advanced Nursing* **25** (6): 1233–40.

Mountain, G. and Pighills, A. (2003) Pre-discharge home visits with older people: time to review practice. *Health and Social Care in the Community* **11** (2): 146–54.

National Council for Ageing and Older People (1998) *Adding Years to Life and Life to Years: a Health Promotion Strategy for Older People.* Dublin: National Council for Ageing and Older People.

Nutbeam, D., Wise, M., Bauman, A., Harris, E. and Leeder, S. (1993) *Goals and Targets for Australia's Health in the Year 2000 and Beyond.* Canberra: AGPS.

Parker, S. G., Peet, S. M., McPherson, A., Cannaby, A. M., Abrams, K., Baker, R., Wilson, A., Lindesay, J., Parker, G. and Jones, D. R. (2002) A systematic review of discharge arrangements for older people. *Health and Technology Assessment* **6** (4): 1–180.

Parkes, J. and Shepperd, S. (2003) Discharge planning from hospital to home. Cochrane Review. In *The Cochrane Library* 4. Oxford: Update Software.

Patterson, C. J. and Mulley, C. P. (1999) The effectiveness of pre discharge home visits: a systematic review. *Clinical Rehabilitation* **13**: 101–4.

Princess Royal Trust for Carers (1998) *Eight Hours a Day and Taken for Granted. You Just Get on With it Don't You*. London: Princess Royal Trust for Carers.

Przybylski, B. R., Durmont, E. D., Watkins, M. E., Warren, S. A., Beauline, A. P. and Lier, D. A. (1996) Outcomes of enhanced physical and occupational therapy in a nursing home setting. *Archives of Physical Medicine & Rehabilitation* 77 (6): 554–61.

Raynes, N. (2000) Quality care: the inside story. *Elderly Care* 11 (10): 8–17.

Tonks, A. (1999) Medicine must change to serve an ageing society. *British Medical Journal* 319: 1450–1.

United Kingdom Parliament (1995) *Carers (Recognition and Services) Act*. London: HMSO.

United Kingdom Parliament (2000) Carers *and Disabled Children's Act*. London: HMSO.

US Department of Health and Human Services (2000) *United States of America. Healthy People 2010. Improving Health and Objectives for Improving Health*. Two vols. Washington, DC: US Government Printing Office.

VanderPloeg, W. (2001) Health promotion in palliative care: an occupational perspective. *Australian Journal of Occupational Therapy* 48 (1): 45–8.

Vetter, N. (2003) Inappropriate delayed discharge form hospital: what do we know? *British Medical Journal* 326: 927–8.

Victor, R. C., Healy, J., Thomas, A. and Sergeant, J. (2000) Older patients and delayed discharge from hospital. *Health and Social Care in the Community* 8 (6): 443–52.

Wang, H.-X., Karp, A., Winblad, B. and Fratiglioni, L. (2002) Late-life engagement in social and leisure activities is associated with a decreased risk of dementia: a longitudinal study from the Kungsholmen Project. *American Journal of Epidemiology* 155 (12): 1081–7.

Waters, K., Allsopp, D., Davidson, I. and Dennis, A. (2001) A sources of support for older people after discharge from hospital: 10 years on. *Journal of Advanced Nursing* 33 (5): 575–82.

Wenger, G. C. (1992) *Help in Old Age: Facing up to Change: a Longitudinal Network Study*. Liverpool: Liverpool University Press.

Wilcock, A. A. (1998a). *An Occupational Perspective of Health*. Thorofare, NJ: Slack.

Wilcock, A. A. (1998b). Occupations for health. *British Journal of Occupational Therapy* 61 (8): 340–5.

Wilcock, A. A (2002) *Occupation for Health, Volume 2: a Journey From Prescription to Self Health*. London: COT.

WHOQOL Group (1995) The World Health Organisation Quality of Life Assessment (WHOQOL): position paper from the World Health Organisation. *Social Science and Medicine* 41: 1403–9.

World Health Organisation (1983) *Objectives of Health Promotion in the Elderly*. European Regional Planning Group. Copenhagen: WHO.

World Health Organisation (1986) *Ottawa Charter for Health Promotion*. Geneva: WHO.

World Health Organisation (2002) *Active Ageing: a Policy Framework*. Geneva: WHO.

CHAPTER 10

Health Promotion in Eating Disorders: the Contribution of Occupational Therapists

PRISCILLA HARRIES

Occupational therapists are one of the professional groups that share a role in researching and promoting the health of individuals with eating disorders (National Institute for Clinical Excellence [NICE], 2003). Occupational therapists view the interaction between the person, their occupations and their environment as being essential to health (Godfrey, 2000). As Wilcock discusses in the overview chapter to this part of this book, occupational engagement can be used as an agent to promote physical, mental and social health and wellbeing. Essential to the focus of that engagement is the individual's choice of occupation. To have health benefits, it must have value and meaning to the individual and provide an appropriate level of challenge (Zemke and Clarke, 1996).

Eating disorders have severe effects on the lives of many individuals and their families. Anorexia nervosa has one of the highest mortality rates of any psychiatric disorder, whilst bulimia nervosa can lower quality of life and cause severe gastrointestinal damage. Eating disorders not otherwise specified (EDNOS) affect up to a third of adolescents in the United Kingdom (UK) (Pratt and Woolfenden, 2003). It is therefore appropriate that the eating disorders field has been identified as an important target for research into risk factors and prevention (Eating Disorders Association, 2002; Key and Lacey, 2002). This chapter will critically assess the occupational therapists' health promotion strategies for clients with anorexia nervosa and bulimia nervosa, focussing on the occupational therapy contribution to secondary and tertiary health promoting strategies and the potential for delivering primary prevention programmes. Interventions relating to the prevention of obesity will not be covered (please see the recent Cochrane Review on this topic, Campbell et al., 2002).

Engaging mental health service users

Since the 1970s mental health services have become more community based. In line with this, many inpatient programmes for anorectic individuals have moved away from the inpatient setting (NICE, 2003). In order to maximise effectiveness, mental health services have aimed to enable individuals to be more involved with managing and improving their own health. For occupational therapists, the move to the community environment has been a positive one, enabling participation in a greater choice of occupations. Occupational therapists view occupation not only as paid employment but also as activities such as socialising, sports, eating, dressing, childcare and money management. Eating disorders can affect functioning in all of these types of occupations. Occupational deprivation and poor occupational balance can then commonly result, which can create additional stress for individuals, thereby reducing their health still further. Occupational therapists aim to enable individuals to use both their occupational capacity and their environment to promote their health and their quality of life.

Promoting access for mental health service users

As identified in Chapter 1, primary health promotion activities have accelerated since the publication of the Ottawa Charter (World Health Organisation (WHO), 1986). Mental health promotion has also been highlighted as the first requirement of the UK National Health Service (NHS) National Service Framework for Mental Health (Department of Health (DoH), 1999). In the UK extensive mental health resources are available for people with eating disorders, but they mainly relate to secondary and tertiary health promotion. Whilst health promotion aims to enable individuals to increase control over and improve their health (WHO, 1986: iii) individuals with eating disorders are commonly resistant to this strategy. Fear of putting on weight can cause individuals to avoid health services, thereby leaving themselves at great psychological and physical risk. Because of this, health professionals including occupational therapists in the eating disorders field have considered ways of engaging these individuals in promoting their own health. One innovative approach has been the development of motivational interviewing (Treasure and Ward, 1997). This is an approach that encourages individuals' capacity for change and is used by occupational therapists to guide therapeutic communications (Orchard, 2003). The approach complements the occupational therapy philosophy, with issues of volition and motivation traditionally recognised by occupational therapists as being central to individuals' potential to change (Kielhofner, 1995). The client centred perspective, which strongly focusses on the individual's needs and motivations, has been internationally recommended in occupational therapy practice (Canadian Association of Occupational Therapists, 1997). Sumsion, in Chapter 8 of this book, examines in detail how occupational therapists support this empowering and enabling model of promoting health. Therapy goals, identified and valued by the individual, are central to client centred practice.

There is one caveat to this practice. In the case of severe anorexia nervosa, decisions have to be made for the client. In the UK, for example, the Mental Health Act (DoH, 1983) is sometimes used if an individual's life is in danger, so that clients at very low weights can be forcibly detained in hospital (Orchard, 2003). Although this action appears to contradict the empowering model, psychological therapy and supported eating programmes are sometimes needed to help individuals return to a level of health that enables them to make their own rationale decisions once again.

Risk and maintenance factors for eating disorders

Essential to any eating disorders health promotion programme is the need to address the stressors that can lead to and maintain anorexia nervosa and bulimia nervosa. Individuals who are at high risk of developing eating disorders have been found to be associated with a higher prevalence of unhealthy weight regulation practices (Killen, 1996, cited in Pratt and Woolfenden, 2003). Focussing interventions only on dietary intake has not been found to be beneficial (Hay et al., 2003). Individuals at high risk are also associated with a higher prevalence of depressive symptoms (Killen, 1996, cited in Pratt and Woolfenden, 2003). There appears to be some evidence that this is the key issue that requires attention. For some clients, depressive symptoms can be a result of low weight; however for anorectic individuals, even when weight levels are restored, poor self-esteem and negative self-image tend to persist (Garner and Garfinkel, 1985). Stice (2002) identified negative affect as a maintenance factor for binge eating. He also identified that perfectionism was a maintenance factor for bulimic pathology. Psychological therapies can address negative self-evaluation and perfectionism, common traits for those with bulimia and anorexia nervosa. Occupational therapists are one of the professions that have been identified as providers of psychological therapies for individuals with eating disorders (NICE, 2003).

Occupational therapists' use of psychological therapies

Bruch (1973) was the first to advocate psychological therapies for eating disorder. She identified that individuals had to find alternative methods of self-expression. As the traditional psychodynamic therapies were costly and lengthy, time limited therapies were developed. A range of health professionals, including occupational therapists, may provide these. The current psychological therapies available to individuals with eating disorders include focal analytic theory (FPT), interpersonal psychotherapy (IPT), cognitive behaviour therapy (CBT), cognitive therapy (CT), motivational enhancement therapies (MET) and cognitive analytical therapy (CAT) (see Hay et al., 2003 for a detailed discussion of these therapies). The most recent Cochrane Review, which evaluated the evidence from randomised controlled trials on several of these key types of therapy, concluded that one particular approach could not yet be recommended (Hay et al., 2003).

The purpose of psychological therapies is to encourage individuals to think and act differently. Occupational therapists also support these approaches through group and individual therapy (Henderson, 1999; Lock, 2000). Cognitive behaviour principles, for example, are used in assertiveness training, stress management and relaxation training. Psychoanalytic principles are used in projective art and drama therapy groups. However for occupational therapists, the benefits of therapy are viewed in terms of the impact they have on an individual's capacity to participate in occupations. It is important therefore to understand how these therapies link to occupational engagement.

Assertiveness training can be used to facilitate a sense of autonomy and self-worth, reduce feelings of guilt and develop coping strategies. Individuals with eating disorders often feel helpless, and ineffective. Assertiveness training can empower individuals to take a more autonomous perspective and can facilitate healthy self-expression. Stress management can equip the individual with physical, cognitive and behavioural methods of coping with stress. Yoga and relaxation can also be used in early sessions, when minimal energy expenditure is required. The practice of positive self-talk can be invaluable for individuals with eating disorders as feelings of inadequacy and self-disparagement are commonly experienced (Casper et al., cited in Garner and Garfinkel, 1985). Sessions that focus on the identification and restructuring of negative thoughts, beliefs and attitudes can be valuable for challenging low self-esteem. Following stress management groups, individuals have reported their increased awareness of their own particular stressors and that they feel more equipped to cope with some of those stressors (Harries, 1992). These group or individual therapies can enable the individual to develop strategies to eliminate the causes of stressors (proactive prevention), as well as improving coping mechanisms to resist stressors (reactive prevention) (Austin, 2000). Essential to the field of eating disorders is the development of the individual's capacity for improved self-esteem and self-expression. As these capacities develop, previous coping mechanisms, and such methods as starvation and purging, can be gradually reduced in favour of healthy coping mechanisms (Harries, 1992).

Occupational therapists use the creative media such as art and drama to improve self-identity and develop effective communication skills. Drama therapy can be empowering for an individual's verbal and non-verbal expression (Creek, 1990). The use of movement can facilitate sensory perception and physical awareness, which are particularly valuable in promoting body image. Issues of control can be explored through trust exercises. The exploratory nature of drama can be used to assist individuals to develop self-awareness. This is valuable as self-awareness is usually overdependent on external measures for self-esteem, such as appearance. Art can be used to facilitate healthy expression of emotions. When severely affected by anorexia nervosa individuals can be very withdrawn and unable to verbalise their feelings. Their body can become the sole focus of their feelings. The art appears to be less threatening as a starting point as it is a pictorial medium rather than a verbal one. As the individual begins to create they are beginning a dialogue with themselves, they can feel in control but they are allowing some of their feelings to be shared. For example one individual, who remained silent during psychotherapy, felt safe to express herself through the projective art (Harries, 1992). Projective art proved to be a catalyst to being able to verbally express feelings.

When art is used in this therapeutic capacity, the aesthetic value of the art is not important, and the individual is actively discouraged from this expectation. The time engaged in the art is valued more highly than the subsequent dialogue that can be developed from it. However the experience of verbalising feelings and the therapeutic support that can be provided by the therapist can lead to greater self-insight and self-knowledge. The painting is unique to the individual. This is an important factor in developing the individual's autonomy. Some therapists choose to direct the topic for the art. Others prefer to allow the individual to chose the focus and not necessarily even verbalise what that may be. In Harries (1992) the examples of individuals' art demonstrate how expression, mood, control and insight are developed, key issues that are needed to promote health in individuals with anorexia. Individuals with bulimia nervosa can have very different needs. Expression can be vented through anger and risk taking and can also be impulsive. Paint can spread off the paper and onto the table and others' artwork may be damaged in the process. This can be seen in contrast to the art of individuals with anorexia nervosa, which is often characterised by neat, small careful drawings. Both art and drama can be used therapeutically to allow each individual to develop greater self-awareness and self-expression.

Proactive and reactive health promoting strategies are also used to enable individuals to engage in occupations. Individuals begin using the coping strategies that have been learnt in therapy. They begin to use these in daily life through gradual engagement in self-care, work and leisure occupations. Through the return to valued occupational engagement, occupational balance and quality of life is promoted. Occupational therapists view health not only as the remediation of the signs and symptoms of illness but also as the restored capacity to engage in a meaningful and satisfying life.

Home management, leisure and work

Previous research (Harries, 1992) has identified home management areas that are stressful for clients with eating disorders, including money management, menu planning, shopping, cooking, eating. Often lifestyles have been adopted where social eating has been avoided. Individuals with anorexia nervosa, for example, sometimes choose shift work where there is less regularity in meal times and therefore less peer awareness of eating habits.

It commonly appears that money has been stringently saved or overspent depending on whether the individual has anorexia nervosa or bulimia nervosa respectively. Budgeting and menu planning for healthy eating have not necessarily been learnt as the individual is most likely to have begun to limit their eating during childhood when a parent may have been preparing food for them. As normal eating is established a higher than expected calorie intake may be needed to maintain a stable weight (Weltzin et al., 1991).

Shopping for clothes can be a high anxiety provoking experience (Martin, 1998). Acceptance of a healthier body shape is challenged as clothes' size alters. Although coping mechanisms have been developed it is the transfer of the use of these coping mechanisms into the individual's lifestyle that is key to enabling health.

Leisure has often become an isolated activity, usually focussed on exercise. The recent media trend toward not only valuing thinness but also physical fitness may have contributed to this (Martin, 1998). Physical exercise is commonly used to lose weight. Exercise addiction is very common and in some studies has been shown to be present in a third of the sample (Kron et al., 1978). The individual who came to see the occupational therapist in Kent, having run from Essex, portrays an extreme example of this. This level of exercise can add severe physiological risks for individuals whose diet is not stable. Advice such as not arriving at the swimming pool until half and hour before it closes can prevent the individual from continuing to exercise for an excessive period (Harries, 1992). Of course, some exercise is important for health but careful thought needs to be given to methods of reducing the risks of overexercising.

It can be valuable to encourage engagement with group sports as this has the benefit of increasing socialisation opportunities as well as encouraging physical exercise that is time limited. If the individual values exercise, a sports group can be identified that would be of interest.

As health is restored one aspect of life that may need reconsideration is the type of paid employment the individual may want to engage in. Identifying work environments that do not cause too much stress to the individual are an important part of preventing relapse. Commonly perfectionism and over-achievement can drive individuals into taking work that is too challenging. This can lead to stress and anxiety and reinforce the feelings of lack of self-worth. If they have previously had difficulty with autonomous decisions they may have chosen a career that others approved of rather than one that they valued themselves. They may also have been drawn to a career that valued physical appearance. They may also have found it satisfying working in catering where they were more aware of their ability to abstain from eating. Occupational therapists are astutely aware of facilitating individuals to find the appropriate challenge, aiming to utilise the individual's optimal level of skill and match it to the optimal level of challenge. In order for individuals to select an appropriate career, occupational therapists can facilitate increased awareness of stressors relating to different types of occupation. Preparation for interview situations can be rehearsed or discussed, giving particular emphasis to the ability to portray a positive self-image, which is a difficult task for individuals who have low self-esteem. The health benefits that can be gained from working in a fulfilling job can sometimes be the sole reason that an individual does not feel the need to return to their former lifestyle. If the mind and body are engaged in meaningful occupation, there is less risk that unhealthy habits and roles will be resumed.

Although eating disorders in men are not common (Olivardia et al., 1995), there are some additional issues that should be considered. Excessive exercise has been found to be more common in men with eating disorders than women with eating disorders (Touyz et al., 1993). Occupational therapists would need to enable the return to healthy levels of exercise and help the individual to identify when they may be at risk of overexercising. It has also been identified that homosexual men or those who are struggling to accept their sexuality can be at risk of eating disorders (Burns and Crisp, 1984). The homosexual community places value on male physical attractiveness, more so than the heterosexual community. A history of childhood sexual abuse is also common in men with anorexia nervosa (Olivardia et al., 1995). Men with eating disorders are also more likely to have an additional mental health problem such as substance misuse, so care must be taken to avoid the adoption of one coping strategy to deal with their eating disorders that might negatively impact on other problems.

Health promotion targeting primary prevention of eating disorders

Intervention programmes aimed at preventing eating disorders in children and adolescents have used a variety of approaches (Pratt and Woolfenden, 2003). These mainly represent primary prevention strategies for school age children. As occupational therapists prepare to support primary health promotion programmes, consideration needs to be given to the nature of effective health promotion programmes in this field. Some of the programmes reviewed by the Cochrane group (Pratt and Woolfenden, 2003) have opted for using media images as a stimulus for discussion on societal attitudes about body size (Neumark-Sztainer et al., 2000). Other programmes have used class discussions in schools on eating disorders, eating behaviours and coping with the demands of growing up (Buddeberg-Fischer et al., 1998). The first of these approaches, the media literacy method, was found to show a statistically significant effect, with the follow up at sixth months identifying less internalisation or acceptance of societal ideals relating to appearance (Pratt and Woolfenden, 2003: 10). This

complements the findings of Stice's (2002) meta-analysis on risk and maintenance factors that identified thin internalisation and body dissatisfaction as key
risk factors for developing eating pathology.

A third type of programme focussed on self-esteem, communication and
stress management skills rather than directly on eating (O'Dea and Abraham,
2000). It could not be included in the Cochrane meta analysis as it was the
only one of its kind. In O'Dea's study, 470 school children participated. It
provided the *Everybody's Different* programme to an intervention group and
the normal personal development and health class to a control group. Body
satisfaction and self-esteem were found to have significantly improved in the
intervention group. It appears that programmes that promote individuality
and awareness of media pressure to fit the thin image can be valuable in eating
disorders prevention. Self-esteem has since been recognised as a key protective
factor against developing eating pathology (Stice, 2002).

In the UK, where thinness is valued, this approach may therefore be
effective. It may be that other approaches may be more valuable in cultures
where thinness is less important such as the black or Arab cultures (Littlewood,
1995). Indeed those screening for anorexia nervosa, particularly in non-white
women, should be aware that the fear of fatness may not be present in these
cultures and that screening tools such as the Eating Attitudes Test may not be
appropriate for the detection of eating problems (Nasser, 1986).

Looking to the future

Building self-image, self-worth, communication skills, stress management
skills and media awareness have been shown to be important when attempting
to reduce the risks of developing or maintaining eating disorders (Harries,
1992; Pratt and Woolfenden, 2003). In the UK, where thinness is often
equated with attractiveness (Martin, 1998), societal attitudes need to shift to
reduce pressures on young people to diet. Media images need to be challenged
through media advocacy programmes and occupational therapists should join
the media advocacy movement to help facilitate these changes.

Young people can easily be led to believe that success in life is related to
body size (Martin, 1998). If the various media persistently portray this image
there is a continued risk of eating disorders. Young people need to be assisted
to value themselves for their personality rather than for their physical attractiveness. Occupational therapists can educate young people to find the level of
life challenge that is rewarding to them but not anxiety provoking. Matching
skill level to task challenge is vital to maintain effective health thereby reducing
risk of depression and psychological distress (Csikszentmihalyi, 1992).

It is also important to note that eating disorders are not solely caused by
societal pressure to be thin as historically they precede this fashion (Lasegue,
1873). As risk factors are wide ranging and include personality traits and
familial predisposition, both the individual's social environment and their

occupational performance skills require consideration. Fairburn et al.'s studies (1997, 1999) have identified that perfectionism traits and overdependence on external approval can lead to eating disorders. Including families in the health promotion process may be valuable in assisting healthy family relationships.

Occupational therapists must continue to develop their secondary and tertiary health promotion services in relation to eating disorders. To assist in the primary prevention strategies meaningful occupational engagement can be utilised as a tool for promoting health. Individuals' self-worth can be fostered through occupational challenges that are well matched to individuals' occupational capacity. Effective occupational engagement can be used to promote autonomy and self-efficacy, thereby helping to reduce some of the risk factors that can lead to the development eating disorders.

References

Austin, S. B. (2000) Prevention research in eating disorders: theory and new directions. *Psychological Medicine* **20**: 1249–62.

Bruch, H. (1973) *Eating Disorders: Obesity, Anorexia Nervosa and the Person Within.* New York: Basic Books.

Buddeberg-Fischer, B., Klaghofer, R., Gnan, G. and Buddeberg, C. (1998) Prevention of disturbed eating behaviour: a prospective intervention study in 14 to 19 year old Swiss students. *Acta Psychiatrica Scandinavica* **98**: 148–55.

Burns, T. and Crisp, A. (1984) Outcome of anorexia nervosa in males. *British Journal of Psychiatry* **145**: 319–25.

Campbell, K., Waters, E., O'Meara, S. and Summerbell, C. (2002) Interventions for preventing obesity in children. Cochrane Review. In *The Cochrane Library 1.* Oxford: Update Software.

Canadian Association of Occupational Therapists (1997) *Enabling Occupation: an Occupational Therapy Perspective.* Ottawa: CAOT Publications.

Casper, R. C., Eckert, E. D., Halmi, K. A., Goldberg, S. C. and Davis, J. M. (1980) Bulimia: its incidence and clinical importance in patients with anorexia nervosa. *Archives of General Psychiatry* **37**: 1030–5.

Creek, J. (1990) *Occupational Therapy and Mental Health.* Edinburgh: Churchill Livingstone.

Csikszentmihalyi, M. (1992) *Flow: the Psychology of Happiness.* London: Rider.

Department of Health (1983) *The Mental Health Act.* London: HMSO.

Department of Health (1999) *National Service Framework for Mental Health.* London: DoH.

Eating Disorders Association (2002) *'It's not about Food It's About Feelings': an Education Resource about Eating Disorders and Related Issues for Teachers and those Working with Young People.* Norwich: Eating Disorders Association.

Fairburn, C. G., Cooper, Z., Doll, H. A. and Welch, S. L. (1999) Risk factors for anorexia nervosa: three integrated case-control comparisons. *Archives of General Psychiatry* **56** (5): 468–76.

Fairburn, C. G., Welch, S. L., Doll, H. A., Davies, B. A. and O'Connor, M. E. (1997) Risk factors for bulimia nervosa: a community based case control study. *Archives of General Psychiatry* **54** (6): 509–17.

136 *Health Promoting Practice*

Garner, D. M. and Garfinkel, P. E. (1985) *Handbook of Psychotherapy for Anorexia Nervosa and Bulimia.* New York: Guildford.

Godfrey, A. (2000) Policy changes in the National Health Service: implications and opportunities for occupational therapists. *British Journal of Occupational Therapy* 63 (5): 218–24.

Harries, P. (1992) Facilitating change in anorexia nervosa: the role of occupational therapy. *British Journal of Occupational Therapy* 55 (9): 334–9.

Hay, P., Bacaltchuk, J., Claudino, A., Ben-Tovin, D. and Yong, P. Y. (2003) Individual psychotherapy in the outpatient treatment of adults with anorexia nervosa. Cochrane Review. in *The Cochrane Library 4.* Chichester: Wiley.

Henderson, S. (1999) Frames of reference utilised in the rehabilitation of individuals with eating disorders. *Canadian Journal of Occupational Therapy* 66 (1): 43–51.

Key, A. and Lacey, H. (2002) Progress in eating disorder research. *Current Opinion in Psychiatry* 15 (2): 143–8.

Kielhofner, G. (1995) *A Model of Human Occupation: Theory and Application.* Baltimore, MD: Williams & Wilkins.

Killen, J. D. (1996) Development and evaluation of a school-based eating disorder symptoms prevention program. In Smolak, L., Levine, M. P. and Striegel-Moore, R. (eds) *The Developmental Psychopathology of Eating Disorders: Implications for Research, Prevention and Treatment.* Mahwah, NJ: Lawrence Erlbaum & Associates.

Kron, L., Katz, J., Gorzynski, G. and Wuner, H. (1978) Hyperactivity in anorexia nervosa: a fundamental clinical feature. *Comprehensive Psychiatry* 19: 433–40.

Lasegue, E. (1873) Translated from 'De l'Anorexia Hystérique'. *Archives of General Medicine* 21: 338.

Littlewood, R. (1995) Psychopathology and personal agency: modernity, culture change and eating disorders in South Asian societies. *British Journal of Medical Psychology* 68: 45–63.

Lock, L. C. (2000) Reoccupying the preoccupied: occupational therapy for sufferers of eating disorders. In Hindharsh, T. (ed.) *Eating Disorders: a Multiprofessional Approach.* London: Whurr.

Martin, J. E. (1998) *Eating Disorders, Food and Occupational Therapy.* London: Whurr.

Nasser, M. (1996) Comparative study of the prevalence of abnormal eating attitudes among Arab female students of both London and Cairo universities. *Psychological Medicine* 16: 621–5.

National Institute for Clinical Excellence (2003) *Eating Disorders: Core Interventions in the Treatment and Management of Anorexia Nervosa, Bulimia Nervosa, and Related Eating Disorders.* NICE Guideline, second draft for consultation. London: NICE.

Neumark-Sztainer, D., Sherwood, N., Coller, T. and Hannan, P. (2000) Primary prevention of disordered eating among preadolescent schoolgirls: feasibility and short-term effect of a community-based intervention. *Journal of the American Dietetic Association* 100 (12): 1466–73.

O'Dea, J. A. and Abraham, S. (2000) Improving body image, eating attitudes and behavior of young male and female adolescents: a new educational approach which focuses on self-esteem. *International Journal of Eating Disorders* 28: 43–57.

Olivardia, R., Pope, H., Mangweth, B. and Hudson, J. (1995) Eating disorders in college men. *American Journal of Psychiatry* 152: 1279–85.

Orchard, R. (2003) With you, not against you: applying motivational interviewing to occupational therapy in anorexia nervosa. *British Journal of Occupational Therapy* 66 (7): 325–7.

Pratt, B. M. and Woolfenden, S. R. (2003) Interventions for preventing eating disorders in children and adolescents. Cochrane Review. In *The Cochrane Library 4.* Chichester: Wiley.

Stice, E (2002) Risk and maintenance factors for eating pathology; a meta-analytic review. *Psychological Bulletin* 5: 825–48.

Touyz, S., Kopec-Schrader, E. and Beumont, P. (1993) Anorexia in males: a report of 12 cases. *Australian and New Zealand Journal of Psychiatry* 27: 512–17.

Treasure, J. and Ward, A. (1997) A practical guide to the use of motivational interviewing in anorexia nervosa. *European Eating Disorders Review* 5 (2): 391–420.

Weltzin, T., Fernstrom, M., Hansen, D. and McConaha, C. (1991) Abnormal calorific requirements for weight maintenance in patients with anorexia and bulimia nervosa. *American Journal of Psychiatry* 148: 1675–82.

World Health Organisation (1986) *Ottawa Charter for Health Promotion.* Geneva: WHO.

Zemke, R. and Clarke, F. (1996) *Occupational Science: the Evolving Discipline.* Philadelphia, PA: F. A. Davis.

CHAPTER 11

Occupational Therapists and the Promotion of Psychological Health in Rheumatoid Arthritis

Jo Adams and Sally Pearce

Traditional approaches to the definition and treatment of rheumatoid arthritis (RA) emphasise the physical and biomedical elements of the disease. In the past psychosocial factors associated with the disease have tended to be marginalised, yet commentators argue that psychosocial factors contribute almost to the same extent as biomedical factors to the impact of disability experienced by individuals with RA (Escalante and del Rincón, 2002; Yelin and Katz, 2002). It is also widely acknowledged that assessment and care of psychological aspects associated with chronic disease are less often addressed than physical symptoms by occupational therapist and other healthcare staff, regardless of healthcare need (Shipley and Newman, 1993; Parker and Wright, 1995; Newbold, 1996).

This chapter will highlight the importance of psychosocial factors in mediating the amount of disability experienced by individuals with RA. Self-efficacy, helplessness, coping skills, depression, social support and the social environment will be discussed in terms of their position as important mediators in individual ability and social participation in RA (Escalante and del Rincón, 1999). The strategies that occupational therapists may utilise to address these are also explored.

Rheumatoid arthritis is a systemic, inflammatory autoimmune disease with an unpredictable course, no known cure and a potentially lifelong duration. Referred to as the commonest potentially treatable cause of disability in many countries (Emery and Salmon, 1995), rheumatoid disease has been shown to have significant physical, social, economic and psychological consequences (Pincus, 1995). The disease can lead to structural impairment (Uhlig et al., 2000), functional disability and restriction in social participation (Mottonen et al., 1998; Kroot et al., 2000; Young et al., 2000).

The exact cause of RA is still unknown. There is, as yet, no evidence to suggest that there are any environmental risk factors associated with the disease. There is also no evidence of any associated socio demographic, occupational or psychological factors in the disease aetiology, although obesity, smoking and recent experience of an emotionally traumatic event may be related to the disease onset (Symmons and Harrison, 2000). The onset of RA most frequently affects people aged 30–50 (Arthritis Research Campaign, 2000). Since its highest point in 1960, there is now a general decline in both the prevalence and incidence of worldwide RA except in some African countries where the rates are rising (Calvo and Alarcón, 2000). It is suggested that 500–600 per 100,000 of the adult population in the United Kingdom (UK) are affected (Silman and Hochberg, 1994) where it is estimated that RA is prevalent in 1.16 per cent of women and 0.44 per cent of men (Symmons et al., 2002).

Most definitions of the disease will concentrate on the physical manifestations of joint structural impairment, pain, localised inflammation, reduction of mobility, deformity and fatigue (see Chapter 16 of this text for further discussion of the symptoms of RA). Despite RA being a chronic painful disease with possible long term reduction in social participation and social roles (Young et al., 2000), there is little acknowledgement of the possible accompanying psychological sequelae in disease definition. However, the psychological status of the individual with RA has been seen as central to mediating the amount of disability individuals can experience (Parker and Wright, 1997; Escalante and del Rincón, 1999). Psychological factors influence the relationship between disease activity and disability in RA and social and psychological factors have been seen to be powerful modulators of disability outcomes (Parker and Wright, 1995). The severity of disease activity does not necessarily predict the level of functional limitations (Scott, 2000) and as medical intervention has been seen to be only partially effective more recently attention has been given to implementing psychosocial strategies for improving health status.

Escalante and del Rincón (2002) provide a clear diagrammatic pathway for understanding the influence of contextual and psychosocial modifiers on the disease disability pathway which serves as a useful model for health professionals developing health promotion practice in RA.

Rheumatoid arthritis and psychological wellbeing

A comment by an anonymous patient, that arthritis may not kill you but it sure as hell makes you wish you were dead (Pigg et al., 1985) encapsulates the impact of RA on psychological wellbeing and quality of life.

RA is a chronic and unpredictable disease with a diagnosis that is potentially lifelong. Following a course of painful relapses and remissions with an evasive prognosis, individuals with rheumatoid arthritis will inevitably respond emotionally to each new progression of their disease. The result is lifelong uncertainty about disease episodes (Hodes and Charles, 1992: 53) and as Persson

PATHOLOGY ➝ IMPAIRMENT ➝ FUNCTIONAL ➝ DISABILITY
                                              LIMITATION

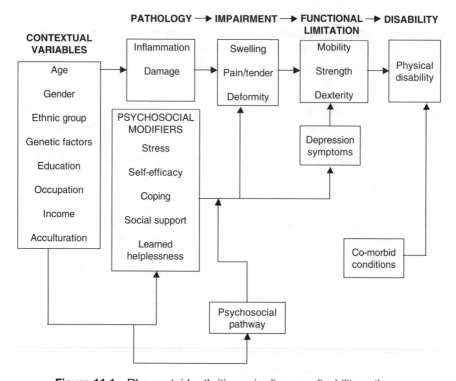

Figure 11.1   Rheumatoid arthritis: main disease–disability pathway

Source: Escalante and del Rincón (2002): 337. Reprinted by permission of Wiley-Liss Inc.,
a subsidiary of John Wiley & Sons, Inc.

et al. (1999: 137) point out there are few other groups of diseases that cause so much pain and disability for so many people over such extended periods of time.

Parker and Wright (1995) report that psychological wellbeing bears a significant relationship to both disability and perceived quality of life for individuals with rheumatoid arthritis, both measures being adversely affected by low mood and low self-esteem. The complex interaction between physical disabilities and perceived quality of life are discussed fully by Diener et al. (1997) and are not dealt with in detail in this chapter. However, feelings of helplessness reported in an RA population have also been seen to significantly affect competency in carrying out daily functional tasks (Serbo and Jajic, 1991). Ryan (1997) also found individuals with rheumatoid arthritis and depressive symptoms performed 12 per cent less daily activity than those patients who did not have any depressive symptoms and she argues that physical symptoms of RA can be limited by preserving psychological wellbeing.

The individual's subjective health beliefs are important in relation to the promotion of health with RA patients (Rotter, 1966). People's belief about whether they can contribute towards the control of their symptoms, their style of coping and their predisposition towards cheerful or depressive moods should all be acknowledged as contributing towards the individual's ability to manage their arthritis (Persson et al., 1999). There are a wide range of significant factors beyond the physical pathology of the disease that are associated with the increased likelihood of individuals with rheumatoid arthritis experiencing depressive symptoms, these include:

- dissatisfaction with personal ability to carry out socially valued roles (Katz and Neugebauer, 2001)
- loss of valued activities (Katz and Yelin, 1995)
- lack of knowledge of coping strategies (Savelkoul et al., 2001), maladaptive coping strategies such as passive coping (Covic et al., 2000) and fantasising and catastrophising (Keefe et al., 1989)
- reduction in social relationships and associated increase in social isolation (Newman, 1996; Ryan, 1997; Zautra et al., 1998)
- poor relationship with, and/or understanding of the disease by the partner (Kraaimaat et al., 1995; Riemsma et al., 2000)
- learned illness avoidant behaviour (Elfant et al., 1999)
- presence of deformity and the alteration of body image and reduced self-esteem (Dumas, 1992)
- belonging to a low socioeconomic class, where integral life experience and possible deprivation may predispose the individual to depression (Hawley and Wolfe, 1988)
- ongoing pain (Young, 1992; Parker and Wright, 1995; Newman, 1996; O'Hara, 1996)
- more severe functional impairment and disability (Young, 1992; Newman, 1996)
- presence of fatigue (Neville et al., 1999).

Newbold (1996) also identified that the greatest emotional disturbance is considered to take place in the initial stages of the disease when a diagnosis is confirmed. In particular the immediate stressors were stated as being:

- informing family of the diagnosis
- management of medication and treatment
- modifying work and social life
- uncertainty about the future.

It is widely acknowledged that assessment and care of psychological symptoms are less often addressed than physical symptoms by occupational therapist and other healthcare staff (Shipley and Newman, 1993; Parker and Wright, 1995; Newbold, 1996). Patients diagnosed with physical disease receive appropriate intervention for the physical component of their disease whilst accompanying psychological and social problems often go unaddressed (Shipley and Newman, 1993; Parker and Wright, 1995; Newbold, 1996). This should be of concern for occupational therapists because there is an increasing body of evidence identifying the differences in psychological status, such as anxiety, negative mood, poor coping strategies and feelings of loss of control or helplessness for the rheumatoid population from that in a healthy population (McEvoy DeVellis, 1995; Persson et al., 1999). Some commentators go as far as suggesting that the psychological burden of dealing with the unpredictable nature of the disease can outweigh the physical burden imposed by it (Neville et al., 1999). There remains controversy, however, about the prevalence of low mood, anxiety and depression in the rheumatoid population (Persson et al., 1999). Various studies estimate that as many as 46 per cent of individuals with RA have depressive symptoms (Frank et al., 1988; Young, 1992; Maisaik et al., 1996; Marks and Wilkins, 1997) compared with 15 per cent of the general population (Ormel and Tiemens, 1997).

It is unsurprising that stress is likely to increase the physical symptoms of the disease (Gio-Fitman, 1996). Reaction to a possible stressful event is individual but an individual's perception can be altered and the effects of stress can be partly influenced. Developing an understanding of disease or disability will also affect illness perceptions, and the extent to which individuals feel that they can influence the course of their illness. Illness perceptions are particularly potent as they have the ability to influence behaviour and coping ability (Smith et al., 1990; Pimm, 1997). Occupational therapists should acknowledge the impact of illness perception and provide assistance to individuals in developing a realistic understanding of their illness, as people who do not receive such assistance are more likely to go on to develop more depressive symptoms and less effective coping strategies than those who do (Katz and Yelin, 1993). Such impact of occupational therapists and other healthcare professionals on psychological, social and physical wellbeing in RA in influencing negative or unrealistic perceptions of the impact of illness has also been seen to be long term (Ryan, 1997).

Promoting psychological health in RA

In attempting to define health promoting strategies to assist in addressing functional ability and wellbeing in a chronic illness such as RA, Haworth (2000) clearly lists the components of any intervention that might be offered by occupational therapists. These include encouraging adaptive coping strategies and sound beliefs of self-efficacy; ensuring that there are appropriate levels of social support available and providing educational programmes on self-management skills. There are further strategies that have been proven to be effective in promoting psychological health in individuals and a discussion of these follows.

Open relationships

There are new developments in the way that individuals with chronic diseases are approached and assisted; fortunately rheumatology teams and the occupational therapists who work with them have already been proactive in seeking non-medical ways to enhance patient care. *The Expert Patient* (Department of Health (DoH), 2001) leads the way in acknowledging that individuals can make a considerable impact on the long term management of their own disease and improve their own quality of life and pain relief. This general approach of patient participation, open disclosure, improving the patient's confidence and understanding in their arthritis and building a sound patient and clinician relationship based on partnership has already clearly produced improved concordance to occupational therapeutic advice (Jensen and Lorish, 1994).

It is also timely for occupational therapists to re-evaluate the personal impact of the disease for the individual. Various studies have shown that both health professionals, including occupational therapists, and family members are not accurate at anticipating or interpreting the amount of personal impact disability has on the individual with RA (Riemsma et al., 2000; Katz and Neugebauer, 2001; Hewlett et al., 2001, 2002). New scales of measuring the personal impact of disability are being developed (Hewlett et al., 2002) and these should be used alongside standardised factual disability scales that record what a person can or cannot do, to more accurately represent the individual's personal experience and assist in more clearly indicating intervention priorities for all team members to work towards.

Improving patient autonomy

Increasing patient confidence and autonomy in managing their own care embraces the recommendations set out in *The Expert Patient* (DoH, 2001) and such a general approach by occupational therapists will encompass health promotion activity. Patient initiated appointments have already been seen to be more effective than more traditional ways of dealing with outpatient appointments. Individuals given the responsibility of using a self-referral system, reported higher self-efficacy and greater satisfaction and confidence than those patients using a more traditional specialist initiated system that was more costly and less effective (Hewlett et al., 2000; Kirwan et al., 2003).

The training of individuals with RA to become patient educators also goes further in improving their own knowledge and understanding of the disease process and helps them to manage their own symptoms more effectively. The training programme has been seen to assist the individual volunteers increase self-efficacy scores and improve effective communication with their physicians (Hainsworth and Barlow, 2001). The impact of patient educators can be higher than that of traditional rheumatology self-management sessions provided by occupational therapists and other health professionals. Branch et al.'s (1999) work highlights the statistically significant impact that patient educators can have over and above traditional healthcare provision in improving patients' knowledge about resources and satisfaction with healthcare services.

Pain management has also been improved with increasing patient autonomy. Gifford's (1998) research summarises succinctly the improvement that chronic pain sufferers can experience when a biopsychological approach is adopted. The use of education strategies, improving patient autonomy in their care and reducing reliance on drug therapy, is better able to address the sensory, cognitive and affective components of pain than a traditional medical approach.

Strengthening self-efficacy belief

Social Learning Theory (Bandura, 1977) forms the basis of self-efficacy work. It refers to strengthening the individual's belief that they can effect a change in pain levels, functioning and behaviours to achieve a positive change in health status. The approach is a cognitive learning one and encourages the individual to perceive their situation from an optimal perspective, and to manage their arthritis and lessen the dependency on healthcare services (Marks, 2001). Perceived self-efficacy can be measured by such tools as the Arthritis Self-efficacy Scale (Lorig et al., 1989).

Levels of self-efficacy have been seen to be important in RA, being associated with chronic pain and predictive of level of pain and functional impairment (Strahl et al., 2000). A high level of self-efficacy is necessary if appropriate, desired behaviour change is to be achieved, for example carrying out exercises as requested or pacing oneself to manage fatigue effectively. Occupational therapists can improve levels of self-efficacy with positive outcomes for health status. A lack of belief in one's own ability to manage the physical manifestations of RA and assist in pain control can lead to a decline in confidence and function. Arnstein et al. (1999) demonstrated that the self-belief in being able to influence pain management acts as a mediator between pain intensity, disability and depression in RA. Cognitive management of the disease can, to some degree, mitigate the potential physiological effects of flareup in the disease. Encouraging the belief that an individual can have some impact on their disease management and progression can assist in raising self-efficacy levels and go some way to improving the initiation of successful coping strategies and sustaining positive behavioural change.

Developing self-management education programmes

Kate Lorig developed the first formal self-management programme in America in the 1980s (Lorig et al., 1985). The Arthritis Self-management Programme was seen to be effective in giving health benefits to people with arthritis whilst reducing healthcare costs and was used as the model for the UK equivalent, Challenging Arthritis. Developed with Arthritis Care, Challenging Arthritis has been seen to be clinically effective in improving health status in arthritis (DoH, 2001). The programmes are based on improving and actualising self-efficacy beliefs to improve self-management of symptoms.

Patient education is primarily given to individuals with chronic conditions and is not the same as health promotion programmes. It has long been acknowledged that patients want to know more about their disease, and believe that the more they understand the better they feel that they can cope with their symptoms and the long term implications of their diagnosis. Participatory self-management education programmes will encourage the individual to change behaviour as well as improve their cognitive understanding of the disease. Straightforward occupational therapy techniques such as appropriate activity analysis, breaking down tasks into manageable components, provision of verbal persuasion and teaching about the physiology of symptomatic presentation in RA can contribute towards effective health and self-management education programmes (Hewlett et al., 2001).

Self-management education programmes are likely to include the following three core elements:

- improving knowledge about anatomy and physiology of the disease, pain mechanisms, pharmacology and drug monitoring, joint protection techniques and community resources
- practising skills and behaviours for joint protection techniques, pain management, work modification and simplification, fatigue management, exercise programmes, altering diet and nutrition
- increasing awareness of psychological coping strategies; communicating with occupational therapists and health professionals, problem solving, goal setting, improving self-efficacy beliefs, dealing with anxiety and depression and maintaining family and social relationships (Lindroth, 2000).

Traditionally these programmes have been seen to be more effective in increasing knowledge than changing behaviour in the long term (Hammond, 1994, 1998, 1999; Hawley, 1995) and more recently cognitive behaviour programmes have been introduced in an attempt to encourage sustained active behavioural change and improve competency and self-efficacy beliefs (Ryan, 1997). However, it appears that the timing of such programmes will be crucial in their ability to effect such change. Providing such programmes within the first six months of diagnosis has not been seen to produce effective therapeutic change in status (Freeman et al., 2002). Nevertheless, the possible impact of such programmes in supporting the individual around the stressful time of diagnosis cannot be disputed and it seems that more work is required on the most effective way to introduce such cognitive behavioural approaches for this population.

Developing effective coping strategies

Coping is a multidimensional construct and cannot be neatly categorised into good or bad coping (Smith et al., 1997). However, Lazarous and

Folkman (1984) provide a clear description of coping as a psychological mechanism for managing stress that incorporates behaviour, feelings and thoughts. Coping mechanisms are a strategy for dealing with stressors in daily life and for an individual with RA the potential stressors highlighted earlier may serve to break down positive coping mechanisms. People's beliefs seem to affect coping strategies indirectly. Those individuals with an internal locus of control and positive health beliefs are able to use problem orientated strategies, whereas those who believe they can exert little influence on their situations tend to revert to emotional avoidant strategies. These avoidant strategies lead to poorer adjustment, lower self-esteem and an increase in depressive symptoms (Newbold, 1996) and are associated with a withdrawal from social contact and the potential for increased disability (Marks, 2001).

Active coping styles are highly relevant to an occupational therapy process as they include positive strategies that encourage the individual to take responsibility for their symptoms, continue to attempt to carry out daily tasks and use such strategies as distraction to manage pain and discomfort. Passive coping is an ineffective style involving withdrawal from functioning, engaging in wishful thinking and relying on others for symptomatic relief. For the healthcare professional it is important to identify what stressors their clients or patients perceive to be most important and their perception of control over these. Through education, individuals' potential stressors can become manageable and this in turn can increase a sense of personal control, promoting active coping strategies enabling the person to regain control. The work of Newbold (1996) suggests that occupational therapists should endorse such positive coping strategies, encouraging the individual to think about solutions for difficulties; practising relaxation to limit the impact of stress; assisting the individual to seek help and encouraging them to take part in direct action and to accept their condition.

Investing time to encourage active coping strategies with individuals seems to be an efficient and effective use of occupational therapists' time. Achieving active coping strategies has already been seen to be effective in significantly reducing pain, overall adjustment to the condition, levels of depression and functional impairment (Manne and Zautra, 1992; Strahl et al., 2000).

Social relationships

It has already been noted above that family members' perceptions of RA can differ and that some of the greatest emotional disturbance around the time of diagnosis involves the individual informing their family of their diagnosis (Newbold, 1996). In general individuals would like their families to understand more about the condition and therefore families should also be involved with education programmes that are offered to the person with RA.

Coping with chronic disease involves social relationships in a special sense. Like the chronically ill person, friends and family are confronted with a whole range of changes and are also expected to provide support for the individual in coping with the disease. Encouraging the support and understanding of the family can be crucial in controlling levels of stress and depression associated with the disease. It is accepted that exacerbation or deterioration of physical symptoms has already been linked to a negative or unbalanced response between the individual and their family, friends and carers (Kraimaat et al., 1995; Ryan, 1997; Neville et al., 1999 and Riemsma et al., 2000). Encouraging the support and understanding of the family can be crucial in controlling levels of stress and depression associated with the disease and the development of effective self-management strategies (Riemsma et al., 2000).

Finally the implications on work relationships should also not be forgotten. It is estimated that up to two thirds of individuals with the disease experience disruption to social relationships, leisure and work activities (Ryan, 1997). Individuals with RA are perceived at work to have poorer interpersonal job skills and lower job performance (McQuade, 2002) and the education programmes and information should ideally go further and involve employers and colleagues as well.

RA is a chronic disabling condition that can cause severe emotional and physical disability. The effects of RA are mediated by contextual, social and psychological factors and management of stressors produce important clinical benefits, both psychologically and physically. Occupational therapists can play an active and effective health promotion role in assisting the individual to understand and manage their condition more effectively. The emphasis on a psychosocial model of care is particularly timely in rheumatology when there is already sound evidence that strategies that employ health promotion principles to improve individual autonomy, responsibility and partnership are more health enhancing than relying on drugs alone.

References

Arnstein, P., Caudill, M., Mandle, C. L., Norris, A. and Beasley, R. (1999) Self-efficacy as a mediator of the relationship between pain intensity, disability and depression in chronic pain patients. *Pain* **80** (3): 483–91.

Arthritis Research Campaign (2000) *Rheumatoid Arthritis: a Handbook for Patients*. Chesterfield: Arthritis and Rheumatism Council.

Bandura, A. (1997) *Social Learning Theory*. Englewood Cliffs, NJ: Prentice-Hall.

Branch, V. K., Lipsky, K., Nieman, T. and Lipsky, P. E. (1999) Positive impact of an intervention by arthritis patient educators on knowledge and satisfaction of patients in a rheumatology practice. *Arthritis Care and Research* **12** (8): 370–5.

Calvo, F. and Alarcón, G. S. (2000) Epidemiology of rheumatoid arthritis. In Firestein, G. S., Panyani, G. S. and Wollheim F. A. (eds) *Rheumatoid Arthritis: New Frontiers in Pathogenesis and Treatment*. Oxford: Oxford University Press.

Covic, T., Adamson, B. and Hough, M. (2000) The impact of passive coping on rheumatoid arthritis. *Rheumatology* **39**: 1027–30.

Department of Health (2001) *The Expert Patient – a New Approach to Chronic Disease Management for the 21st Century*. London: HMSO.

Diener, E., Suh, E. M., Lucas, R. E. and Smith, H. L. (1997) Subjective wellbeing: three decades of progress. *Psychological Bulletin* **125** (2): 276–302.

Dumas, L. (1992) Arthritis in women: social considerations in the clinical management of rheumatoid arthritis. *Journal of Home Healthcare Practitioners* **4** (2): 42–52.

Elfant, E., Gall, E. and Perlmuter, L. C. (1999) Learned illness behaviour and adjustment to arthritis. *Arthritis Care and Research* **12**: 411–16.

Emery, P. and Salmon, M. (1995) Early rheumatoid arthritis: time to aim for remission? *Annals of Rheumatic Diseases* **54**: 944–7.

Escalante, A. and del Rincón, I. (1999) How much disability in rheumatoid arthritis is explained by rheumatoid arthritis? *Arthritis and Rheumatism* **42** (8): 1712–21.

Escalante, A. and del Rincón, I. (2002) The disablement process in rheumatoid arthritis. *Arthritis Care and Research* **47** (3): 333–42.

Frank, R., Beck, N., Parker, J., Kashani, J., Elliot, T., Haut, A., Smith, E., Atwood, C., Brownlee-Duffeck, M. and Kay, D. (1988) Depression in rheumatoid arthritis. *Journal of Rheumatology* **15** (6): 920–5.

Freeman, K., Hammond, A. and Lincoln, N. B. (2002) Use of cognitive behavioural arthritis education programmes in newly diagnosed rheumatoid arthritis. *Clinical Rehabilitation* **16**: 828–36.

Gifford, L. (1998) Pain, the tissues and the nervous system: a conceptual model. *Physiotherapy* **84** (1): 27–36.

Gio-Fitman, J. (1996) The role of psychological stress in rheumatoid arthritis. *MEDSURG Nursing* **5** (6): 422–5.

Hainsworth, J. and Barlow, J. (2001) Volunteers' experience of becoming arthritis self-management lay leaders: 'It's almost as if I've stopped ageing and started to get younger!'. *Arthritis Care and Research* **45**: 378–83.

Hammond, A. (1994) Joint protection behaviour in patients with rheumatoid arthritis following an education programme. *Arthritis Care and Research* **7**: 5–9.

Hammond, A. (1998) The use of self-management strategies by people with rheumatoid arthritis. *Clinical Rehabilitation* **12**: 81–7.

Hammond, A. (1999) The effect of a joint protection education programme for people with rheumatoid arthritis. *Clinical Rehabilitation* **13**: 392–400.

Hawley, D. J. (1995) Psycho educational interventions in the treatment of arthritis. *Baillière's Clinical Rheumatology* **9**: 803–23.

Hawley, D. and Wolfe, F. (1988) Anxiety and depression in patients with rheumatoid arthritis: a prospective study of 400 patients. *Journal of Rheumatology* **15** (6): 932–41.

Haworth, R. (2000) Aspect group 5: psychological wellbeing and self-management. *Journal of Rheumatology Occupational Therapy* **14** (2): 41–5.

Hewlett, S., Cockshott, Z., Kirwan, J., Stamp, J. and Haslock, I. (2001) Development and validation of a self-efficacy scale for use in British patients with rheumatoid arthritis (RASE). *Rheumatology* **40**: 1221–30.

Hewlett, S., Mitchell, K., Haynes, J., Paine, T., Korendowych, E. and Kirwan, J. (2000) Patient initiated hospital follow up for rheumatoid arthritis. *Rheumatology* **39**: 990–7.

Hewlett, S., Smith, A. P. and Kirwan, J. R. (2002) Measuring the meaning of disability in rheumatoid arthritis: the Personal Impact Health Assessment Questionnaire (PI HAQ). *Annals of the Rheumatic Diseases* **61**: 986–93.

Hodes, D. and Charles, C. (1992) Psychosocial manifestations of arthritis for the individual and family. *Journal of Healthcare Practice* **4** (2): 53–63.

Jensen, G. M. and Lorish, C. D. (1994) Promoting patient co-operation with exercise programmes: linking research theory and practice. *Arthritis Care and Research* 7: 181–9.

Katz, P. P. and Neugebauer, A. (2001) Does satisfaction with abilities mediate the relationship between impact of rheumatoid arthritis on valued activities and depressive symptoms? *Arthritis Care and Research* 45: 263–9.

Katz, P. P. and Yelin, E. (1993) Prevalence and correlates of depressive symptoms among persons with rheumatoid arthritis. *Journal of Rheumatology* 20: 790–6.

Katz, P. P. and Yelin, E. H. (1995) The development of depressive symptoms among women with rheumatoid arthritis: the role of function. *Arthritis and Rheumatism* 38: 49–56.

Keefe, F. J., Brown, G. K., Wallston, K. A. and Caldwell, D. S. (1989) Coping with rheumatoid arthritis pain: catastrophising as a maladaptive strategy. *Pain* 37: 51–6.

Kirwan, J. R., Mitchell, K., Hewlett, S., Hehir, M., Pollock, J., Memel, D. and Bennett, B. (2003) Clinical and psychological outcome from a randomised controlled trial of patient initiated direct access hospital follow up for rheumatoid arthritis extended to 4 years. *Rheumatology* 42: 422–6.

Kraaimaat, F. W., van Dam-Baggen, R. M. J. and Bijlsma, J. W. J. (1995) Association of social support and the spouse's reaction with psychological distress in male and female patients with rheumatoid arthritis. *Journal of Rheumatology* 22: 644–8.

Kroot, E. J. A., van Leeuwen, M. A., van Rijswijk, M. H., Preevoo, M. L. L., Van't Hof, M. A., van de Putte, L. B. A. and van Riel, P. L. C. M. (2000) No increased mortality in patients with rheumatoid arthritis: up to 10 years of follow up from disease onset. *Annals of the Rheumatic Diseases* 59: 954–8.

Lazarous, R. and Folkman, S. (1984) *Stress, Appraisal and Coping.* New York: Springer.

Lindroth, Y. (2000) Patient education. In Friestein, G. S., Panayi, G. S. and Wollheim, F. A. (eds) *Rheumatoid Arthritis: New Frontiers in Pathogenesis and Treatment.* Oxford: Oxford University Press.

Lorig, K., Lubeck, D., Kraines, R. G., Seleznick, M. and Holman, H. R. (1985) Outcomes of self help education for patients with arthritis. *Arthritis and Rheumatism* 28: 680–5.

Lorig, K., Chastain, R., Ung, E., Shoor, S. and Holman, H. (1989) Development and evaluation of a scale to measure perceived self-efficacy in people with arthritis. *Arthritis and Rheumatism* 32: 37–44.

Maisaik, R., Austin, J., West, S. and Heck, L. (1996) The effect of person centred counselling on the psychological status of persons with systemic lupus erythematosus or rheumatoid arthritis. *Arthritis Care and Research* 9 (1): 60–6.

Manne, S. L. and Zautra, A. J. (1992) Coping with arthritis current status and critique. *Arthritis and Rheumatism* 35 (11): 1273–80.

Marks, R. (2001) Efficacy theory and its utility in arthritis rehabilitation: review and recommendations. *Disability and Rehabilitation* 27 (7): 271–80.

Marks, C. and Wilkins, R. (1997) Depression in rheumatoid arthritis: recognition and intervention. *Journal of Musculoskeletal Medicine* 14 (3): 52–60.

McEvoy DeVellis, B. (1995) The psychological impact of arthritis: prevalence of depression. *Arthritis Care Research* 8: 279–83.

McQuade, D. V. (2002) Negative social perception of hypothetical workers with rheumatoid arthritis. *Journal of Behavioural Medicine* 25 (3): 205–17.

Mottonen, T., Paimela, L., Leirisalo-Repo, M., Kautiainen, H., Ilonen, J. and Hannonen, P. (1998) Only high disease activity and positive rheumatoid factor indicate poor prognosis in patients with early rheumatoid arthritis treated with 'sawtooth' strategy. *Annals of Rheumatic Diseases* 57: 533–9.

Neville, C., Fortin, P. R., Fitzcharles, M.-A., Baron, M., Abrahamowitz, M., Du Berger, R. and Esdaile, J. M. (1999) The needs of patients with arthritis: the patients perspective. *Arthritis Care and Research* **12**: 85–95.

Newbold, D. (1996) Coping with rheumatoid arthritis: how can specialist nurses influence it and promote better outcomes? *Journal of Clinical Nursing* **5**: 373–80.

Newman, S. (1996) Psychological assessment in rheumatic diseases. *Arthritis Research Council Topical Review* Series **3** (9 September).

O'Hara, P. (1996) *Pain Management for Health Professionals.* London: Chapman and Hall.

Ormel, J. and Tiemens, B. (1997) Depression in primary care. In Honig, A. and van Praag, H. M. (eds) *Depression: Neurobiological, Psychopathological and Therapeutic Advances.* Chichester: Wiley.

Parker, J. C. and Wright, G. E. (1995) The implications of depression for pain and disability in rheumatoid arthritis. *Arthritis Care and Research* **8** (4): 279–83.

Parker, J. C. and Wright, G. E. (1997) Assessment of the psychological outcomes and quality of life in the rheumatic diseases. *Arthritis Care and Research* **10**: 406–12.

Persson, L.-O., Berglund, K. and Sahlberg, D. (1999) Psychological factors in chronic rheumatoid diseases: a review. *Scandinavian Journal of Rheumatology* **28**: 137–44.

Pigg, J., Driscoll, P. and Caniff, R. (1985) *Rheumatology Nursing: a Problem Orientated Approach.* New York: Wiley Medical.

Pimm, T. (1997) Self regulation and psycho educational interventions for rheumatic disease. In Petrie, K. J. and Weinman, J. A. (eds) *Perceptions of Health and Illness.* Amsterdam: Harwood Academic.

Pincus, T. (1995) The underestimated long term medical and economic consequences of rheumatoid arthritis. *Drugs* **50** (Suppl 1): 1–14.

Riemsma, R. P., Taal, E. and Rasker, J. J. (2000) Perceptions about perceived functional disabilities and pain of people with rheumatoid arthritis: differences between patients and their spouses and correlates with wellbeing. *Arthritis Care and Research* **13**: 255–61.

Rotter, J. B. (1966) Generalised expectancies for internal versus external control of reinforcement. *Psychology Monographs* **80** (1): 609.

Ryan, S. (1997) How rheumatoid arthritis affects patients' families. *Nursing Times* **93** (18): 48–9.

Savelkoul, M., De Witte, L. P., Candel, M. J. J., Van der Tempel, H. and Van den Borne, B. (2001) Effects of a coping intervention on patients with rheumatic diseases: results of a randomised controlled trial. *Arthritis Care and Research* **45**: 69–76.

Scott, D. L. (2000) The diagnosis and prognosis of early arthritis: rationale for new prognostic criteria. *Arthritis and Rheumatism* **46** (2): 286–90.

Serbo, B., and Jajic, I. (1991) Relationship of the functional status, duration of the disease and pain intensity and some psychological variables in patients with rheumatoid arthritis. *Clinical Rheumatology* **10** (4): 419–22.

Shipley, M. and Newman, S. (1993) Psychological aspects of rheumatic diseases. *Baillière's Clinical Rheumatology* **7** (2): 215–19.

Silman, A. J. and Hochberg, M. C. (1994) *Epidemiology of the Rheumatic Diseases.* Oxford: Oxford University Press.

Smith, C., Wallston, K. A., Dwyer, K. A. and Dowdy, S. W. (1997) Beyond good and bad coping: a multidimensional examination of coping with pain in persons with rheumatoid arthritis. *Annals of Behavioural Medicine* **19** (1): 11–21.

Smith, T., Peck, J. and Ward, J. (1990) Helplessness and depression in rheumatoid arthritis. *Health Psychology* **9** (4): 377–89.

Strahl, C., Klienknecht, R. A. and Dinnel, D. L. (2000) The role of pain anxiety, coping and pain self-efficacy in rheumatoid arthritis patient functioning. *Behaviour Research and Therapy* **38**: 863–73.

Symmons, D. and Harrison, B. (2000) Early inflammatory polyarthritis: results from the Norfolk Arthritis Register with a review of the literature, I: Risk factors for the development of inflammatory polyarthritis and rheumatoid arthritis. *Rheumatology* **39**: 835–43.

Symmons, D., Turner, G., Webb, R., Asten, P., Barrett, E., Lunt, M., Scott, D. and Silman, A. (2002) The prevalence of rheumatoid arthritis in the United Kingdom: new estimates for a new century. *Rheumatology* **41**: 793–800.

Uhlig, T., Smedstad, L. M., Vaglum, P., Moum, T., Gerard, N. and Kvien, T. K. (2000) The course of rheumatoid arthritis and predictors of psychological, physical and radiographic outcome after 5 years of follow up. *Rheumatology* **39**: 732–41.

Yelin, E. H. and Katz, P. P. (2002) Focusing interventions for disability among patients with rheumatoid arthritis. *Arthritis and Rheumatism* **47**: 231–3.

Young, A., Dixey, J., Cox, N., Davies, P., Devlin, J., Emery, P., Gallivan, S., Gough, A., James, D., Prouse, P., Williams, P. and Winfield, J. (2000) How does functional disability in early rheumatoid arthritis (RA) affect patients and their lives? Results of 5 years of follow-up in 732 patients from the early RA study (ERAS). *Rheumatology* **39**: 603–11.

Young, L. (1992) Psychological factors in rheumatoid arthritis. *Journal of Consulting and Clinical Psychology* **60** (4): 619–27.

Zautra, A. J., Hoffman, J. M., Matt, K. S., Yocum, D., Potter, P. T. and Castro, W. L. (1998) An examination of individual differences in the relationship between interpersonal stress and disease activity among women with rheumatoid arthritis. *Arthritis Care and Research* **11**: 271–9.

PART III
PROMOTING HEALTH THROUGH PHYSIOTHERAPY

CHAPTER 12

The Culture and Context for Promoting Health through Physiotherapy Practice

SALLY FRENCH AND JOHN SWAIN

The profession of physiotherapy has largely taken a biomedical approach to patient and client care. This is strongly reflected in physiotherapy literature and research and undergraduate curricula. Over the years, however, education in the social sciences has been included in initial training and more physiotherapists now work in the community rather than hospitals, reflecting changes in National Health Service (NHS) structure and policy in the United Kingdom (UK) (Department of Health (DoH), 2000). Physiotherapy has until recent times been under the control of doctors and physiotherapy practice, and its biomedical orientation, have reflected this control. Many authors (see for example Tones and Tilford, 2001) point out that medicine has focussed on the individual and that this has been perpetuated by the greater power of medical professionals when compared with those who work in health promotion. Looking outwards to wide social, political and economic factors that may impact on people's health and wellbeing has not been encouraged and, even today, education in the social sciences within physiotherapy is marginalised and has tended to focus on micro issues such as interpersonal communication (Swain et al., 2004a).

This chapter aims to uncover the meaning of health promotion in physiotherapy practice. Health promotion is a complex and contested concept. Different authors and professional groups define health promotion in diverse ways, which is not surprising given that the notion of health itself has different interpretations (see Jones, 2000; Tones and Tilford, 2001: 2; Tones and Green, 2004).

In providing this overview of health promotion in physiotherapy, in-depth interviews were conducted with a small sample consisting of two physiotherapy lecturers, four clinical physiotherapists and two people who have received physiotherapy as patients and clients. Quotations from these interviews are used to illustrate some of the issues facing physiotherapists in promoting health. The first section explores the meaning of health and health promotion, approaches to health promotion in physiotherapy practice, and some of the complex and difficult challenges facing physiotherapists in adopting health promoting principles and applying these to practice. From this basis the discussion turns to questions of physiotherapy education. The conclusion draws the analysis together with particular emphasis on the central implications for physiotherapist and client relationships.

Defining health, wellbeing and health promotion

In 1948 the World Health Organisation (WHO) defined health as a state of complete physical, psychological and social wellbeing and not merely the absence of disease or infirmity (WHO, 1948). Although this definition helped to move the concept of health towards a more holistic understanding, it was criticised for being idealistic and unrealistic and for failing to recognise that people define their health in a variety of ways based on their knowledge, values and expectations and whether or not they can fulfil roles of importance to them (Jones, 2000; Ewles and Simnett, 2003). The WHO later expanded and redefined its description of health by stating that it included the extent to which individuals or groups are able to realise aspirations and satisfy needs and to change or cope with the environment. Health, therefore, became seen as a resource for everyday life, not the objective of living. It emerged as a positive concept emphasising social and personal resources as well as physical capacities (WHO, 1984).

The term health promotion is essentially a contested concept, but generally refers to strategies that not only attempt to prevent ill health and disease in its broadest sense but also to improve quality of life and wellbeing (Bunton and Macdonald, 2002; Seedhouse, 2004 and Chapter 1 of this text). This is in contrast to the biomedical approach where the emphasis is on finding a cure or managing a condition once it has occurred (Waddell and Peterson, 1994). Although there is no widely adopted definition of health promotion, the various explanations, models and frameworks emphasise the need to empower people to have more choice and control over those aspects of their lives which affect their health including the communities in which they live (see Chapter 1 for further discussion of definitions and explanations of health promotion). There is also a recognition that medicine and professional practice have had little effect on health and that health can be improved far more successfully by investing in the social fabric of society and reducing inequalities (Marmot and Wilkinson, 1999; Adams et al., 2003). Tones (2001) argues that medical services need to be reshaped and reorientated, as a fundamental aim of health promotion is demedicalisation.

Some authors, such as Naidoo and Wills (1998) have provided a kind of typology of health promotion, dividing it up into set functions encompassing disease prevention, health education and health information, public health reform, and community development. The fundamental set of principles to guide practice are also clearly recognised as those provided by Naidoo and Wills (1998) that include a focus on health not illness, the empowerment of clients, recognising that health is multidimensional, and acknowledging the influence of factors external to the individual which impinge upon their health. There is also the notion that the implementation of health promotion is multidimensional and can be applied at the individual, community, policy and structural levels (see Chapter 1 of this text and also Katz et al., 2000).

Broad, or more holistic, views of health and wellbeing were apparent in the interviews. A physiotherapy lecturer, for instance, stated:

I see it from a more holistic viewpoint. It's not just the absence of disease. There has been a tendency in healthcare to view it as that especially in Westernised healthcare. Eastern healthcare has a different viewpoint, it's more that the person feels good about themselves, they feel good about their life, how they're running their life, their lifestyle and what they're doing. There's the physical aspect with them actually being physically well, but also in terms of psychosocial and mental health.

A service user indicated a similar view, though obviously from a different standpoint:

Health is whether I'm in a state to do things. I'm ill when I'm stuck to my bed ... wellbeing is when I'm allowed to get on with living without anybody impacting on my ability to do what I want so that rest isn't a word that is in my wellbeing.

A holistic view of health and wellbeing can be seen as a concept that has many different connotations for physiotherapists. First, it challenges a medicalised view of individuals which is clearly expressed by the two lecturers in relation to disability and old age:

Someone with a disability can have a high level of health and wellbeing because it's a personal state and that's a different interpretation from the medical viewpoint. With old age we're going to have to move more to the Eastern viewpoint of old age as part of life and that it shouldn't be medicalised.

Second, this notion of health and wellbeing extends thinking beyond the individual to the social context, however it is defined. A clinical physiotherapist and visiting lecturer turned this into a question for self-reflection:

I used to teach the students in the first year ... I gave an example of somebody moving away from home, coming into a new environment, maybe different forms of study, so their workload changes, their social circle would change, and with that they may be doing things we wouldn't promote as being good for your health, such as smoking and drinking and also that that might have an implication on how much physical activity they are doing. That was an example I used to use with the students, saying 'are you physically, mentally and socially well?'

Such considerations underpin the approaches adopted for health promotion in physiotherapy practice.

Approaches to health promotion

Nutbeam and Harris (1999) emphasise the diverse range of information and theories needed in the practice of health promotion, including epidemiological and demographic information; information from the behavioural and social sciences; and knowledge of community needs and priorities. Ewles and Simnett (2003) list the following approaches to health promotion that are not necessarily mutually exclusive:

1. The medical approach, which values preventative measures and patient compliance
2. The behavioural change approach, which seeks to change people's attitudes and behaviour in ways defined by the professional
3. The educational approach, in which people are given information but their values and choices are respected. The role of the professional is to help people to gain the skills to make well informed decisions and to offer their help and support
4. The client centred approach, in which clients identify what they want to know and what actions, if any, to take. Self-empowerment is central and the professional acts as a facilitator
5. The social change approach, in which the focus is on changing society not on changing individuals. (See also Katz at al., 2000 for further discussion of approaches.)

All the five approaches above were apparent in the views expressed in the interviews. The literature and the views expressed by physiotherapists suggest, however, that the overall orientation to health promotion within physiotherapy practice reflects the medical, behavioural change and educational approaches listed above. The provision of information is certainly a key strategy, even defining health promotion in therapy practice, as illustrated by the following quotations:

> And this is where I start asking myself, what is health promotion? And I suppose all of it is, even small amounts of education informing the person how to manage their condition and how to get more well.
>   I'll give you examples of what I feel is health promotion. One way would be by doing health education talks, with a group of people talking about whatever subject related to health. So we do one in the cardiac group on how exercise can not only help your heart it can benefit your joints and muscles as well.

Aligned with the educational approach is the notion of the self-management of health and wellbeing by patients and clients, though, as illustrated by the following quotation, the role of the physiotherapist can be one of instigating and enabling the process:

> I think our priority in health promotion is self-management, about personal responsibility and allowing people to be able to look after themselves. Like with smoking you're giving people the tools to come off cigarettes. The research that I've read suggests that the best way to promote people's health is to get them to decide that they want to do it.

The interviews reflected a range of developing strategies such as the use of the Internet to disseminate information, and work in the community such as collaboration between medical professionals and staff in leisure centres.

Another theme given heavy emphasis by physiotherapists was working as members of multiprofessional teams (Payne, 2000), with interprofessional collaboration seen as fundamentally important. As is evident in the following quotations, this seemed to relate mostly to the medical and behavioural change approaches:

> We run the exercise group but part of that is an information session where we have other health professionals coming to talk to the patients such as the pharmacist, the dietitian, the cholesterol nurse. We do stress and relaxation classes, there's a smoking cessation nurse. So there's lots of different professions so if we want to we can refer them to the relevant health professionals to look at certain aspects of lifestyle change. We do an eight week programme.

The physiotherapists did sometimes mention the importance of the broader social context:

> We work with occupational therapists and speech therapists and that has been very helpful to us. OTs work with social services and speech and language therapists work with the educational services so it's widened our experience of working in a multiagency way and has helped us to think about wider aspects of health promotion.

The focus for change, however, largely remains with the individual:

> A person who has a long term medical condition is certainly restricted in many, many ways. Their horizons can be lifted tremendously if they are enabled to be taken out of the house, either with or without a carer, and to have some sort of initiative of their own to go to a centre, for example, to learn different things and participate in the world.

Disabled people, on the other hand, have generated a social model of disability that clearly sites the focus for change within society (Swain et al., 2004b). This would involve the removal of attitudinal, environmental and structural barriers to full participatory citizenship. The need for a social change approach was apparent in both the interviews with disabled clients, who saw this approach as enabling people to make personal choices about their health and their functional ability, even if that involved making mistakes.

Tones (2001) stresses the political nature of health promotion and believes that health education should include critical consciousness raising and challenging false consciousness in order to generate pressure for change (see also Tones and Green, 2004).

The physiotherapists were, however, generally cautious about becoming overtly political in their health promotion work though opinions were mixed. This reticence is illustrated in one respondent's view. They felt it appropriate to be politically aware, but that they would not be involved in campaigning for disabled rights, for example. They regarded their professional role as giving information to clients, pointing them to website information but not campaigning. A recent article (Limb, 2004) also demonstrates this lack of political endeavour, whilst advocating a leading role in health promotion for the profession does not mention any intervention beyond the level of health education.

Some disabled people have questioned such apolitical stances. Ken Davis (2004), a disabled activist, is fervent in his criticism of health professionals' lack of political commitment and the disabled people's movement has strongly criticised professional practice, viewing it as oppressive and abusive (Swain et al., 2003). There do seem to be possibilities for change, however, particularly with the growing impact of the social model of disability and the implementation of the Disability Discrimination Act (website address in References under *Disability*). In this light, physiotherapists may work towards a much broader brief. They would need to recognise the political nature of disability and work together with disabled people to break down disabling barriers and to promote the struggle for full citizenship for all disabled people (French, 2004).

Questions of health promotion

While it was evident within the interviews that physiotherapists can put a high priority on health promotion in their work, it was also clear that it posed some complex and fundamental challenges. At the heart of these questions is the traditional approach and role of physiotherapy. One lecturer summarised this as follows:

> The problem is that physios tend to work in tertiary care and the role there is very much rehabilitation, getting back to a level or potential, and physios get locked into seeing themselves in that role, making people better. It's much more collaborative these days but my sense is that they don't see beyond getting someone better ... It's very much an illness service. We're not in the right place and we're not there at the right time.

Along the same lines, one physiotherapist posed the issues as questions:

> I start asking myself, what is health promotion? What can we do to stay well? What can we do to become more well? And I think the type of people that we engage tend to be the ones that have a problem. So then is it health promotion or rehabilitation, and where does rehab end and where does further health promotion start?

An immediate concern, then, has to be defining the client group to whom health promotion is directed. Is the prime client group people who may be at risk but who have no diagnosed condition, therefore requiring a primary health promotion approach, or clients who have already, for instance, experienced a heart attack, or developed diabetes, or back pain, or have sustained an injury, requiring secondary health promotion skills and interventions? As one physiotherapist asked:

> But what about the people who haven't had a heart attack, don't have angina, but are overweight, don't do any exercise, smoke and drink and all those things? And how do we engage people with all the risk factors for heart disease?

Perhaps not surprisingly, this immediately begs questions of time implications, resources, workforce capacity and capability for such a possible broadening of the role of physiotherapists. Questions also arise concerning the venue for health promoting physiotherapy facilities. A health promotion approach suggests that physiotherapy needs to be based in community facilities, such as fitness and leisure centres, rather than within medical institutions.

Another inherent set of issues relates to, at its broadest, the human relations between physiotherapists and their clients. Essentially, this can be seen as moving away from what can be characterised as a paternalistic relationship. The challenge to physiotherapists is in engaging in a more facilitatory role that enables clients to promote their own health and wellbeing. One lecturer emphasised this as a key development:

> There are so many legal challenges to the paternalistic model going on now, that I think that the idea that patients are responsible for their own care and their own health and their own wellbeing, and that we need to look much more at self-management of health, will become much more important.

The main issue for physiotherapists can become one of motivating or engaging people in self-management within both primary and secondary prevention. This can be seen as a continuous problem of maintaining motivation, as indicated in the following quotation:

> ... people lapse. Sometimes you win a battle but lose another battle. Some people who stop smoking put on weight. Once they're out of the loop of the health service there's a problem. The secondary prevention group tend to be highly motivated

because they've already had heart problems but it's difficult to start it with those who haven't had problems yet. There's a drive to try and improve primary prevention. That's a big issue of trying to get into the whole community and to change people's mind sets.

This physiotherapist felt that information is being filtered too slowly to the public and it is now the time to be more aggressive in marketing terms in order to ensure the health messages are being received. Other problems with the behavioural change approach, through the dissemination of information, include the changing nature of information and its variability. Information on diet, for instance, can vary depending on the source or which professional is imparting the information. It is also known to change over time as further evidence becomes available. The accessibility of information can also be problematic, for instance for people with visual impairments (French et al., 1997) and learning difficulties (Walmsley, 1999; Shaughnessy and Cruse, 2001). One physiotherapist added to this:

> We also have people of different nationalities [sic] and that is another problem of trying to impart information. There is also a problem with literacy and also the people who know it all.

Furthermore, as the following story from a physiotherapist illustrates, the information that is given is not necessarily the information received:

> There's so much ignorance around, they don't really understand a lot of what's going on. For example we've got a diabetic lady who was told by a dietitian at the initial diagnosis not to eat this, that and the other. It was completely misunderstood by the patient who virtually eats nothing and she's on insulin. She was so muddled that she wouldn't eat rice and protein and now her digestive system can't seem to accept enough food to keep her going.

It can be argued that the most fundamental difficulty with the medical and behavioural approaches to health promotion is that they can build on and maintain the unequal power relations between physiotherapists and patients and clients. The balance of power needs to be shifted from professionals to patients and clients. Emphasising the difficulties of establishing such changes in relationships, a lecturer traced the origins of the more traditional relationship back to recruitment:

> It's something about the ethos, physio is lodged in the biosciences. When physio candidates come for interview they say 'I love sports'. They have an image of physios as 'doing unto', they've often had a sports injury themselves. They're attracted to the 'hands on'.

The fundamental challenge is underlined too by analyses of professional–client relationships in the literature (French and Swain, 2001), particularly drawing on the experiences of disabled clients. There is evidence to suggest that clients experience a lack of control within physiotherapy and can become demoralised, rather than empowered (Middleton, 1999: 18).

A disabled client spoke of the depersonalisation she felt in relationships with healthcare professionals:

> Healthcare professionals can make you angry and depressed. They can treat you like a child ... They can belittle me by talking down to me – I lose my identity. I become a 'we'. They ask, 'How are we today?' 'Are we going anywhere?' And I've suddenly multiplied – I'm no longer a single person and I'm not me I'm just a 'we'. And that happens quite a lot. Another one keeps calling me 'darling'. Ungenuineness in healthcare. I have no identity, I am just someone who gets my butt washed.

Her advice to physiotherapists seems to call for more client centred and social change approaches to health promotion:

> Health promotion should be about listening as well as giving information, they should listen ... If they're going to promote health, they need to listen to disabled people, but also be more aware of the social implications of disability. It's all very well them putting a ramp into the surgery, but if their mentality is the same, then the barriers won't be broken down.

A lecturer emphasised the difficulties of turning principles of health promotion into practice:

> It's always got to be applied. I think that's the only way they're going to recognise that it's a lot harder than they realise.

Health promotion and physiotherapy education

The Chartered Society of Physiotherapy (CSP) espouses the importance of health promotion in physiotherapy education and practice but has little to say about the particular approaches or philosophical underpinnings adopted or how they should be taught or practised. They argue that physiotherapists play a broad role in health promotion, health education and self-care which extends to advising and teaching patients' and clients' carers, other healthcare professionals and support workers, the aim being to provide a coherent approach to maintaining individuals' independence and wellbeing (CSP, 2002: 19). Moreover, the promotion of good health and the use of preventative approaches are presented as key aspects of physiotherapy practice. The CSP recommend that students should develop their understanding of issues relating to health promotion, health education, self-care and illness prevention through their initial training (CSP, 2002: 49).

Given the priority afforded to health promotion, and the complexity of the whole arena, it is not surprising that the physiotherapists and lecturers saw education as a key area of concern. Two main issues recurred. The first was the priority, or rather lack of priority, given to health promotion in physiotherapy education. There was a consensus of opinion that health promotion was generally not a major focus, and for some participants, though not all, had been given less priority in recent years. In such circumstances, education in health promotion had been experiential rather than part of the formal education and training process.

> I don't think that we are taught about health promotion so it's something we pick up on the job from a variety of other health professionals. I've learned an awful lot from the nurses.
>
> No, I don't believe we got very much. I felt that it had a low priority. I don't recall doing much directly on health promotion. We didn't do much on health education. There was no focus on health promotion. A lot of my learning has been 'on the job' learning really. I sometimes think, 'Am I really qualified to be discussing diet with somebody or smoking cessation?' Your instincts tell you that you shouldn't just be telling people, 'That's bad, stop' but you are never taught how to approach it. Apart from that there isn't time to sit down and talk to people about it. It's all very ad hoc.

For one lecturer, the lack of focus on health promotion is a reflection of the reactive rather than proactive nature of physiotherapy education:

> At the moment it doesn't have a great priority although I think we touch on it all the time. The big problem here is the 'chicken and egg' thing. We're currently preparing physiotherapists for the current NHS and the current NHS hasn't got a big push for physiotherapists in health promotion.

The second major issue is whether health promotion should be a topic in its own right in the curriculum, or whether it is a theme that is integral to all the areas covered in the curriculum. As the following quotations illustrate, there was a division of opinion over this issue:

> I think there should definitely be a designated module on health promotion so that it doesn't get lost. If it's integrated with everything else it gets too watered down and the students won't remember it.
>
> I think that if you teach it as a separate entity then it is a separate entity. If it's integrated it's seen as part of your practice.

Many skills pertaining to research, communication, management, publicity and the media are needed to work successfully in the field of health promotion.

To conclude, the physiotherapists expressed some enthusiasm about health promotion and gave it a high priority in developing their work. One who was working in the community said:

> The importance of health promotion should never be underestimated. At the present time I feel that the necessary information, re various pathological conditions, is not reaching the customer, i.e. the potential patient.

They spoke of various developments that indicate both a changing context for developing health promotion and the importance of physiotherapy within this. These developments included clinical governance, *The Expert Patient* programme promoted by government (DoH, 2001), the development of community facilities in, for instance, community clinics and gymnasiums, the changing legal context, and demographic and economic factors. Demographic trends are an important factor in indicating the need for physiotherapists to adopt a more pronounced health promotion philosophy and approach (WHO, 2002).

The development of health promotion approaches, however, requires the balance of power to be shifted from professionals to patients and clients. In WHO health promotion directives (see, for example, WHO, 1986, 1997) and recent UK public health policy developments (see DoH, 1999, 2004; Wanless, 2004), partnership has been a dominant concept signifying the attainment of greater equality not only in interprofessional but also in professional–client relations. In a partnership, the persons or groups who traditionally have exercised control need to change the way they have worked in the past. As Standing (1999) points out working in partnership with clients involves far more than learning new techniques of treatment. It involves a willingness and capacity to respond imaginatively to every person as a unique individual and to help and support each person in the achievement of his or her own aspirations and desired lifestyle. Enabling and empowering approaches (Tones, 2001) are crucial to this changing paradigm.

Power relations, organisational and professional structures are, by their nature, deeply ingrained, and cosmetic alternations can mask a lack of fundamental change. Central to moving towards more health promoting practice is shifting emphasis from medical and behavioural change approaches towards more client centred (see Chapter 8) and social change (see Chapter 1) approaches and, with this, possibilities for physiotherapists to work for and with clients in creating the contexts and relationships that facilitate clients in empowering themselves to improve their own health and wellbeing at every level.

References

Adams, L., Amos, M. and Munro, J. (eds) (2003) *Promoting Health: Politics and Practice*. London: Sage.

Bunton, R. and Macdonald, G. (2002) *Health Promotion: Disciplines, Diversity and Developments*. London: Routledge.

Chartered Society of Physiotherapy (2002) *Curriculum Framework for Qualifying Programmes in Physiotherapy.* London: CSP.

Davis, K. (2004) The crafting of good clients. In Swain, J., French, S., Barnes, C. and Thomas, C. (eds) (2004) *Disabling Barriers – Enabling Environments,* second edition. London: Sage.

Department of Health (1999) *Saving Lives: Our Healthier Nation.* London: HMSO.

Department of Health (2000) *The NHS Plan: a Plan for Investment. A Plan for Reform.* London: HMSO.

Department of Health (2001) *The Expert Patient: a New Approach to Chronic Disease Management for the 21st Century.* London: DoH.

Department of Health (2004) *Choosing Health: Making Healthier Choices Easier.* London: The Stationery Office.

Disability Discrimination Act. www.dda-centre.co.uk (accessed 22 December 2004).

Ewles, L. and Simnett, I. (2003) *Promoting Health: a practical guide,* fifth edition. London: Baillière Tindall.

French, S. (2004) Defining disability: implications for physiotherapy practice. In French, S. and Sim, J. (eds) *Physiotherapy: a Psychosocial Approach,* third edition. Oxford: Butterworth-Heinemann.

French, S., Gillman, M. and Swain, J. (1997) *Working with Visually Disabled People: from Theory to Practice.* Birmingham: Venture Press.

French, S. and Swain, J. (2001) The relationship between disabled people and health and welfare professionals. In Albrecht, G. L., Seelman, K. D. and Bury, M. (eds) *Handbook of Disability Studies.* Thousand Oaks, CA: Sage.

Jones, L. (2000) Promoting health: everybody's business? In Katz, J., Peberdy, A. and Douglas, J. (eds) *Promoting Health: Knowledge and Practice,* second edition. Basingstoke: Palgrave (now Palgrave Macmillan).

Katz, J., Peberdy, A. and Douglas, J. (2000) *Promoting Health: Knowledge and Practice.* Basingstoke: Palgrave (now Palgrave Macmillan)/Open University.

Limb, M. (2004) Driving the public health agenda. *Physiotherapy Frontline* **10** (4): 7.

Marmot, M. and Wilkinson, R. G. (1999) *Social Determinants of Health.* Oxford: Oxford University Press.

Middleton, L. (1999) *Disabled Children: Challenging Social Exclusion.* Oxford: Blackwell Science.

Naidoo, J. and Wills, J. (1998) *Practising Health Promotion: Dilemmas and Challenges.* London: Baillière Tindall.

Nutbeam, D. and Harris, E. (1999) *Theory in a Nutshell: a Guide to Health Promotion Theory.* London: McGraw-Hill.

Payne, M. (2000) *Teamwork in Multiprofessional Care.* Basingstoke: Palgrave (now Palgrave Macmillan).

Seedhouse, D. (2004) *Health Promotion: Philosophy, Prejudice and Practice,* second edition. Chichester: Wiley.

Shaughnessy, P. and Cruse, S. (2001) Health promotion with people who have a learning disability. In Thompson, J. and Pickering, S. (eds) *Meeting the Health Needs of People Who Have a Learning Disability.* London: Baillière Tindall.

Standing, S. (1999) The practice of working in partnership. In Swain, J. and French, S. (eds) *Therapy and Learning Difficulties.* Oxford: Butterworth-Heinemann.

Swain, J., Clark, J., French, S., Parry, K. and Reynolds, F. (2004a) *Enabling Relationships in Health and Social Care: a Guide for Therapists.* Oxford: Butterworth-Heinemann.

Swain, J., French, S., Barnes, C. and Thomas, C. (eds) (2004b) Disabling Barriers – Enabling Environments, second edition. London, Sage.

Swain, J., French, S. and Cameron, C. (2003) *Controversial Issues in a Disabling Society*. Buckingham: Open University Press.

Tones, K. (2001) Health promotion: the empowerment imperative. In Scriven, A. and Orme, J. (eds) *Health Promotion: Professionals Perspectives*, second edition. Basingstoke: Palgrave (now Palgrave Macmillan).

Tones, K. and Green, J (2004) *Health Promotion: Planning and Strategies*. London: Sage.

Tones, K. and Tilford, S. (2001) *Health Promotion: Effectiveness, Efficiency and Equity*, third edition. Cheltenham: Nelson Thormes.

Waddell, C. and Petersen, A. R. (1994) *Just Health: Inequalities in Illness, Care and Prevention*. Edinburgh: Churchill Livingstone.

Walmsley, J. (1999) Community and people with learning difficulties. In Swain, J. and French, S. (eds) *Therapy and Learning Difficulties*. Oxford: Butterworth-Heinemann.

Wanless, D. (2004) *Securing Good Health for the Whole Population: Final Report*. London: HMSO.

World Health Organisation (1948) *Preamble of the Constitution of the World Health Organisation*. Geneva: WHO.

World Health Organisation (1984) *Report of the Working Group on Concepts and Principles of Health Promotion*. Copenhagen: WHO.

World Health Organisation (1986) *Ottawa Charter for Health Promotion*. Geneva: WHO.

World Health Organisation (1997) *The Jakarta Declaration on Health*. Geneva: WHO.

World Health Organisation (2002) *Active Ageing: a Policy Framework*. Geneva: WHO.

CHAPTER 13

Client Health Education and Empowerment through Physiotherapy in Neurorehabilitation

STEPHEN ASHFORD

Neurological rehabilitation refers to interdisciplinary work with individuals following central nervous system damage to address the physical, emotional, cognitive and communication issues that can result. In this chapter the focus will be primarily on brain injury. Physiotherapy is one of the professions involved with assisting an individual to deal with the health related consequences of neurological injury. Neurological rehabilitation is an interdisciplinary approach and does not implement intervention from a single professional perspective. However the following chapter will consider specifically the role of physiotherapy in promoting health through the empowerment of clients in this area of practice. Neurological physiotherapy has developed over time; having traditionally focussed on specific impairment, it has begun to concentrate more on empowering the individual to achieve functional and health outcomes while still continuing to address specific impairment issues. The following chapter will examine the empowerment of clients through physiotherapy and the possible barriers to this objective. The role of the client in rehabilitation will be examined in conjunction with the need for the physiotherapist to promote health and independence.

The International Classification of Diseases (ICD) is a system used to identify specific diseases and medical conditions, which is widely applied in health related fields such as medicine. This system was designed by the World Health Organisation (WHO) to classify pathological conditions such as head injury or stroke. The ICD serves this function effectively but does not classify the consequences of these conditions. In 1980 the World Health Organisation produced the International Classification of Impairments, Disabilities and Handicaps (ICIDH). This classification was produced to attempt to redress this imbalance and classify the consequences associated with disease.

In 2001 the ICIDH was updated in terms of its terminology and was then renamed the International Classification of Functioning, Disability and Health (ICF, sometimes referred to as the ICIDH-2). The aim of the ICF as with the ICIDH is to provide a standard language to discuss the consequences of health conditions (WHO, 2001). The ICF identifies function at the following three different levels, all of which relate to health:

1. system function – functioning of the body system
2. activity – functioning in the physical environment
3. participation – functioning within wider society and culture.

The ICF has been identified as important and useful by a number of professions in neurorehabilitation. Edwards (2002) has identified the ICF as a conceptual and operational model for physiotherapy intervention in neurorehabilitation practice that is useful in the measurement of outcome and can also be used in exploring goal achievement. Wade and de Jong (2000) also contend that the ICF model fosters more consistent communication between rehabilitation medicine professionals, as it provides a common language.

WHO has defined health in a number of ways but the one that has meaning for neurorehabilitation concerns the extent to which an individual or group is able to realise aspirations and satisfy needs and to change or cope with the environment (WHO, 1984). This identifies a perspective on health that goes beyond addressing ill health or disease and is more intent on considering the wellbeing and empowerment of the individual and communities.

Whilst physiotherapists in neurorehabilitation emphasise the importance of client involvement in the rehabilitation process, physiotherapy as a profession has perhaps been slow in addressing issues of wider participation in rehabilitation, but is now beginning to redress this imbalance. The incorporation of the ICF into rehabilitation practice has emphasised the importance of considering function at not just a system function (impairment) level, but also in respect of activity and participation. Physiotherapy with its biomedical origins has perhaps not always placed the relative importance on these areas that they deserve, particularly as they relate to general health and wellbeing. The use of the ICF in this area, therefore, is one factor that is prompting physiotherapists to consider the broader health promoting implications of their intervention.

In neurorehabilitation, physiotherapists adopting a health promotion approach must address issues of client empowerment and participation in their own rehabilitation process. The health promotion principle of empowering people to sustain and/or increase their level of wellbeing (Downie et al., 1996) and independence is fundamental to rehabilitation in general, but particularly to neurorehabilitation physiotherapy, where physical intervention provided by the therapist in the short term is expected to have impact for the client in the long term. Independence can be defined as the individual's ability to undertake a physical task without assistance. However a return to the person's pre-injury state in its entirety is often not possible and independence can then be achieved through other means such as assistive technology or directing a carer to meet the individual's needs.

Physiotherapy practice in neurorehabilitation

Physiotherapy with its biomedical origins focusses in neurorehabilitation on the client's motor control abilities (Stokes, 1998; Shumway-Cook and Woollacott, 2001; Edwards, 2002). Motor control is defined as the individual's ability to control specific movements of the body. Movement of the body is key to function, as human beings require movement in order to fully participate in a normal social role. Motor control is often disrupted by central nervous system damage and is therefore of concern when considering the function of the individual client.

Rehabilitation of motor control involves working with the body system to mediate the neurological damage. This can be identified from key physiotherapy literature in the neurorehabilitation area (Carr and Shepherd, 1998, 2003; Stokes, 1998; Shumway-Cook and Woollacott, 2001; Edwards, 2002), which tends to focus on making changes at the system level of function with some consideration given to activity limitation but much less so to participation restriction. Activity and participation, however, and physiotherapy as a profession are seen to work towards developing the independence of the client in these areas also. Despite developments in treatment perspectives the focus of intervention is still often directed towards system impairment as is indicated by key authors in the field (see for example, Edwards, 2002; Carr and Shepherd, 2003). A focus on impairment seems appropriate for the profession, but must be balanced with an awareness of activity and participation restriction so that these broader health promoting issues may be addressed.

Different rationales and approaches to physiotherapy practice in neurorehabilitation have developed and changed over time, manifest in the amount of control the client is given in terms of their own rehabilitation. Motor control, defined by Shumway-Cook and Woollacott (2001) as the ability to regulate or direct mechanisms essential to movement, is fundamental to client independent function. Mathiowetz and Haugen (1994) with further elaboration by Shumway-Cook and Woollacott (1995) and Plant (in Stokes, 1998) identify three classic models of motor control and associated physiotherapeutic approaches: reflex, hierarchical and systems.

The reflex model was initially based on the observations of Sherrington (1906) and is focussed around a system that relies on reflex arc activity to perform movement. Therefore movement is dictated before it actually takes place and is unlikely to change during performance but can be altered in relation to feedback. A key treatment approach based on this model is proprioceptive neuromuscular facilitation (PNF) developed by Knott and Voss (1968). The approach is based on observations by Kabat (cited in Knott and Voss, 1968) that movement patterns in normal individuals occur in a spiral or diagonal pattern and are purposeful in nature. Physiotherapy using this approach will focus on passive movement initially, progressing to active movement in spiral and diagonal patterns. This approach has limited focus on issues such as task practice and the practical integration of the intervention into specific functional settings.

The hierarchical model as the title implies is based on the concept of a hierarchical model of control within the central nervous system (CNS). The concept implies that higher centres in the CNS will control lower centres. It is based on an open loop system where movement programmes are stored centrally and then influence the expression of movement distally but do not have total control over it. Therefore if central programmes for movement are disrupted in some way then control distally will be altered and more reflexive activity may be observed. A widely used treatment approach originating in this model is that of Bobath (1990). The aim is to inhibit unwanted reflex activity and facilitate more normal movement, which in this context is equated to energy and task efficient movement seen in the population without impairment. The approach emphasises the importance of correct handling and facilitation by the therapist to allow normal movement and that one level of functioning should be achieved before progression to the next, for example ability to sit before ability to stand. This approach gives much of the control for rehabilitation to the therapist and can only allow for more direct client control once they have achieved a higher level of functional ability.

The systems model has developed to a certain extent from the open loop model of motor control but incorporates other perspectives such as learning theory and biomechanics that are important in the development of normal movement. The model originally developed for the work of Schmidt (1975) with schema theory and has been built upon by authors such as Mulder (1993), Mathiowetz and Haugen (1994) and Shumway-Cook and Woollacott (1995). A treatment approach based on this model is motor relearning (Carr and Shepherd, 1980) which emphasises the importance of relearning normal movement with an emphasis on practice of specific tasks and then incorporation of training into the functional setting. Thus in this approach the therapist has control of the assessment and analysis of the intervention but at an early stage responsibility for functional practice is transferred to the client.

Movement emerges from an interaction between the individual, the task and the environment (Shumway-Cook and Woollacott, 2001) suggesting that systems function impairment is only one factor that should be targeted for intervention. Gillen and Burkhardt (1998), writing from an occupational therapy perspective, target their intervention at the activity level as well as the systems level. They feel that practice of the whole activity provides a better environment for learning than practice of components of the activity. Shumway-Cook and Woollacott (2001) emphasise the importance of task specific practice that targets more specifically the activity level. Similarly, Carr and Shepherd (1980) advocate the practice of tasks in the situation in which they must be performed thereby ensuring that learning is task specific. They also advocate reduction of hands-on therapist intervention and more specific client individual practice. Client self-practice can then afford the individual more power and responsibility over the rehabilitation they are receiving and possibly its outcome.

Empowerment versus disempowerment: the role of the physiotherapist

A fundamental principle of health promotion is to empower individuals and communities thus enabling them to increase control over their level of health and wellbeing (Tones, 2001). De Vito (1988) describes rehabilitation as aiming to enable disabled clients to achieve the highest functional ability that they are capable of. The emphasis here is on the client as an active participant in the rehabilitation process. This would suggest that one role of the rehabilitation physiotherapist might be to enable the client to increase control over the rehabilitation process through empowering methodologies.

Self-efficacy theory (Bandura, 1982) is one methodological approach to health promotion that presents the need to empower individuals to enable change in behaviour and is concerned with perception of individual efficacy or ability to control an action. Self-efficacy influences an individual's ability to perceive their true situation and ability to influence it, in the face of obstacles. Empowerment from the health professional to the client involves the health professional not simply transferring power to the client, which is sometimes referred to as impowerment (MacDonald, 1998; see also Chapter 2 in this text) but awareness and skill development that enable them to take control of their rehabilitation. In subacute rehabilitation the physiotherapist is in an ideal position to facilitate the transfer of power or in the management of long standing impairment, in facilitating the maintenance of empowerment. (For further discussion of client empowerment in physiotherapy practice see Chapter 14.)

Impowerment and empowerment of the client are fundamental to physiotherapy practice in all rehabilitation settings and are implicit in rehabilitation practice. Impowerment aims to relinquish power that the professional in a medical setting might hold and allow the client to take the lead role. Client empowerment seems to be more developed in spinal cord injury rehabilitation, with more of a focus on individual activity and the aim of useful occupation following system impairment. However some of the lessons learned in this area have not necessarily transferred to rehabilitation in stroke and head injury.

French (1994) discusses empowerment in terms of the role of the ICD and ICIDH (now the ICF) and how this relates to the practice of health professionals, particularly therapists. She reinforces the view that the ICIDH takes a broader view of disease and system impairment than the ICD and allows the examination of the results of disease from the individual's perspective in terms of the impact of the disease on general health and wellbeing. The ICIDH therefore allows the consequence of disease to be seen in terms of its implications for social and physical functioning within the individual's social and physical environment.

The ICIDH, however, has been criticised by organisations representing disabled people, and was rejected by Disabled People's International (IDP) (French, 1994). The criticism is directed at the ICIDH because it still suggests that disability and handicap arise from impairment rather than from social and environmental causes. The ICF goes some way to addressing these criticisms because it has moved further away from the medical model and towards a more social model of health. In the ICF activity and participation look much more at the different constraints in society that may limit social functioning irrespective of reduced function at systems level. Nonetheless, alterations in function at systems level are still a significant factor.

Physiotherapeutic practitioners with biomedical backgrounds need to consider classification systems such as the ICF when contemplating how to practise in a rehabilitation setting. This is particularly the case in neurorehabilitation where the physiotherapist has to take account of factors involved in a client's ability to function and needs to go beyond the impairment of the system and consider wider function. If the focus of intervention is purely on the system impairment then even when improvement is achieved this may not lead to improvement at a functional activity level. It is also much harder for the client to become responsible for their rehabilitation if it has no functional significance for them. Empowerment is enabled when the clients are able to take more responsibility for their own rehabilitation. A focus on activity and participatory function is one factor in achieving this.

The intervention of single professionals in assisting in the empowerment of individual clients has some support in the literature. Tones (1991) argues that a critical part of empowering individuals is to teach them the relevant skills required in the particular situation they face. He asserts that professionals are generally well placed to do this with an emphasis on interventions such as teaching (for example, exercise to be carried out by the client) that assists in enabling the individual to promote their own health and wellbeing. Physiotherapy despite having a focus on system impairment is in a prime situation to take on this role. Labonte (1994) also emphasises the need for intervention to encourage and develop empowerment at both an individual and a small group level, which is often the setting in which physiotherapy practice takes place. Physiotherapy as a profession is therefore in an ideal situation to promote health through processes of empowerment of those clients undergoing rehabilitation following brain injury.

In neurorehabilitation practice, however, physiotherapists are not usually working independently, but as part of an interdisciplinary team consisting of other therapy professions such as occupational therapy (see contributions in Part II), speech and language therapy (see Chapter 18) as well as nursing (see Part I) and medicine. Therefore physiotherapy should not be considered as a stand-alone profession in the neurorehabilitation context but as one factor in the whole rehabilitation programme.

While physiotherapists may have an ideal opportunity to empower the clients that they work with, certain barriers exist. Some of the treatment approaches as previously discussed include strategies for treatment that may, dependent on interpretation by individual clinicians, lead to disempowerment rather than empowerment of the client.

Treatment approaches such as proprioceptive neuromuscular facilitation (PNF) (Knott and Voss, 1968) are based on the reflexive model of motor control. PNF begins with the physiotherapist maintaining control of treatment intervention and does not allow the client to direct or control the exercise programme initially. However the approach quite quickly allows the client to take responsibility for their own progression with assisted practice with the therapist and then independent practice. However the exercises to be practised are abstract and the approach does not directly address integration into meaningful function. So while the approach does allow for some client involvement, the control is still predominantly with the physiotherapist.

From the hierarchical model a widely used treatment approach in the United Kingdom (UK) is that of Bobath (1990). This approach relies heavily on the analytical skill and the hands-on facilitation ability of the physiotherapist. The control in terms of the intervention is with the physiotherapist. The approach focusses on the quality of movement performance, but does not directly address issues of task practice. This approach has undergone significant development in recent years but these changes in perspective are poorly represented in the literature and therefore their impact on client empowerment is difficult to assess. However with the current documented evidence available, the approach is very much physiotherapist led and directed.

The systems model has led to the development of models of treatment such as motor relearning (Carr and Shepherd, 1980). This approach emphasises the importance of the relearning of normal movement but also has a heavy emphasis on practice of specific tasks and then incorporation of training into the functional setting. This approach while initially being physiotherapist directed allows for significant client control and involvement during rehabilitation, incorporating task practice and self-directed practice by the client.

To an extent it is essential that the physiotherapist take a role in directing intervention at the initial stages because they are the specialists in the field of physical rehabilitation. However the skill is in transferring control to the client using an empowering approach. This process will involve health education so that the client understands the principles they are working towards and are enabled to perform component or task practice. This approach is very dependent on the extent to which the client is able to take responsibility for his or her own intervention. In the case of clients who have significant cognitive impairment or cognitive impairment linked with profound physical impairment this may be very difficult. However it is possible in the majority of cases, even in severe complex impairment following brain injury, for the client to take elements of control for themselves. Even in these cases, or perhaps especially in these cases, the physiotherapist needs to consider ways in which power can be transferred from the professional to the client.

Health promotion and health education through physiotherapy practice

The health promotion principle of empowerment has developed from a number of WHO declarations, particularly the Ottawa Charter (WHO, 1986) (see Chapter 1 for further discussion of the WHO health promoting principles). Tones (2001) stresses that empowerment has the primary concern of assisting people to obtain control over their own lives and as a result health. Rehabilitation contributes positively to health promotion at a secondary level as it attempts to empower and improve quality of life (Brown et al., 1996).

Physiotherapy in neurological rehabilitation could also be seen as having a wider role to play in health promotion. In the UK this is primarily through organisations such as the physiotherapy professional body's (Chartered Society of Physiotherapy's) special interest groups (Association of Chartered Physiotherapists Interested in Neurology) and involvement of these organisations in influencing governmental policy as represented for example by the National Institute for Clinical Excellence (NICE) and National Service Frameworks (NSFs) for healthcare provision. It therefore becomes apparent that the role of physiotherapy in neurological rehabilitation is not as simple as that of pure client interaction, but also involves broader influence on policy and provision of rehabilitation services for neurologically impaired adults. Health policy is therefore crucial in the development of public health and will affect certain groups of the population in different ways. Some health policy will focus specifically on certain groups within the population, for example those with neurological impairment or brain injury. Physiotherapists need to continue to be involved in influencing policy at this level.

Health promotion is also concerned with sustaining or increasing an individual's level of wellbeing. A number of authors have identified that health promotion may involve different strategies to achieve the goals of empowering individuals to maintain their own health (Tones, 1983; Tannahill, 1990). Latter (1998) identifies health education as one component part of health promotion practice essential in empowering individuals. Health education with individual clients is generally encapsulated as teaching and information giving activity aimed at helping them achieve and maintain physical, mental and social wellbeing, and at a primary level free from disease or infirmity (Jones and Douglas, 2000). Physiotherapists therefore have a role in the empowerment of the individual in rehabilitation. From a physiotherapy perspective this will be in terms of facilitating the client in taking responsibility for areas of their own physical rehabilitation and ongoing physical management (for further discussion of health promotion through physiotherapy practice see Chapter 12).

Rehabilitation practice goes beyond health education and is often on an individual client basis with each rehabilitation programme specifically tailored to the individual. The physiotherapy programme will involve aspects of health education that will lead to empowerment. However the intervention will also need to go beyond this to produce changes at the systems function level, and improvement in the system impairment, which are then incorporated into functional activity. In subacute rehabilitation it is often not possible for the client to feel fully empowered in the initial phases of the rehabilitation process. If an individual has undergone a stroke, for example, then initially they may well have restricted understanding about its pathology or related physiology and anatomy. They will also have limited knowledge of how to physically rehabilitate themselves. This is where the physiotherapist is the expert in the client's physical rehabilitation and will provide intervention aimed at both the impairment of systems function and the activity restrictions. An explanation of why intervention is undertaken, and the reasons behind specific techniques or exercises would be given. Education regarding the pathology, intervention and prognosis would also be provided. However even at this stage of the rehabilitation process effort needs to be made to actively involve the client, and carer when appropriate, in the rehabilitation programme. One way in which this can be done is through the goal setting process.

Goal setting takes place in neurological rehabilitation in order to set realistic targets for the outcome of the rehabilitation process. The physiotherapist in conjunction with the rest of the therapy team and the patient will set the goals for the rehabilitation programme. One method of goal setting used in neurological rehabilitation for example is Goal Attainment Scaling (GAS). Goal attainment scaling is an individualised health outcome measure that was first introduced in the 1960s by Kirusek and Sherman (1968) for assessing outcomes in mental health settings. It has been shown to be suitable for health problems which warrant a multidimensional and individualised approach to treatment planning and outcome measurement and has been used to demonstrate clinically important change in a variety of settings including elderly care (Schultz, 1977 cited in Kiresuk et al., 1994), neurological management in children (Maloney et al., 1978) and rehabilitation counselling (Goodyear and Bitter, 1974). GAS is useful when considering the empowerment of the client, because it directly involves the client in the identification, setting and scoring of their rehabilitation goals. The process of setting the goals involves the client in scoring how important the goal is to them, while the rehabilitation team score how difficult it might be to achieve the goal. This process in itself gives the client significant power at an early stage to direct their own rehabilitation, albeit with the advice and input of the rehabilitation team (for further discussion and examples of client centred practice see Chapters 4 and 8).

In subacute rehabilitation the aim is to progress to the point where the client becomes an expert in their own rehabilitation and management. The time taken for individuals to achieve control over their rehabilitation may vary considerably depending on the impairments to body system function and activity restrictions they face. There is also a significant period of psychological adjustment to a new situation, within which they now need to function. This adjustment period will vary greatly between different individuals even when they seem to the outside observer to have very similar system impairment. For example following a stroke resulting in hemiplegia (loss of sensory and motor function down one side of the body) improvements in the system impairment may be seen. However recovery of hand function may not be possible because of the initial pathology. The individual then has to adjust to the physical situation of performing activities with a single functioning hand. They also need to adjust psychologically to this new situation.

Physiotherapists need to ensure that they enable and empower, rather than allow clients to become dependent on them for intervention and psychological support in the long term. In the majority of cases following a neurological insult the client must progress past the need for physiotherapy input and become functional in their social setting even if the system impairment is not fully resolved. In the majority of cases it is not possible for the client's system to function at the level it had prior to the neurological insult. French (1994) identifies that while individuals may not have an impairment free body at the system level, this does not mean they have to necessarily suffer from activity restriction or limitation in their participation. It is therefore important for the client to understand this and become the expert in their own rehabilitation, so that at the right point in time they go beyond rehabilitation and are just living life.

Case example

John is a 36 year old man who suffered a traumatic brain injury six years ago. He has had a period of subacute rehabilitation and now lives in his own home with a live-in carer. Initially following his head injury he was unable to sit, stand, transfer or feed himself. However following rehabilitation he is now able to sit and propel himself in a manual wheelchair and transfer chair to chair by standing with assistance from his carer. He has a modified vehicle, which his carer drives, has a busy social life and is also involved in some part time work with support from his employer. He has made improvements in his system impairments and has also made large progress in terms of his activities and participation in the wider community. However he is still unhappy with his inability to walk and makes constant requests for more physiotherapy to address this. His previous physiotherapist feels that he will be unable to make further progress with walking because the area of brain damage has resulted in limited control of his leg movement, which has not improved. John is unwilling to accept this and still seems to be adjusting psychologically to his altered physical situation and is having difficulty coming to terms with a different way of functioning. Despite appearing to have an active and interesting lifestyle, John may feel that his quality of life is very limited because of his inability to walk. Napolitano (1996) makes the point that in modern Western societies inability to walk does not have to be a significant activity limitation. She identifies that, subject to the physical environment, it is possible to function at a high level. However many restrictions to full participation in society still exist for individuals with system impairment. Many public buildings still lack equity of access for wheelchair users when compared to that provided for those without impairment. Nevertheless it is still possible for John to participate in an active lifestyle but his inability to make the psychological adjustment is currently limiting his progress.

In a minority of patients following a neurological insult continued physiotherapy is required just to prevent deterioration in their physical condition. However clients in this position can still move beyond rehabilitation and accept that physiotherapy intervention may not be about producing improvement to system impairment or even an activity restriction but is provided to prevent deterioration or secondary complications of the neurological insult. However in the majority of cases, clients need to be empowered to take an active role in partnership with their interdisciplinary team to promote their own rehabilitation. This should lead to positive gains in physical rehabilitation, but more importantly to an adjustment to functioning and engaging in wider society when professional support is withdrawn.

Physiotherapy as a profession has a significant role to play in promoting health in the field of neurological rehabilitation, particularly through individual empowerment, but also in wider healthy public policy. Physiotherapists are in an ideal position through their professional body and special interest groups to positively influence policy making so that the physical rehabilitation requirements of clients are taken into account. The physiotherapist is actively engaged in the secondary heath promotion of clients through empowerment approaches, particularly those that relate to health education and the development of personal skills. The physiotherapist assists the individual to make functional improvement at the level of system impairment and has a key role in enabling the client to take responsibility for their own rehabilitation and adjusting to a different way of functioning. This should eventually lead to the client becoming expert in his or her own condition.

Neurological rehabilitation is an interdisciplinary occupation with the client at the centre. This should place physiotherapy practice in this speciality, in an ideal position to consider the empowerment of clients and their involvement in the rehabilitation process. The physiotherapy profession has influence at a strategic or policy level, but it is at the specific client interaction level that physiotherapy seems to have the greatest potential for promoting the health of individuals.

References

Bandura, A. (1982) Self-efficacy mechanism in human agency. *American Psychologist* **37** (2): 122–47.

Bobath, B. (1990) *Adult Hemiplegia: Evaluation and Treatment*, third edition. Oxford: Butterworth-Heinemann.

Brown, I., Renwick, R. and Nagler, M. (1996) The centrality of quality of life in health promotion and rehabilitation. In Renwick, R., Brown, I. and Nagler, M. (eds) *Quality of Life in Health Promotion and Rehabilitation: Conceptual Approaches, Issues and Applications*. London: Sage.

Carr, J. and Shepherd, R. (1980) *Physiotherapy in Disorders of the Brain*. London: Heinemann.

Carr, J. and Shepherd, R. (1998) *Neurological Rehabilitation – Optimising Motor Performance*. Oxford: Butterworth-Heinemann.

Carr, J. and Shepherd, R. (2003) *Stroke Rehabilitation*. Oxford: Butterworth-Heinemann.

De Vito, A. J. (1988) Documenting client education in rehabilitation: an interdisciplinary approach. *Rehabilitation Nursing* 13 (1), 26–8.

Downie, R. S., Tannahill, C. and Tannahill, A. (1996) *Health Promotion: Models and Values*, second edition. Oxford: Oxford University Press.

Edwards, S. (2002) *Neurological Physiotherapy*, second edition. Edinburgh: Churchill Livingstone.

French, S. (1994) *On Equal Terms: Working with Disabled People*. Oxford: Butterworth-Heinemann.

Gillen, G. and Burkhardt, A. (1998) *Stroke Rehabilitation: a Functions-Based Approach*. London: Mosby.

Goodyear, D. L. and Bitter, J. A. (1974) Goal attainment scaling as a programme evaluation measure in rehabilitation. *Journal of Applied Rehabilitation Counselling* 5: 19–26.

Jones, L. and Douglas, J. (2000) The rise of health promotion. In Katz, J., Peberdy, A. and Douglas, J. (eds) *Promoting Health: Knowledge and Practice*. Basingstoke: Palgrave (now Palgrave Macmillan)/Open University.

Kiresuk, T. and Sherman, R. (1968) Goal Attainment Scaling: a general method for evaluating community mental health programmes. *Community Mental Health Journal* 4: 443–53.

Knott, M. and Voss, D. E. (1968) *Proprioceptive Neuromuscular Facilitation*, second edition. London: Harper and Row.

Labonte, S. (1994) Health promotion and empowerment: reflections on professional practice. *Health Education Quarterly* 21: 253–68.

Latter, S. (1998) Health promotion in the acute setting: the case for empowering nurses. In Kendall, S. (ed.) *Health and Empowerment: Research and Practice*. London: Arnold.

Macdonald, T. H. (1998) *Rethinking Health Promotion: a Global Approach*. London: Routledge.

Maloney, F. P., Mirrett, P., Brooks, C. and Johannes, K. (1978) Use of the Goal Attainment Scale in the treatment and ongoing evaluation of neurologically handicapped children. *American Journal of Occupational Therapy* 32: 505–10.

Mathiowetz, V. and Haugen, J. B. (1994) Motor behaviour research: implications for therapeutic approaches to central nervous system dysfunction. *American Journal of Occupational Therapy* 48: 733–45.

Mulder, T. (1993) Current topics in motor control: implications for rehabilitation. In Greenwood, R., Barns, M. P., McMillan, T. M. and Ward, C. D. (eds) *Neurological Rehabilitation*. Edinburgh: Churchill Livingstone.

Napolitano, S. (1996) Mobility impairment. In Hales, G. (ed) *Beyond Disability – Towards an Enabling Society*. London: Sage.

Schmidt, R. A. (1975) A schema theory of discrete motor learning. *Psychology Review* **82**: 225–60.

Schultz, P. R. (1977) Primary health care to the elderly: an evaluation of two health manpower patterns. Reprinted in Kiresuk, T. J., Smith, A. and Cardillo, J. E. (eds) (1994) *Goal Attainment Scaling: Applications, Theory and Measurement.* Totowa, NJ: Lawrence Erlbaum Associates.

Sherrington, C. (1906) The interactive action of the nervous system. Reprinted in Kandel, E. R., Schwartz, J. H. and Jessell, T. M. (eds) (1991) *Principles of Neural Science*, third edition. Stamford, CT: Appleton Lange.

Shumway-Cook, A. and Woollacott, M. H. (1995) *Motor Control: Theory and Practical Applications.* Baltimore, MD: Williams and Wilkins.

Shumway-Cook, A. and Woollacott, M. H. (2001) *Motor Control: Theory and Practical Applications*, second edition. Philadelphia, PA: Lippincott, Williams and Wilkins.

Stokes, M. (1998) *Neurological Physiotherapy.* London: Mosby.

Tannahill, A. (1990) Health education and health promotion: planning for the 1990s. *Health Education Journal* **49** (4): 194–8.

Tones, K. (1983) Education and health promotion: new direction. *Journal of the Institute Health Education* **21** (4): 121–31.

Tones, K. (1991) Health promotion, empowerment and the psychology of control. *Journal of the Institute of Health Education* **29**: 17–26.

Tones, K. (2001) Health promotion: the empowerment imperative. In Scriven, A. and Orme, J. (eds) *Health Promotion: Professional Perspectives*, second edition. Basingstoke: Palgrave (now Palgrave Macmillan).

Wade, D. T. and de Jong, B. A. (2000) Recent advances in rehabilitation: clinical review. *British Medical Journal* **320**: 1385–8.

World Health Organisation (1984) *Health Promotion: a WHO Discussion Document on the Concepts and Principles.* Geneva: WHO.

World Health Organisation (1986) *Ottawa Charter for Health Promotion.* Geneva: WHO.

World Health Organisation (2001) *International Classification of Functioning, Disability and Health, Short Version.* Geneva: WHO.

CHAPTER 14

Physiotherapists Promoting Health in Cardiac Rehabilitation

JENNI JONES AND SALLY HINTON

Cardiovascular disease (CVD) encompasses all disorders of the heart and blood vessels and accounts for almost a third of global deaths. Coronary heart disease (CHD) mortality rates worldwide have varied greatly over the past few decades highlighting the important contribution of changing environmental factors alongside the involvement of genetic factors (Hardman and Stensel, 2003). The United Kingdom (UK) currently has one of the highest mortality rates in the world with the exception of some Eastern and Central European countries, for example Romania (Hardman and Stensel, 2003). In the UK, CHD is the most common cause of premature death accounting for 125,000 deaths in 2000 (Office for National Statistics, 2001) and although mortality rates have been declining over the last 30 years, the overall burden of CHD on health resources is now far greater due to the advances in diagnostic techniques and surgical interventions.

Cardiac rehabilitation is now considered an integral part of the regular medical management of patients with CHD with increasing numbers of registered programmes in the UK over the past decade (Horgan et al., 1992). In 1997 Bethell et al. (2000) identified 300 programmes, of varying structure and service provision, in a large national audit. Cardiac rehabilitation aims to achieve improved recovery from myocardial infarction (MI), coronary artery bypass surgery/graft (CABG), or angioplasty and reduce the risk of recurrent cardiac events, and as such is seen as secondary prevention. Originally cardiorehabilitation addressed only patients recovering from acute myocardial infarction and focussed on supervised exercise sessions and return to work. More recently, however, the rehabilitation process has evolved into a more comprehensive lifestyle intervention programme as reflected in the Task Force report of the Working Group on Cardiac Rehabilitation of the European Society of Cardiology (Tavazzi et al., 1992). This approach has been echoed in the World Health Organisation (WHO) revised definition (WHO, 1993) of cardiac rehabilitation and was further reinforced by the Second Joint Task Force of the European and other Societies' recommendations on prevention of CHD in clinical practice (Wood et al., 1998). To reflect the increased focus on secondary prevention Goble and Worcester (1999) defined cardiac rehabilitation as the coordinated sum of interventions required to ensure the best physical, psychological and social conditions so that patients with chronic or post acute cardiovascular disease may, by their own efforts, preserve or resume optimal functioning in society and, through improved health behaviours, slow or reverse progression of disease.

Comprehensive cardiac rehabilitation typically encompasses exercise training, health education about risk factor modification and counselling and is delivered ultimately by a variety of healthcare professionals who together offer a wide and specialised skill base. The overall effectiveness in regard to mortality has been well documented, where early meta-analyses demonstrated that patients who attended exercise based cardiac rehabilitation after a myocardial infarction had a statistically significant reduction in all cause and cardiac mortality of 20–25 per cent compared to those patients who did not attend (Oldridge, 1988; O'Connor et al., 1989). A more recent meta-analysis (Jolliffe et al., 2000a) stated that all cause mortality reduced by 27 per cent with those patients who attended an exercise based cardiac rehabilitation programme. The trials included in this review however mainly enrolled white middle aged males with very few trials enrolling women and the elderly and the ethnic origin of the participants was seldom reported.

The risk factors for CHD are well established, with substantial scientific evidence to support the finding that lifestyle interventions including smoking cessation, healthy food choices and increased physical activity, control of blood pressure, cholesterol and diabetes, and the selective use of prophylactic drug therapies (aspirin and other antiplatelet therapies, beta blockers, ACE inhibitors, lipid lowering drugs and anticoagulants) can reduce morbidity and mortality in patients with established coronary disease and can also help to reduce the risk of developing this disease in high risk individuals (Wood et al., 1998). Comprehensive cardiac rehabilitation aims to address all modifiable risk factors (Figure 14.1), which are susceptible to intervention, for example by a person changing their attitude, lifestyle or behaviour patterns, or through administration of drugs (Brodie, 2000).

A variety of expertise is required for a comprehensive cardiac rehabilitation, typically that of a cardiac specialist nurse, physiotherapist, occupational therapist, dietitian, exercise professional, member of the medical team and psychologist. The contribution in terms of patient contact hours and administration time of each team member will vary greatly along with the profession of the coordinator of the service, although most commonly the coordinator is a specialist nurse or physiotherapist. This multidisciplinary team achieve lifestyle targets through behaviour change strategies, using a number of possible theoretical approaches or models that attempt to describe the factors that are important in changing and maintaining health behaviour. These approaches

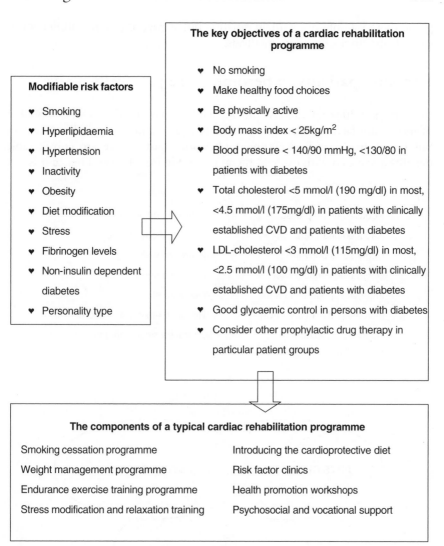

Figure 14.1 The contribution of a cardiac rehabilitation programme in the management of modifiable risk factors for CVD

Sources: Brodie (2000); European Society of Cardiology (2003)

are applied by all disciplines, for example smoking cessation interventions by the nurse specialist, stress management by the occupational therapist and dietary modification by the dietitian. The physiotherapist also uses behaviour change strategies to support patients in becoming physically active and although this will be discussed in more detail it is essential to recognise that the physiotherapist does not work in isolation but as part of an integrating coordinated team employing these methods.

Enabling patients to become more physically active

Over the past 20 years, exercise therapy has become a fundamental component of most multifactorial cardiac rehabilitation programmes, typically delivered, but by no means exclusively, by a physiotherapist. There are considerable benefits associated with exercise therapy (see Figure 14.2) and hence it is not

Reduced blood pressure   Improved quality of life

Reduced heart rate   Increased confidence

Reduced % body fat   Improved wellbeing

Decreased fibrinogen levels   Improved self-efficacy

Improved lipoprotein profile   Reduced stress

Increased insulin sensitivity   Reduced anxiety and depression

Reduced symptoms   Improved sleep patterns

Decreased risk of arrhythmia

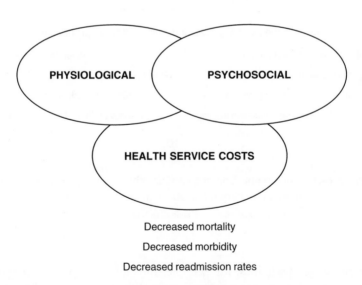

Decreased mortality

Decreased morbidity

Decreased readmission rates

Figure 14.2   The benefits of exercise training in cardiac rehabilitation

Sources: Astrand (1987); Biddle (1995); Bouchard and Despres (1995); Ferguson et al. (1987);
Manson et al. (1992); Martinsen et al. (1985)

difficult to justify its inclusion in this population group, who as a result of CVD often present with physical, cognitive and social problems. Some of these benefits are associated with physical activity whilst others are associated with greater intensities and increasing levels of physical fitness.

The problems associated with physical inactivity are significant and hence the challenge for the physiotherapist is to get patients to participate in sufficient amounts of exercise and physical activity to confer the benefits outlined in Figure 14.2, as well as provide strategies to maintain these changes in exercise behaviour in the longer term. Currently few people across Europe participate in the recommended levels of physical activity to benefit health (EUROASPIRE Study Group, 1997, 2001). This is further supported by a UK study that found that although 80 per cent of participants considered themselves to be fit, one third of men and two thirds of women were unable to continue walking at three miles per hour up a 1 in 20 slope without becoming uncomfortably breathless (Health Education Authority (HEA)/Sports Council, 1992). In recognition of the increasing proportions of the population categorised as sedentary more recent public health messages have moved away from the traditional emphasis on formal exercise prescription and now highlight the health benefits conferred by daily participation in general physical activity. The change was prompted by the need to increase professional and public awareness that relatively moderate physical activity will still confer significant health benefits, even when peak aerobic capacity, a measure of physical fitness, remains unchanged. As a consequence, the current public health messages recommend that adults should accumulate at least 30 minutes of moderate intensity physical activity on most, preferably all, days of the week (Pate et al., 1995; Physical Activity and Cardiovascular Health, 1996; US Department of Health and Human Services, 1996). It is important to recognise that these public health messages are associated with primary prevention and illness prevention, whereas in individuals with established heart disease the health related benefits are supported by cardiovascular endurance training exercise programmes, resulting in potentially greater workloads. The health and fitness benefits associated with physical activity follow a dose response relationship, in that some activity is better than none and in most circumstances more confers greater benefit. Hence, cardiac rehabilitation physiotherapists who, by definition, are working more in the context of secondary prevention, will not only be involved in motivating patients to develop an habitually physically active lifestyle, for example, using the stairs rather than a lift, but also in prescribing and delivering moderate intensity endurance exercise training which will confer measurable physiological changes known to reduce symptoms and mortality (Leon, 2000).

A key element in the success of an exercise intervention is the use of a client centred approach by the physiotherapist, where exercise prescription is highly individualised and a variety of options are offered to provide a menu based approach to cater for differing needs. The physiotherapist is able to use their knowledge and skills in assessing fitness and interpreting clinical exercise test results to synthesise assessment findings into safe and effective exercise and physical activity plans, sensitive to each individual patient's physical, psychosocial, cognitive and behavioural capabilities and needs. The physiotherapist also uses extensive background knowledge in pathophysiology in order to adapt exercises to patients with co-morbidities to CVD, thus individualising the exercise to be both clinically effective as well as sensitive to these limitations (Association of Chartered Physiotherapists Interested in Cardiac Rehabilitation (ACPICR), 2003). Providing options allows a more client centred approach and although the exercise programme is predominantly outpatient and group based it may be provided in a range of settings, such as hospitals, community health centres, leisure centres and general medical practices, or a combination of these. Outpatient cardiac rehabilitation may also be provided on an individual basis in the patient's home after a thorough assessment and with regular reviews. The length, content and type of programme will vary according to the specific needs of the individual and the available resources. Generally, these outpatient programmes commence after the patient has spent a short period of time at home following discharge from hospital, and last until optimal recovery is achieved, typically in six to 12 weeks (New Zealand Guideline Group (NZGG), 2002). This structured outpatient cardiac rehabilitation is a recognised focal point for the development of a lifelong approach to prevention and hence empowering the patient to adopt self-management strategies is a key objective during this time. Ongoing maintenance of behaviour change beyond the period of inpatient and outpatient rehabilitation is crucial if long term health benefits are to be realised.

Enabling people to make behaviour change is a difficult and dynamic process but is essential if lifestyle interventions are to be effective and long term. Each cardiac patient will enter into the programme with a different combination of feelings, support, motivation and goals and it is therefore difficult to prescribe a single methodology (NZGG, 2002). A variety of sociocognitive models are utilised in supporting patients in becoming more physically active whilst participating in cardiac rehabilitation. The health belief model (Becker et al., 1979) states that a person is likely to become physically active if they perceive a threat to their personal health and this behaviour change is influenced by a combination of triggers to action and beliefs. Hence the patient must also believe that making changes will result in a reduction of risk. As part of the assessment process the physiotherapist assesses the patient's perception of the risk of physical inactivity and health beliefs using a series of questions relating to illness perception. Another important concept used by physiotherapists in cardiac rehabilitation, which relates to empowerment approaches, is self-efficacy theory, where the individual patient has to judge their ability to devise and execute strategies of action to successfully perform the desired behaviour (NZGG, 2002). The patient is more likely to sustain a physically active lifestyle if they feel it is within their capabilities. Regular contact with the patient during the outpatient programme allows the physiotherapist to reinforce the benefits and individual achievements, provide the patient with personal experiences and the opportunity to compare with others as well as provide the patient with valuable feedback. These factors as well as the use of counselling techniques to identify strategies to overcome perceived barriers and build confidence all potentially increase self-efficacy and lead to greater ability to sustain positive behaviour changes in the longer term.

The theory of planned behaviour (Azjen, 1991) is another model commonly used by the physiotherapist in cardiac rehabilitation to assist patients in becoming more physically active. This model is concerned with behavioural intention, involving attitudes and social norms, and is incorporated by the physiotherapist identifying at the initial assessment the patient's attitude towards being active and the influences of the patient's social conditions, as knowledge of these will provide a framework in planning a feasible exercise plan. The final model that will be discussed and that is commonly implemented clinically within cardiac rehabilitation is the transtheoretical model or stages of behaviour change model (Prochaska and DiClemente, 1984) in which patients are seen as moving through a series of stages to change behaviour. Marcus et al. (1992) described this model as the Stages of Exercise Behaviour Change (SEBC) when they used it within the area of health related physical activity. SEBC enables a client centred approach where the physiotherapist identifies the stage of change that the patient currently is at and subsequently responds with an appropriate exercise intervention for this stage. For example with a patient who is contemplating whether to take up exercise the physiotherapist will provide health education, written and verbal, assisting the patient in their decision making process, formed from weighing up the advantages and disadvantages to change. Positive features for exercising could include enhanced confidence, increased self-esteem and having more energy for one's family and friends. Negative factors could include being too tired to exercise, feeling uncomfortable and breathless, and not having sufficient time. Knowledge of individuals' perception of advantages and disadvantages to increasing physical activity levels is essential to any effective exercise programme. Health promotion interventions, therefore, need to focus on increasing the advantages that the participants might feel about increasing their exercise levels, in order for movement to occur through the stages. Patients who attend outpatient cardiac rehabilitation are usually in the action stage and may be new to this exercise behaviour and hence need support, positive reinforcement and techniques to increase self-efficacy. Once effective exercise behaviour has been maintained for longer than six months, the individuals will have reached the maintenance stage of this model and will therefore need assistance by the physiotherapist in identifying triggers that may result in relapse and possible strategies to overcome these triggers. The movement through this model is dynamic and recognises that an individual can easily regress out of a stage as well as move forwards. The presence of the relapse stage and the spiral design of the model is especially pertinent to exercise behaviour as maintaining regular exercise can require a lot of effort in terms of time and money and therefore relapse can easily occur, so the physiotherapist prepares the patient for this possibility, highlighting this as a learning experience rather than a failure to succeed.

Finally following the assessment process, goal setting, according to the patient's priority, forms a fundamental component in planning the exercise intervention. The inclusion of motivational counselling techniques, a directive client centred counselling style that is designed to assist clients in exploring and resolving ambivalence to increase motivation for change often supports this agenda setting process. The emphasis therefore is on facilitating physical activity to become a relatively permanent lifestyle choice by helping the patients to help themselves. The physiotherapist should actively listen, reflect back to the patient key messages, paraphrase and summarise in order to guide the patient in becoming physically active.

In summary cardiac rehabilitation provides the opportunity for physiotherapists to coach and encourage patients and their families to participate in sufficient amounts of exercise and physical activity to benefit health. However to achieve this each individual needs to have a belief that change is possible, be motivated to make the change and have a support network and personal capacity to enact and sustain change. The exercise intervention delivered should be client centred and matched to the patient's specific circumstances, readiness to change and process of change. The physiotherapist further encourages a client centred approach by demonstrating empathy and through the use of motivational counselling techniques aims to build the individual's belief that becoming more active is possible both now and in the longer term outside of the programme. Furthermore a proactive approach, where barriers are identified and responding to these barriers is practised as well as identifying coping strategies to become active again as quickly as possible should the individual experience a relapse will in addition facilitate maintenance of long term behaviour change.

Factors affecting long term compliance with exercise

There are many barriers to individuals attending their first appointment and consequently adhering to completing the whole programme, alongside factors which will affect the long term compliance with lifestyle changes recommended by cardiac rehabilitation professionals. Attendance at outpatient cardiac rehabilitation programmes may be restricted due to the limited accessibility of services in terms of the venue, time of day, transport, the low socioeconomic status of the patient and lack of referral or non-recommendation from medical staff (Jolliffe et al., 2000b). Greenfield et al. (2004) conducted a qualitative study of reasons for non-participation and non-adherence in 40 patients. Reasons for non-attendance were multifactorial and individualistic and included social characteristics, individual patient needs and location of programmes. Glazer et al. (2002) highlighted that those patients who had poorer psychological functioning at the start of a cardiac rehabilitation programme were less likely to adhere to the exercise sessions and more likely to drop out of rehabilitation. These results reinforced the importance of evaluating psychological functioning in patients entering cardiac rehabilitation services. Other studies have highlighted recruitment issues and identified women and the elderly as less likely than men to be invited to attend cardiac rehabilitation programmes (Gavin and Gavin, 1995).

Physiotherapists need to be aware of factors that are strongly related to poor adherence so that any health promoting strategies can be appropriately targeted. Daly et al. (2002) identified these factors as strength of physician's referral, being female, being older, having a lower education status, and having a poor functional capacity. King et al. (1997) studied healthy individuals in order to identify the best combination of predictors of long term compliance with exercise and found that initial Body Mass Index (BMI), fitness and perceived stress levels were predictive variables.

Compliance, which is an individual's adherence to a medical regimen or health advice, will be affected by a person's motivation and how important the individual perceives the lifestyle change to be in reducing their health problem. Individuals under close supervision in a structured exercise programme were found to quickly quit exercise when the supervision was discontinued (Ice, 1985). Dorn et al. (2000) also stated that compliance with an exercise training programme in myocardial infarction patients decreased over time and that individuals who were at high risk for repeat events were the ones most likely to show low compliance. The more information is given to an individual regarding an intended behaviour change the more likely the long term compliance for that particular behaviour, for example informing exercise participants in advance of the possible side effects of exercise may prevent a patient associating increased levels of activity with discomfort and accept symptoms as a sense of increasing exertion.

Regular exercise is time consuming, inconvenient, possibly costly and therefore adherence to an exercise programme is often lower than to other medical regimens, such as prescribed medication. Exercise adherence rates in cardiac patients are similar to that of the general population, reported at around 50 per cent dropout within the first six months (Buckley et al., 1999). Dishman (1986) explored long term compliance with exercise and identified factors influencing dropout rates. Medical reasons or ill health were stated as the most prominent factors and the avoidable reasons identified included inconvenient time, inaccessible location of sessions, insufficient time and lack of partner support. Other studies have described work, financial reasons and lack of motivation or commitment as reasons for dropout from a cardiac rehabilitation before rehabilitation goals have been met (Evenson and Fleury, 2000). Physiotherapists aiming to improve the individual's success in maintaining regular physical activity could target the inhibiting factors identified in the studies above.

A negative attitude to rehabilitation from partner and family will also affect those who attend (Scottish Intercollegiate Guidelines Network (SIGN), 2002) and effective health promotion interventions should include both the individual and their family as the impact of CHD is substantial and both patients and families collectively have to cope with the rehabilitation process. Difficulties may be experienced due to an anxious, overprotective or unsupportive partner, that may affect attendance. With interventions which target behaviours such as cardio-protective diet and regular exercise, therefore, it would be important to address the specific concerns of close family members (McGee, 1999). Some lifestyle changes require more family involvement than others. Maintaining a cardiopro-tective diet, for example, may rely on other family members who buy and prepare the patient's meals. Moreover, a spouse continuing to smoke when individuals are trying to give up reflects the importance of early partner involvement in the reha-bilitation process, encouraging their participation in exercise, as appropriate, and health education sessions. Partners can be involved to a varying degree through all the stages of recovery in increasing the likelihood of long term compliance (NHS Centre for Reviews and Dissemination, 1998) and support networks for families introduced at an early stage. The social influence of family and friends can have a positive impact on health by enhancing an individual's motivation to con-tinue an exercise regime and the presence of an effective support network is an important factor in preventing relapse from the desired lifestyle change.

Once the outpatient phase of cardiac rehabilitation is complete, in order for individuals to comply with long term exercise behaviour a seamless pathway of care from acute to community services which closely follows the individual's recovery is vital. Effective two way communication between all health profes-sionals in primary and secondary care and between health and leisure services is essential to allow this seamless care of the individual with coronary disease, which should begin immediately after the acute cardiac event or when the pro-fessional is made aware of the individual with CHD, which could be on diag-nosis prior to an acute event.

Physiotherapists play a key role in undertaking the exercise consultation prior to individuals safely exercising in the community independently and also in transferring information regarding an individual's clinical history and exer-cise prescription to community exercise instructors (Hughes et al., 2002). These consultations should be client centred, involving the evaluation of stage of change, the potential barriers to increasing physical activity, the presence of positive social support and finally, individual goal setting.

As identified in the evidence based guidelines produced jointly by the New Zealand Guideline Group and the Heart Foundation (NZGG, 2002) adopting a patient centred approach involves heightened sensitivity to social and environ-mental pressures on individual patients (Chapters 8 and 13 for further discussion of client centred approaches to promoting health). The behaviour change process should be specific to the personal and social context of the patient. As highlighted by these groups achieving a patient centred approach involves:

- negotiation
- reflective listening
- simple open ended questions
- the avoidance of confrontation

- increasing self efficacy
- clarifying and summarising
- working at the patients pace, respecting their autonomy
- being empathetic
- listening and encouraging with verbal and non-verbal cues
- belief that low motivation is not lack of power but the lack of a pathway.

Physiotherapists who provide exercise training in a client centred approach will promote health by improving the functional capacity of patients with cardiac disease, lessen the symptoms of angina and shortness of breath and hence make an important contribution to cardiac rehabilitation. The aim of exercise prescription is to provide individual advice on the level and type of exercise needed to improve functional capacity and increase energy expenditure without compromising safety or detracting from enjoyment. The physiotherapist has the challenge of providing a progressive individualised and client centred exercise plan that confers benefit but also considers clinical characteristics, lifestyle, attitudes, available social support, culture and environment. Assessment of the patient's beliefs, stage of change, motivation to change and self-efficacy are fundamental to supporting individuals to sustain behaviour change. Cardiac patients will face a number of barriers to behaviour change. To promote health effectively the physiotherapist must identify potential barriers and enable the patient to practise coping strategies to overcome these barriers, if changes are to be adhered to in the longer term. In order for the person to be empowered to adopt positive lifestyle change, the home environment and family relationships must be considered and the person given the tools to be resilient to the inhibiting factors to change. If there are barriers to attendance, the physiotherapist can provide home based cardiac rehabilitation hence advocating a menu based approach, with choices depending on patients' varying needs.

In conclusion, during the outpatient cardiorehabilitation programme patients are provided with the knowledge of lifestyle behaviours associated with a reduced risk of further cardiac disease that relate to their individual health concerns. Positive behaviour changes are enabled and most importantly patients are equipped with the necessary skills and confidence to sustain these changes in the longer term. The overall health promoting goal of the physiotherapist within cardiac rehabilitation, in conjunction with the other members of the multidisciplinary team, is to positively influence confidence, attitudes, beliefs, social efficacy and resilience in an approach designed to empower individuals and enable long term exercise behaviour.

References

Association of Chartered Physiotherapists Interested in Cardiac Rehabilitation (ACPICR) (2003) *Standards for the Exercise Component of Phase III Cardiac Rehabilitation*. London: Chartered Society of Physiotherapy.

Astrand, P. O. (1987) Exercise physiology and its role in disease prevention and in rehabilitation. *Archives of Physical Medicine and Rehabilitation* 68: 305–9.

Azjen, I. (1991) The theory of planned behaviour. *Behaviour and Human Decision Process* 50: 179–211.

Becker, M. H., Kirsch, J. P., Hafner, D. P., Drachman, R. H. and Taylor, D. W. (1979) Patient perceptions and compliance. In Haynes, R. B., Taylor, D. W. and Sackett, D. L. (eds) *Compliance in Health Care*. Baltimore, MD: Johns Hopkins University Press.

Bethell, H., Turner, S., Flint, E. J. and Rose, L. (2000) The BACR database of cardiac rehabilitation units in the UK. *Coronary Health Care* 4: 92–5.

Biddle, S. (1995) Exercise and psychosocial health. *Research Quarterly for Exercise and Sport* 66 (4): 292–7.

Bouchard, C. and Despres, J. (1995) Physical activity and health: atherosclerotic, metabolic, and hypertensive diseases. *Research Quarterly for Exercise and Sport* 66 (4): 268–75.

Brodie, D. (2000) *Cardiac Rehabilitation: an Educational Resource*. London: British Association of Cardiac Rehabilitation.

Buckley, J., Holmes, J. and Mapp, G. (1999) *Exercise on Prescription: Cardiovascular Activity for Health*. Oxford: Butterworth-Heinemann.

Daly, J., Sindone, A. P., Thompson, D. R., Hancock, K., Chang, E. and Davidson, P. (2002) Barriers to participation in and adherence to cardiac rehabilitation programs: a critical review. *Progress in Cardiovascular Nursing* 17: 8–17.

Dishman, R. K. (1986) Exercise compliance: a new view for public health. *Physician and Sports Medicine* 14: 5.

Dorn, J., Naughton, J., Imamura, D. and Trevisan, M. (2000) Correlates of compliance in a randomised exercise trial in myocardial infarction patients. *Medicine and Science in Sports and Exercise* 33 (7): 1081–9.

EUROASPIRE Study Group (1997) A European Society of Cardiology survey of secondary prevention of coronary heart disease: principal results. *European Heart Journal* 18: 1569–82.

EUROASPIRE Study Group (2001) Lifestyle and risk factor management and use of drug therapies in coronary patients from 15 countries: principal results from EUROASPIRE II, Euro Heart Survey Programme. *European Heart Journal* 22: 554–72.

European Society of Cardiology (2003) *Guidelines on CVD Prevention: Third Joint European Societies Task Force on Cardiovascular Disease Prevention in Clinical Practice*. Sophia Antipolis, France: European Society of Cardiology.

Evenson, K. and Fleury, J. (2000) Barriers to outpatient cardiac rehabilitation participation and adherence. *Journal of Cardiopulmonary Rehabilitation* 20: 241–6.

Ferguson, E. W., Bernier, L. L., Banta, G. R., Yu-Yahiro, J. and Schoomaker, E. B. (1987) Effects of exercise and conditioning on clotting and fibrinolytic activity in man. *Journal of Applied Physiology* 62: 1416–21.

Gavin, J. and Gavin, N. (1995) *Psychology for Health Professionals*. Leeds: Human Kinetics.

Glazer, K., Emery, C., Frid, D. and Banyasz, R. (2002) Psychological predictors of adherence and outcomes among patients in cardiac rehabilitation. *Journal of Cardiopulmonary Rehabilitation* 22: 40–6.

Goble, A. J. and Worcester, M. U. (1999) *Best Practice Guidelines for Cardiac Rehabilitation and Secondary Prevention: a synopsis*. Melbourne: Heart Research Centre/Department of Human Services.

Greenfield, S., Jones, M., Jolly, K. and Raftery, J. (2004) A qualitative study of reasons for non-participation and non-attendance at cardiac rehabilitation (abstract).

European Journal of Cardiovascular Prevention & Rehabilitation 11 (1, Supplement): 13.

Hardman, A. E. and Stensel, D. J. (2003) *Physical Activity and Health*. London: Routledge.

Health Education Authority/Sports Council (1992) *Allied Dunbar National Fitness Survey*. London: Health Education Authority.

Horgan, J., Bethell, H., Carson, P., Davidson, C., Julian, D., Mayou, R. A. and Nagle, R. (1992) Working Group of the British Cardiac Society. *British Heart Journal* 67: 412–18.

Hughes, A., Gillies, F., Kirk, A., Mutrie, N., Hillis, W. and MacIntyre, P. (2002) Exercise consultation improves short term adherence to exercise during phase IV cardiac rehabilitation. *Journal of Cardiopulmonary Rehabilitation* 22: 421–5.

Ice, R. (1985) Long term compliance. *Physical Therapy* 65 (12): 1832–9.

Jolliffe, J. A., Rees, K., Taylor, R. S., Thompson, D., Oldridge, N. and Ebrahim, S. (2000a) Exercise-based rehabilitation for coronary heart disease. Cochrane Review. In *The Cochrane Library 4*. Oxford: Update Software.

Jolliffe, J. A., Taylor, R. and Ebrahim, S. (2000b) A *Report on the Clinical and Cost Effectiveness of Physiotherapy in Cardiac Rehabilitation*. London: Chartered Society of Physiotherapists.

King, A. C., Kiernan, M., Oman, R. F., Kraemer, H. C., Hull, M. and Ahn, D. (1997) Can we identify who will adhere to long-term physical activity? Signal detection methodology as a potential aid to clinical decision making. *Health Psychology* 16 (4): 380–9.

Leon, A. S. (2000) Physical exercise following myocardial infarction. *Sports Medicine* 29 (5): 301–11.

Manson, J. E., Nathan, D. M., Krolewski, A. S., Stampfer, M. J., Willett, W. C. and Hennekens, C. H. (1992). A prospective study of exercise and incidence of diabetes among US male physicians. *Journal of the American Medical Association* 268: 63–7.

Marcus, B. H., Selby, V. C., Niaura, R. S. and Rossi, J. S. (1992) Self-efficacy and the stages of exercise behaviour change. *Research Quarterly for Exercise and Sport* 63: 60–6.

Martinsen, E., Medhus, A., Sandvik, L. (1985) Effects of exercise on depression: a controlled trial. *British Medical Journal* 292: 109.

McGee, H. M. (1999) Psychosocial issues for cardiac rehabilitation with older individuals. *Coronary Artery Disease* 10 (1): 47–51.

New Zealand Guideline Group (NZGG) (2002) Cardiac rehabilitation best practice evidence based guideline. Wellington: NZGG.

NHS Centre for Reviews and Dissemination (1998) *Effective Health Care: Cardiac Rehabilitation*, York: University of York.

O'Connor, G. T., Buring, J. E., Yusuf, S., Goldhaber, S. Z., Olmstead, E. M., Paffenbarger, R. S. and Hennekens, C. H. (1989) An overview of randomised trials of rehabilitation with exercise after myocardial infarction. *Circulation* 80: 234–44.

Office for National Statistics (2001) *Mortality Statistics: Series DH2 no. 28*. London: The Stationery Office.

Oldridge, N. B. (1988) Cardiac rehabilitation after myocardial infarction. *Journal of the American Medical Association* 260: 945–50.

Pate, R. R., Pratt, M. and Blair, S. N. (1995) Physical activity and public health: a recommendation from the Centres for Disease Control and Prevention and the American College of Sports Medicine. *Journal of the American Medical Association* 273: 402–7.

194 *Health Promoting Practice*

Physical Activity and Cardiovascular Health (1996) National Institute of Health Consensus Developmental Panel on Physical Activity and Cardiovascular Health. *Journal of the American Medical Association* **276**: 241–6.

Prochaska, J. and DiClemente, C. (1984) *The Transtheoretical Approach: Crossing Traditional Foundations of Change.* Homewood, IL: Dow Jones-Irwin.

Scottish Intercollegiate Guidelines Network (2002) *Cardiac Rehabilitation: a National Clinical Guideline.* Edinburgh: Royal College of Physicians.

Tavazzi, L., Boszormeny, E., Broustet, J. P., Denolin, H., Dorossiey, D., Cobelli, F., Gattone, M., Giordano, A., Horgan, J. H., Kellermann, J. J., Koenig, K., Mathes, P., Opasich, C., Langosh, W., Lewin, B., Maiani, G., Zotti, A. M., Brochier, M. and Sanchin, N. (1992) for the Task Force of the Working Group on Cardiac Rehabilitation of the European Society of Cardiology. Definition of cardiac rehabilitation. *European Heart Journal* **13** (Supplement C): 1–45.

US Department of Health and Human Services (1996) *Physical Activity and Health: A Report of the Surgeon General.* Atlanta, GA: US Department of Health and Human Services, Centres for Disease Control and Prevention, National Centre for Chronic Disease Prevention and Health Promotion.

Wood, D., De Backer, G., Faergeman, O., Graham, I., Mancia, G. and Pyörälä, K. (1998) Prevention of coronary heart disease in clinical practice: recommendations of the Second Joint Task Force of European and other Societies on coronary prevention. *European Heart Journal* **19**: 1434–1503.

World Health Organisation (1993) *Needs and Action Priorities in Cardiac Rehabilitation and Secondary Prevention in Patients with CHD.* Geneva: WHO.

CHAPTER 15

Promoting Health through a Self-help Care Model for the Management of Multiple Sclerosis

LORRAINE DE SOUZA, LORELY IDE AND CLAUDIUS NEOPHYTOU

Multiple sclerosis (MS) is the most common neurological condition resulting in disability in young adults. It has no known cause and there is no cure. The course of the disease is characterised by unpredictable attacks, interspersed by periods of remission, and by fluctuations in symptoms even in the absence of disease activity. MS can affect any centrally controlled neural system and progressive central nervous system (CNS) damage commonly leads to loss of movement, sensory impoverishment, and autonomic dysfunctions. The sensorimotor problems of MS are those most readily identified for intervention by therapists. However, the psychosocial impact of the disease on individuals and their carers is equally important for successful management in the long term. Promoting a self-help model of care places the person with MS and their carers at the centre of decision making and managing change in their lives. Access to, and support from, the health professional network of care is essential, together with the provision of accurate, timely, and appropriate information. It underpins the successful empowerment of individuals in developing self-help strategies, and is reflective of a number of health promotion principles. The successful long term management of MS relies on the broader health promoting role of therapists. The centrality of the person with MS and their carer in the context of managing change due to MS is essential to developing expertise in living successfully with this unpredictable and distressing condition.

What is multiple sclerosis?

MS is a chronic, progressive disease of the CNS affecting predominantly young adults. It is a disease of unknown aetiology, unpredictable prognosis, and has

195

no known cure or demonstrably effective treatment. The disease produces lesions of the protective covering around CNS nerve fibres (myelin) resulting in failure of conduction of nerve impulses (see De Souza and Bates, 2004). MS is problematic to diagnose as it has a variable onset and the remitting nature of early symptoms in the majority of patients often leaves no clinically detectable abnormalities. There is much medical uncertainty, debate, and dispute about the nature of MS, and the prevailing content and tone of this debate often dictates the trends in clinical diagnosis, management and research into all aspects of the disease. Because of the progressive nature of the disease those who have MS will experience increasing neural damage, with resultant disability that may proceed to profound incapacitation that can last a lifetime. The median life expectancy from the time of diagnosis for those with MS is estimated to be about 35 years (Kurtzke, 1970).

The spectre of this worst case scenario has in the past often resulted in reluctance on the part of medical practitioners to provide a confirmation of the diagnosis (Elian and Dean, 1985). Diagnosing MS is not straightforward and can often take time due to the variation of presenting neurological problems and the sporadic nature of exacerbations interspersed by periods of remission when no objective neurological dysfunction may be found. There is no single, simple diagnostic test available. Because of the seriousness of MS as a disease, physicians are generally extremely careful to obtain sufficient evidence for the diagnosis. This may involve patients having to undertake several tests. Despite advances in technology providing better diagnostic tools, a definite diagnosis of MS has to be made clinically based on a history of two exacerbations and evidence of two separate lesions (Poser et al., 1983). In addition, other diagnoses have to be excluded as several diseases can mimic MS (see Matthews, 1991).

Once a diagnosis of MS has been confirmed, current guidelines recommend that the individual affected should be told, preferably by the consultant (National Institute for Clinical Excellence (NICE), 2003). The majority of people with MS prefer to know their diagnosis (Elian and Dean, 1985) although disclosure may be painful and unexpected for some, but a relief for others (Koopman and Schweitzer, 1999).

Accurate descriptions of symptoms and signs may only be compiled from studies of patient series from geographically diverse populations of clinically definite and laboratory confirmed cases (Matthews, 1991). Such studies inevitably suffer from a variety of sources of error, the most important being the retrospective nature of the data gathered about the early and initial stages of the disease. As the definite diagnosis is not permissible until at least two episodes have occurred, or the course has shown progression over at least six months, documentation of the early stages relies on the individual's ability to recall events. As some symptoms may have been so mild or transient that they were too insignificant to be remembered, the exact time of the onset of symptoms cannot be accurately determined. However, the commonest presenting symptom is sensory impairment, followed by optic neuritis and insidious motor deficit (Matthews, 1991). Optic neuritis and sensory impairment are found more commonly in patients with a younger age of onset, and motor deficit more commonly in those with an older age of onset (Koch-Henriksen, 1989; Weinshenker et al., 1989).

Nearly all surveys agree that MS occurs more frequently in women than in men (for example see Acheson, 1977; Kurtzke et al., 1979). However, a sex linked difference in onset symptoms has not been found (Koch-Henriksen, 1989) while the sex of the patient seems to have no influence in the development of the disease (Matthews, 1991). The occurrence of MS is rare before puberty, then increases rapidly to reach a peak at around 30 years, remains high during the fourth decade of life, and then declines rapidly. From the sixth decade of life, the incidence is negligible. The mean age of onset appears to be 29–33 years (Matthews, 1985: 49). It seems, therefore, that MS predominantly affects people in the prime of life when they are entering the period of increased earning power or career advancement and, for women, their peak child bearing years.

In the United Kingdom (UK) approximately 120 per 100,000 people have MS, giving a prevalence of about 80,000 (O'Brien, 1987). It is estimated to cost the UK about £1.2 billion per year (Holmes et al., 1995), not counting the economic burden borne by family members and by the person with MS through loss of earnings (O'Brien, 1987; Hakim et al., 2000). The most common pattern of the disease, affecting almost 90 per cent of cases, is one of unpredictable attacks (relapses or exacerbations) and remissions (Swingler and Compston, 1992), which in some cases becomes progressive as remissions cease (secondary progressive) (Confavreux et al., 1980). A minority of cases experience progression from onset without remission (primary progressive) (Matthews, 1991). The main problems with MS include weakness and fatigability, loss of sensation, visual impairment, incoordination, spasticity, bladder and bowel dysfunction, sexual dysfunction, and intellectual changes affecting memory, concentration and abstract thinking (Matthews, 1998). The resultant spectrum of functional disabilities limits people with MS in all activities of daily living as well as their familial, economic and social roles (Murray, 1995).

Care of people affected by multiple sclerosis

People with MS do not require active intervention at every stage of the disease. However all, even those with mild symptoms, benefit from support and advice from appropriate professionals according to their individual needs (De Souza and Bates, 2004). Specific interventions are usually targeted at symptom management and the effects of relapses. Treatments generally consist of a mixture of appropriate drug therapy and physical therapies, supported by the provision of aids and appliances, psychosocial support, and advice.

More recently, disease modifying drugs have been investigated for their effectiveness in reducing the severity and frequency of relapses and delaying the progression of disability in people with the relapsing remitting form of MS (reviewed by Corboy et al., 2003). Two such therapies, beta-interferon and glatiramer acetate, have been recommended for selected people with MS who fit the criteria for treatment (NICE, 2003) but neither have been recommended for people with progressive MS. Given the complexity and inherent uncertainty of MS and the lack of disease modifying drugs available the major programme for management is one of comprehensive care (De Souza, 1990) involving many disciplines. Therapists, nurses, doctors, social workers, psychologists and counsellors typically provide a range of services in a coordinated fashion. The aim is to maximise ability while minimising further deterioration within the biological limits of the MS (De Souza, 1990; LaRocca et al., 1994). Best practice, however, does not consist of a series of interventions, but embodies a cohesive care plan that enables the person with MS to develop skills for living with the disease (De Souza, 1990; De Souza and Bates, 2004) and recommendations have been published on what provision healthcare services need to make available for people with MS (NICE, 2003).

The philosophy of care from the physiotherapy perspective has been described elsewhere (Ashburn and De Souza, 1988; De Souza, 1990; De Souza and Bates, 2004), as have the timing and types of physiotherapy interventions recommended for use with people with MS (De Souza and Bates, 2004). The emphasis for intervention is on functional activity, active exercises, including walking, and the management of fatigue. An equally important role for the physiotherapist to undertake is a consultative one for the provision of accurate and appropriate information, the education of people with MS and their carers about the disease and its effects, and support and advice about managing the lifestyle changes that living with MS will inevitably bring. It encompasses an understanding that functions such as walking and transferring reach far beyond the physical issues, and extend to social, cultural, psychological and emotional effects of loss and limitation (De Souza and Bates, 2004).

Due to the relatively early onset and unpredictable nature of MS, it is reasonable to expect that the disease will have a considerable impact within a person's social, psychological and emotional health, wellbeing and functioning (Barnwell and Kavanagh, 1997). One area where this is apparent is the reported increase in depression experienced by people with MS (Acorn and Anderson, 1990). These factors need to be considered by all health professionals involved in the care of people with MS and their families. It is essential that professionals appreciate that while their intervention is important and the time available needs to be used to full effect, it is the person with MS and their informal carers who will be the key facilitators of living with MS successfully throughout the 30–40 years of the disease trajectory. For this to be achieved people with MS and their carers need to be actively involved in the planning and decision making regarding their care, including participating in the development of healthcare services and the availability and access to services that are responsive to their needs.

The self-help approach

It is well known that people with MS have a predisposition to seek out and engage in a number of health practices, many unorthodox and some that are not beneficial to their health (Sibley, 1988). However, it is debateable whether or not people with MS behave any differently to the general population in doing so. What is different, however, is that people with MS decide to pursue their own health practices because they have MS, thus indicating a need to take action in the face of an incurable disease.

Orthodox medicine has acknowledged that self-help constitutes 'the fourth estate of medicine' (Lock, 1986) and thus places self-help in parallel with existing healthcare practice rather than in opposition to it. In addition, the self-help expertise of people with chronic conditions is now seen as a major resource for formal healthcare services (Department of Health (DoH), 2003).

The concept of self-help, and what it consists of, is varied. Definitions range from general concepts such as self-help groups, help seeking behaviour and self-care, and health promoting practices, to narrower meanings such as media based materials like books and videos that individuals chose to use without any advice from a health professional (Dean, 1989; Gould and Clum, 1993; Stuifbergen and Roberts, 1997). The most useful approach is a pragmatic one that considers self-help as incorporating a range of health behaviours that aid general wellbeing (Connelly, 1987; Dean, 1989;) or, the things people do to help themselves because they have multiple sclerosis (O'Hara et al., 2000: 63).

People with MS engage in self-help practices seemingly to gain some control and independence in the face of the uncertainty of their illness (McLaughlin and Zeeberg, 1993). It has been suggested that there is a direct relationship between quality of life and satisfaction with self-care and leisure activities of people with MS (Lundmark and Branholm, 1996). Although the need for professional support is reported by a wide range of people undertaking self-help for their health needs, they are more likely to discuss their self-help actions with friends and relatives, or other people with MS, rather than with a health professional (Trojan, 1989; McLaughlin and Zeeberg, 1993). In addition when making choices about which self-help strategies to carry out, they are as likely to seek information from the media or other non-professional sources as to consult a health professional (De Souza, 1990).

People with MS living in the community have been found to engage in many and diverse self-help practices. A Delphi study of self-care in MS found that three quarters of a community sample of respondents reported ten or more self-help practices covering all aspects of living from the physical to the social and psychological (O'Hara et al., 2000). The study revealed the extent to which people with MS are left to their own devices when dealing with daily living and reported the respondents' ten most important self-care practices. In rank order these were: coping (cognitive or behavioural strategies to deal with stress), maintaining independence in activities of daily living, maintaining and developing social networks, rest, mobility (using aids to maximise mobility), taking dietary supplements, medication (prescribed), taking exercise, leisure (including outings, hobbies and holidays), and lastly, conventional therapies normally available from health services. People with MS appear to have more satisfaction in life when they have good emotional health, maintain valued roles with friends and family, engage in meaningful leisure activities and make a contribution to others, such as caring for children or within voluntary organisations (Reynolds and Prior, 2003).

The ranking of conventional therapy last in the priority list above may be interpreted as therapy being of little importance to people with MS. However, this is unlikely to be the case, but rather a reflection of the extent of the unmet need for rehabilitation services experienced by people with MS (Kersten et al., 2000), and an indication of the difficulties they encounter in accessing health services, including therapy (Elian and Dean, 1983; Nodder et al., 2000; O'Hara et al., 2004).

A professionally guided self-care programme for the management of MS in the community based on the above priorities of people with MS has demonstrated small positive health benefits, and significant maintenance of independence (O'Hara et al., 2002). The programme incorporates self-care strategies into professional interventions, and thus focusses rehabilitation on consumers' needs and priorities. This research provides a useful model of how professionals can guide and support self-care in MS in a way that promotes and empowers the role of the individuals concerned (O'Hara et al., 2002).

Information, knowledge and self-reliance

Many people with MS and their carers experience difficulties with obtaining appropriate information about MS (Kersten et al., 2000). Voluntary agencies, such as the MS Society, provide comprehensive material that addresses many problems of MS, and health professionals also provide information when approached. Yet despite these services there still seems to be an information gap. It could be that the priorities of people with MS and professionals are divergent (De Souza, 1990; McLaughlin and Zeeberg, 1993) or that the information available, of necessity, deals with MS in general rather than with the individual seeking specific information to meet his/her precise needs.

One area where information giving has far reaching implications is at time of diagnosis. The recent NICE (2003) guidelines for the management of MS recommend that the individual should be told once the diagnosis has been confirmed. This advice is congruent with the findings that the majority of people with MS prefer to know their diagnosis (Elian and Dean, 1985). In contrast to this advice, it is also reported (Elian and Dean, 1985) that health professionals often try and avoid telling people with MS of their diagnosis, probably with the assumption of not further burdening them with this news. Sometimes healthcare professionals place the onus upon family members of carrying this information in secrecy. This creates the psychological tension of knowing the diagnosis and keeping it secret, which can later have detrimental manifestations upon family relationships once the MS sufferer finds out. The burden of secrecy also denies families the chance to experience the emotions of what receiving a diagnosis of MS means for them together and it can destroy trust.

Another detrimental impact is that the person with MS is denied a central role in decisions about their care. This marginalises and disempowers the person most concerned with the health issues to be addressed by professional intervention. Health professionals need to acknowledge individual differences in attitudes to receiving information and should try to clarify each person's individual preference instead of assuming a particular attitude and generalising it to everyone.

Miller (1987) has identified two independent informational styles for which people have a general preference when receiving and coping with threatening health information: monitors and blunters. Monitors like to find out all they can about their health state and show active information seeking behaviour such as looking up information on the Internet, getting books from the library and asking lots of questions. Blunters, however, prefer not to know the details and take on denial and avoidance strategies to help them cope. However, a person's health status can be improved if the information they receive is congruent with their preferred health information receiving style (Miller and Mangan, 1983; Bonk et al., 2001) and health professionals should become aware of these differences between people and target the information they give to an individual's preferences.

It could be argued that there is too much information for one individual to deal with, sift through, access and successfully use aspects that relate to their particular needs. Here professional guidance can be valuable in helping people with MS find and use appropriate information in a timely way. In order to fulfil this role therapists need to have up to date and accurate information about MS, be able to interpret it, and apply it with skill and precision to the specific needs of the individual concerned.

The NICE guidelines (2003: 13) highlight good practice in communicating information to people with MS, stating that '... the healthcare professional should find out what and how much information the individual wants to receive. (This should be reviewed on each occasion.) ...' It is noteworthy that the guidelines include principles such as making information relevant to the person's specific situation, considering the benefits and risks of giving information as once given information cannot be withdrawn, and only providing information that the professional is certain about within their own knowledge and expertise (NICE, 2003).

Therapists need to be aware of the impact of information on the individual and their family. Good communication skills are essential when giving bad news or unwelcome information in a sensitive and supportive manner. Therapists must be prepared to continue to support the person with MS after providing information, especially if emotional distress has been caused, and to check that those concerned have understood the information correctly as information may be forgotten in whole or in part. Good communication is thought to improve an individual's health outcomes (Stewart, 1995), having a positive influence on emotional health, symptom resolution, functional and physiological status and pain control. Including individuals in making decisions about the management of their illness, and providing emotional support, are recommended. In addition, giving written information limits the problems associated with forgetting and misinterpreting what for most would be new information (Stewart, 1995). Similar guidance is given to healthcare professionals communicating with people with MS (NICE, 2003: 6), to be straightforward, to check the person has understood, to back up the communication with written and other source materials, and to reinforce it if required.

Accessing the network of care

Despite a shift of emphasis from hospital to community care, and the establishment of standards of care for MS, many people with moderate or severe disability fail to receive the assistance they are entitled to.

The UK study by Elian and Dean (1983) showed that people with MS living in the community, were frequently unaware of available services and were not receiving essential services such as cash benefits, house alterations, and home help. Sadly at the moment there is little evidence to demonstrate that this situation has improved. Current use of services and home modifications in people with a broad range of disease severity in the UK has shown that a large proportion, including those severely disabled, failed to receive any community service, thus suggesting that many of their needs were unmet by current practice. The percentage reaching a physiotherapist was 23 per cent and only 21 per cent reached an occupational therapist (Freeman and Thompson, 2000).

This situation is further verified by a recent study (O'Hara et al., 2004), which examined the way in which informal care fitted into the formal care system. People with MS were asked to keep a diary about the nature of care received over a 24 hour period, or a typical day. Just 15 per cent of respondents received visits from health/social service professionals during the documented 24 hours and most of the care was being provided by family or friends in the form of personal care, help with mobility, household tasks, leisure and employment. Therefore, therapists need to be aware that any new professional engagement with those living with MS is likely to be supplementary to an existing complex care network. Professionals need to be attentive to existing strategies and intervene to support and enhance these practices.

The emphasis on care in the community in recent years brings concerns as to what support people living with MS are receiving and to what extent their needs are being met. If family members and friends are providing most of the care, this gives rise to questions about how they are being supported with services in their own right. Healthcare professionals can work with informal carers not only to support them in their caring roles, but also to provide professional input to safeguard their wellbeing and to promote their continuing health.

There have been few studies of carers of people with MS in the UK. A recent review (McKeown et al., 2003) showed that caring for a person with MS has a detrimental effect on carers' physical and psychological wellbeing, social life, work life and financial situation. It provided a number of messages for health professionals including a need to be aware that all areas of caregivers' lives are seriously affected as a result of providing care for a person with MS, and that carers' needs should be regularly and routinely assessed in their own right.

Health professionals need to be aware that caring is performed in a relationship over a normal lifespan and that the relationships that last the course cope with the effects of the disease and develop expertise (Ide and De Souza, 2003).

Quote from a husband carer: '... we have found ways of coping. That is in fact the truth of the whole picture. We haven't resolved it. We have found ways of managing it better. That is what we do – that is exactly what we do.'

Carers often report depression, ill health and living with unresolved problems. There were very few reports of services to these family units and virtually no reports of services offered directly to the carer (Ide and De Souza, 2003; McKeown et al., 2003).

The provision of respite care attempts to alleviate the psychological and physical consequences of caring. This involves the person with MS being supported in a hospital or nursing home environment for a short period of time, with the main aim of giving the prime carer a break from caring responsibilities and time to prepare for another period of care.

However, there seems to be low use of respite services despite an identified need for long-term breaks (Aronson et al., 1996). Cockerill and Warren (1990) found that about half of their respondents had used some form of respite care, mostly family and friends. Some had been admitted to hospital temporarily, and one or two had hired assistants at home. However overall these carers did not seem to be using the respite options offered to them and appeared to have some resistance to them. Reasons may be that the benefits are short lived and although respite can offer immediate relief for carers, it does not help to maintain the longer term social support networks that are important once the respite care has ended (McNally et al., 1999).

Negotiations and reconciliations: managing changes in role and lifestyle

As MS develops in the prime child rearing years there will be a number of people with MS involved in caring for others, especially rearing children. These roles, due to the positive enhancement and regard that they bring to a person, should be of prime interest to health professionals. It is also an area where a person with MS's activity within the family can be enhanced, when other areas naturally deteriorate. For example they can take a more advanced role in meeting their child's developmental needs, especially their emotional and psychological needs.

It is important to recognise that functional disability and independence are not associated with self-assessed quality of life and that people can have positive satisfaction with their quality of life despite their physical and independence status (Albrecht and Devlieger, 1999). Goals, hopes and aspirations are important factors within this status and can change over time with chronic illness triggering new priorities (Reynolds and Prior, 2003). Reprioritising within the course of the disease trajectory can allow people to engage with valued activities, allowing them to maintain their identity and self-esteem as well as providing them with a form of control within a chronic illness that has a high level of uncontrollability associated with it (Reynolds and Prior, 2003). Achieving a sense of control has been associated with a number of positive outcomes and protects against depression and feelings of helplessness (Abramson et al., 1978; Marks et al., 1986; Kamen and Seligman, 1989).

Further areas where people with MS can gain control are the development and maintenance of their physical fitness, the establishment and maintenance of a healthy diet and the minimisation of their stress (Rigby, 2001). Health professionals can negotiate with and support people with MS and their families within all of these areas.

As the majority of people with MS are young adults, the issue of work and remaining in employment is significant. Being out of work, and/or receiving benefits instead of earning a wage, can be both socially and financially devastating. Helping those with MS who want to stay in employment, or retrain for other appropriate employment should be a high priority for healthcare professionals. A proactive approach that draws on multidisciplinary and multiagency expertise is recommended (NICE, 2003), and health professionals need to be fully aware of local and national vocational support services in order to provide appropriate information. Therapists are well placed to use their skills in the assessment of movement, posture, mobility and occupational activities to advise people with MS and employers on appropriate strategies, equipment, adaptations, and the types of reasonable adjustments that may be necessary to comply with the Disability Discrimination Act (www.disability. gov.uk/dda).

Being employed provides people with MS not just with money, but also a sense of identity, status, personal satisfaction and a role of participating in and contributing to society at large (Graham and Roberts, 2000). For those who can no longer stay employed, alternative roles that fulfil their personal needs should be suggested as options, and healthcare professionals can provide information on available choices (NICE, 2003).

Role changes within the family unit can bring challenges as well as rewards. Therapists can help families to adapt to MS so it becomes a part of daily living within normal family life. Informal carers of people with MS often pick up more of the previously shared activities within their relationship. People with MS can be encouraged to take on other roles within the family that they had not previously carried out, so as to maintain some reciprocity within their relationships. For example, whilst giving up some manual jobs, they may take up some non-manual jobs such as the finance and paperwork, or home making tasks (Ide and De Souza, 2003). In essence, therapists can help families living with MS to negotiate and facilitate role changes to the benefit of the family and to enhance the emotional wellbeing of the person with MS.

The complexity and variability of MS challenges those who have the disease, their families and healthcarers alike. Progression of service provision from a medically orientated model towards a biopsychosocial model of care can facilitate self-help and the promotion of health and quality of life for those who live with MS. However, this does not provide all the solutions. Self-help needs to be viewed as a commitment to the long term support of people with MS by health professionals and not a means by which responsibility for care is abrogated by statutory services. The success of the self-help approach to management of MS will require a cultural change in the way health services are perceived and operated by both those who provide the services and those who need to use them.

References

Abramson, L. Y., Seligman, M. E. P. and Teasdale, J. D. (1978) Learned helplessness in humans: critique and reformulation. *Journal of Abnormal Psychology* **87**: 49–74.

Acheson, E. D. (1977) Epidemiology of multiple sclerosis. *British Medical Bulletin* **33**: 9–14.

Acorn, S. and Anderson, S. (1990) Depression in multiple sclerosis: critique of the research literature. *Journal of Neuroscience Nursing* **2**: 209–14.

Albrecht, G. L. and Devlieger, P. J. (1999) 'The disability paradox': high quality of life against all odds. *Social Science and Medicine* **48**: 977–88.

Aronson, K. J., Gleghorn, G. and Goldenberg, E. (1996) Assistance arrangements and use of services among persons with multiple sclerosis and their caregivers. *Disability and Rehabilitation* **18**: 354–61.

Ashburn, A. and De Souza, L. H. (1988) An approach to the management of multiple sclerosis. *Physiotherapy Practice* **4**: 139–45.

Barnwell, A. M. and Kavanagh, D. J. (1997) Prediction of psychological adjustment to multiple sclerosis. *Social Science and Medicine* **45** (3): 411–18.

Bonk, V. A., France, C. R. and Taylor, B. K. (2001) Distraction reduces self-reported physiological reactions to blood donation in novice donors with a blunting coping style. *Psychosomatic Medicine* **63** (3): 447–52.

Cockerill, R. and Warren, S. (1990) Care for caregivers: needs of family members of multiple sclerosis patients. *Journal of Rehabilitation* **56** (1): 41–4.

Confavreux, C., Aimard, G., and Devic, M. (1980) Course and prognosis of multiple sclerosis assessed by the computerised data processing of 349 patients. *Brain* **103**: 281–300.

Connelly, C. (1987) Self-care and the chronically ill patient. *Nurse Clinics of North America* **22**: 621–9.

Corboy, C. J., Gooodin, D. S. and Frohman, E. M. (2003) Disease-modifying therapies for multiple sclerosis. *Current Treatment Options in Neurology* 5: 35–54.

Dean, K. (1989) Conceptual, theoretical and methodological issues in self-care research. *Social Science and Medicine* 29: 117–23.

Department of Health (2003) *The Expert Patient: a New Approach to Chronic Disease Management for the 21st Century.* London: DoH. www.doh.gov.uk/healthinequalities

De Souza, L. H. (1990) *Multiple Sclerosis: Approaches to Management.* London: Chapman and Hall.

De Souza, L. H. and Bates, D. (2004) Multiple sclerosis. In Stokes, M. (ed.) *Physical Management in Neurological Rehabilitation*, second edition. London/Edinburgh: Harcourt Health Sciences/Elsevier.

Elian, M. and Dean, G. (1983) Need for and use of social and health services by multiple sclerosis patients living at home in England. *The Lancet* 1: 1091–3.

Elian, M. and Dean, G. (1985) To tell or not to tell: the diagnosis of multiple sclerosis. *The Lancet* 2: 27–8.

Freeman, J. and Thompson, A. (2000) Community services in multiple sclerosis: still a matter of chance. *Journal of Neurology Neurosurgery and Psychiatry* 69: 728–32.

Gould, R. A. and Clum, G. A. (1993) A meta-analysis of self-help treatment approaches. *Clinical Psychology Reviews* 13: 169–86.

Graham, J. and Roberts, G. (2000) *Making the Most of Multiple Sclerosis: Adjusting to And Coping with Change.* London: MS Society.

Hakim, E. A., Bakheit, A. M. O., Bryant, T. N., Roberts, M. W. H., McIntosh-Michaelis, S. A., Spackman, A. J., Martin, J. P. and McLellan, D. L. (2000) The social impact of multiple sclerosis – a study of 305 patients and their relatives. *Disability and Rehabilitation* 22 (6): 288–93.

Holmes, J., Madgewick, T. and Bates, D. (1995) The cost of multiple sclerosis. *British Journal of Medical Economics* 8: 181–93.

Ide, L. and De Souza, L. H. (2003) A qualitative investigation into the needs of informal caregivers of people with multiple sclerosis living in the community. In *Proceedings of the 14th International Congress of the World Confederation for Physical Therapy*, Barcelona 7–12 June.

Kamen, L. P. and Seligman, M. E. P. (1989) Explanatory style and health. In Johnston, M. and Marteau, T. (eds) *Applications in Health Psychology.* New Brunswick, NJ: Transaction.

Kersten, P., McLellan, D. L. and Gross-Paju, K. (2000) A questionnaire assessment of unmet needs for rehabilitation services and resources for people with multiple sclerosis: results of a pilot study in five European countries. *Clinical Rehabilitation* 14: 42–9.

Koch-Henriksen, N. (1989) An epidemiological study of multiple sclerosis. *Acta Neurologica Scandinavica* 80 (supplement 124): 1–123.

Koopman W. and Schweitzer A. (1999) The journey to multiple sclerosis: a qualitative study, *Journal of Neuroscience Nursing* 31: 17–26.

Kurtzke, J. F. (1970) Clinical manifestations of multiple sclerosis. In Vliken, D. J. and Bruyn, G. W. (eds) *Handbook of Clinical Neurology, Vol. 9, Multiple Sclerosis and other Demyelinating Diseases.* Amsterdam: North-Holland.

Kurtzke, J. F., Beebe, G. W. and Norman, J. E. (1979) Epidemiology of multiple sclerosis in US veterans 1: race, sex and geographic distribution. *Neurology* 29: 1228–35.

LaRocca, N. C., Schapiro, R. T., Scheinberg, L. C. and Kraft, G. H. (1994) Comprehensive care in multiple sclerosis: the whole vs. the parts. *Journal of Neurological Rehabilitation* 8: 95–8.

Lock, S. (1986) Self-help groups: the fourth estate in medicine? *British Medical Journal* **293**: 1596–1600.

Lundmark, P. and Branholm, I. (1996) Relationship between occupation and life satisfaction in people with multiple sclerosis. *Disability and Rehabilitation* **18** (9): 449–53.

Marks, G., Richardson, J. L., Graham, J. W. and Levine, A. (1986) Role of health locus of control beliefs and expectations of treatment efficacy in adjustment to cancer. *Journal of Personality and Social Psychology* **51**: 443–50.

Matthews, W. B. (1985) Clinical aspects: course and prognosis. In: Matthews, W. B., Acheson, E. D., Batchelor, J. R. and Weller, R. O. (eds) *McAlpine's Multiple Sclerosis*. Edinburgh: Churchill Livingstone.

Matthews, W. B. (1991) Symptoms and signs. In Matthews, W. B., Compston, A., Allen, I. V. and Martyn, C. N. (eds) *McAlpine's Multiple Sclerosis*, second edition. Edinburgh and London: Churchill Livingstone.

Matthews, W. B. (1998) Symptoms and signs of multiple sclerosis. In Compston, A., Ebers, G., Lassmann, H., McDonal, I., Matthews, W. B. and Wekerle, H. (eds) *McAlpine's Multiple Sclerosis*, third edition. London: Churchill Livingstone.

McKeown, L. P., Porter-Armstrong A. P. and Baxter, G. D. (2003) The needs and experiences of caregivers of individuals with multiple sclerosis: a systematic review. *Clinical Rehabilitation* **17**: 234–48.

McLaughlin, J. and Zeeberg, I. (1993) Self-care and multiple sclerosis: a view from two cultures. *Social Science and Medicine* **37**: 315–29.

McNally, S., Ben-Shlomo, Y., and Newman, S. (1999) The effects of respite care on informal carers' wellbeing: a systematic review. *Disability and Rehabilitation* **21**: 1–14.

Miller, S. M. (1987) Monitoring and blunting: validation of a questionnaire to assess styles of information seeking under threat. *Journal of Personality and Social Psychology* **52**: 345–53.

Miller, S. M. and Mangan, C. E. (1983) The interacting effects of information and coping style in adapting to gynecological stress: should the doctor tell all? *Journal of Personality and Social Psychology* **45**: 223–36.

Murray, T. J. (1995) The psychosocial aspects of multiple sclerosis. *Neurologic Clinics* **13** (1): 197–233.

National Institute for Clinical Excellence (2003) *Multiple Sclerosis: Management of Multiple Sclerosis in Primary and Secondary Care, Clinical Guideline 8*. London: NICE.

Nodder, D., Chappell, B., Bates, D., Freeman, J., Hatch, J., Keen, J., Thomas, S. and Young, C. (2000) Multiple sclerosis: care needs for 2000 and beyond. *Journal of the Royal Society of Medicine* **93**: 219–24.

O'Brien, B. (1987) *Multiple Sclerosis*. London: Office of Health Economics.

O'Hara, L., Cadbury, H., De Souza, L. H. and Ide, L. (2002) Evaluation of the effectiveness of professionally guided self-care for people with multiple sclerosis living in the community. *Clinical Rehabilitation* **16**: 119–28.

O'Hara, L., De Souza, L. H. and Ide, L. (2000) A Delphi study of self-care in a community population of people with multiple sclerosis. *Clinical Rehabilitation* **14**: 62–71.

O'Hara, L., De Souza, L. H. and Ide, L. (2004) The nature of care giving in a community sample of people with multiple sclerosis. *Disability and Rehabilitation* **26**: 1401–10.

Poser, C. M., Paty, D. W. and Scheinberg, L. (1983) New diagnostic criteria for multiple sclerosis: guidelines for research protocols. *Annals of Neurology* **13**: 227–31.

Reynolds, F. and Prior, S. (2003) 'Sticking jewels in your life': exploring women's strategies for negotiating an acceptable quality of life with multiple sclerosis. *Qualitative Health Research* **13** (9): 1225–51.

Rigby, S. (2001) Living with multiple sclerosis: the potential role of health psychology. *Health Psychology Update* **10** (2): 14–17.

Sibley, W. A. (1988) *Therapeutic Claims in Multiple Sclerosis*, second edition. Basingstoke and London: Macmillan (now Palgrave Macmillan).

Stewart, M. A. (1995) Effective physician–patient communication and health outcomes: a review. *Canadian Medical Association Journal* **152** (9): 1423–33.

Stuifbergen, A. K. and Roberts, G. J. (1997) Health promotion practices of women with multiple sclerosis. *Archives of Physical Medicine and Rehabilitation* **78** (suppl.): S3–S9.

Swingler, R. J. and Compston, D. A. S. (1992) The prevalence of multiple sclerosis in South East Wales. *Quarterly Journal of Medicine* **83**: 325–7.

Trojan, A. (1989) Benefits of self-help groups: a survey of 232 members from 65 disease-related groups. *Social Science and Medicine* **29**: 225–32.

Weinshenker, B. G., Bass, B., Rice, G. P. A., Noseworthy, J. H., Carriere, W., Baskerville, J. and Ebers, G. C. (1989) The natural history of multiple sclerosis: a geographically based study, I: clinical course and disability. *Brain* **112**: 133–46.

CHAPTER 16

Promoting the Health of People with Arthritis: Physiotherapy Approaches

JILL LLOYD

The many different types of arthritis can be reduced to two main categories, those of inflammatory and non-inflammatory. The main inflammatory arthritis is rheumatoid arthritis (RA) but the most prevalent arthritis is osteoarthritis (OA), which is generally non-inflammatory, is the result of a combination of factors and affects mainly elderly people. This chapter will consider methods available to physiotherapists in promoting the health of the person with arthritis.

The health impact of RA and OA

OA will effect approximately 10 per cent of the United Kingdom (UK) population in the later years of their life (Peat et al., 2001). Since incidence increases with years it is expected that with the current demographic trends it will become more prevalent in the UK (Felson, 2000). The processes of OA are those of cartilage destruction and bony overgrowth with consequent effects on other periarticular soft structures. There may also be a mild and possibly short lived inflammatory component (Kuettner and Goldberg, 1995). The condition affects people of both genders, usually above the age of 55 years (Peat et al., 2001) and starts insidiously. The joints affected by OA are mainly the weight bearing joints, the hip, knee and foot and toe joints, but also the small joints of the hands, particularly the thumb. There is also a secondary and similar OA that may start following some injury or alteration in body biomechanics. A huge spectrum of disease severity is possible and some people will become fairly disabled whilst others will remain active and mobile. The clinical features of OA are pain during and after activity which is improved by rest; short duration early morning stiffness, possible minor deformity, decreased range of movement, reduced muscle power and functional impairments. There are no systemic effects, apart perhaps from the secondary effect of sedentary behaviour due to pain.

Management of OA is a mixture of symptom control and health promotion. This can consist of a mixture of specific exercise therapy, disease education, analgesia and surgery. The outcomes following surgery are usually enabling and promote a fresh quality of life.

Rheumatoid arthritis (RA) is a chronic progressive condition with an unpredictable course. It is the most common form of inflammatory arthritis, affecting approximately 1 per cent of the world's population and is estimated to have an economic impact similar to that of coronary heart disease (Callahan, 1998). It affects mainly the joints, but also in more severe disease it can have an effect on internal organs. RA starts in the small joints of the hands and feet, it may then spread to almost all the joints in the body. The joint lining becomes inflamed and swells. Eventually the surfaces of the joints are eroded and characteristic structural deformities may be developed. Within 20 years of onset there is evidence that around 90 per cent of people will have some disability (Buckley, 1997). In certain people organs such as the lungs, heart and kidneys may be involved. This will impair their function causing systemic upset. In addition due to the chronic nature of the inflammation there may be anaemia and fatigue with possibly depression and anxiety (see Chapter 11 for a discussion of the occupational therapy health promoting role in dealing with depression in RA).

The condition affects women more than men in a 2.5:1 ratio (Pincus, 1996). It tends to start insidiously, but the onset may also be sudden or palindromic. The spectrum varies from very mild to severe joint destruction. It affects all age groups but the peak decade of onset is the sixth decade. There are no known predisposing factors currently identified, but work is underway investigating the role of infection as a trigger.

The person with RA may present with pain in many joints, which tends to be worse in the morning and after rest. It may be eased by drug therapy (American College of Rheumatology, 2002). Swelling of many joints is also demonstrated, but particularly of the visible joints in the hands and knees. Examination may reveal decreased range of movement in affected joints and reduced muscle power in the same areas. One of the main symptoms of which the patient complains is stiffness; this is worse in the morning but can be reduced by effective and early drug management (Emery et al., 2002) Stiffness correlates closely with disease activity (Jansen et al., 2000). In addition the patient may have considerable difficulty with performing normal functional daily activities such as getting dressed and undertaking household tasks (Hallert et al., 2003).

Effective management of RA requires early diagnosis and early drug management (Emery et al., 2002). Erosions tend to develop within the first two years of onset (van der Heide, 1995). The correct administration of drugs and monitoring of any side effects will become a task for the multidisciplinary team. Since the condition is chronic, disabling and rarely completely disappears, the person with RA will have met and worked with many health professionals, including physiotherapists. These professionals thus play a key role in facilitating the promotion of the health of persons with RA. These interactions offer ideal opportunities for health promotion, which included health education to increase understanding about the condition. These approaches are designed to empower individuals to manage themselves and achieve an improved health status. Certainly it is now possible for people with arthritis to be referred directly to physiotherapists with an interest in arthritis. This may facilitate the possibility of the patient receiving a more holistic service.

Health promotion strategies available to the physiotherapist

Health promotion strategies in arthritis have not been specific and overt, however with current UK government targets, development of health promotion programmes will be enhanced (Department of Health (DoH), 1999).

Rehabilitation in arthritis is designed to enable the person to function as independently as possible, if that is what they desire. This is very similar to the concept of some health promotion approaches that seek to emphasise self-care and an independent attitude (Stuifbergen and Rogers, 1997; see also Chapter 15 in this text). Adapting and managing chronic and disabling illness is an unending process where the demands alter. The role of the physiotherapist in promoting health is key. There are many strategies available although most of these are currently without effective evaluation.

Pain management

In terms of managing oneself and one's health, one of the major determinants of wellbeing in arthritis sufferers will be freedom from pain. In a recent study in Ireland of women with established RA of more than three years' duration the dominant impairment was pain, with 52 per cent of the sample perceiving their health status as fair, poor or very poor compared with a similar cohort. Moreover, 25 per cent expected poor future health, with only 2 per cent expecting health gains in the future (Minnock et al., 2003). In providing the diagnosis to patients at the start of the disease, reassurance concerning the mildness of the disease raised implications for the patients concerning possible deterioration and likely future pain (Donovan and Blake, 2000). It is regrettable that despite current drug management and advances in health professionals' management of the condition, people with RA still complain of pain as their major limiting factor. It is known that constant pain certainly has a debilitating effect that could lead to depression and other confounding factors (see Chapter 11). Studies have confirmed a cognitive impairment is often apparent in people with chronic pain independent of the intensity of the pain (Hart et al., 2003). Concerns and interest in learning more about the condition seem to be predicted by pain and disability (Neville et al., 1999) whilst it is known that self-management programmes assist in decreasing pain levels and also healthcare costs (Solomon et al., 2002). The development of confidence and motivation to use their own learned skills for effective control of their condition is a primary factor in promoting health and wellbeing in people with RA.

Depression is more common in individuals with RA than in healthy individuals (Dickens et al., 2002). It has been suggested that this may be partly due to the constant pain. A recent study examined the association of depression and RA. Social difficulties and depression were evaluated by examining RA activity, RA damage, and subjective functional disability. The finding indicated a correlation between these three, with over a third of the patients diagnosed as depressed. The recommendations suggested that increased recognition of depression should lead to more appropriate management (Dickens et al., 2003).

Patient and health education

Multidisciplinary teamwork relating to people with RA has led to many health education programmes being developed. The purpose of RA focussed health education is to fully inform patients about their arthritis and enable them to be more involved in management decisions that may affect their future life. The decisions a person with RA may be required to make can be extensive and comprehensive, with the potential to make significant impacts on their life and the way it is lived. Drug treatments for instance may have many benefits and also considerable side effects and health risks attached. Health education is best delivered along with standard medication and other interventions to the person with RA. These planned health promoting activities might involve several different health professionals, including physiotherapists suggesting instructions to assist people to adjust their daily activities according to their arthritis. The aim would be to support and improve health behaviours and coping strategies, all of which is beneficial in enabling patients to cope with their disease (Taal et al., 1997).

It is now well established that health education in disease process and intervention are beneficial in the short term. In a recent Cochrane Review, for example, 24 randomised controlled trials evaluating patient education were examined (Riemsma et al., 2003). There were short term but no long term benefits of these health education initiatives. However in measuring the benefits, outcome measures designed for drug trials were used. These were very disease orientated and did little to consider other more holistic psychosocial aspects of living with RA. Other reports from patients have indicated that enhanced knowledge of their disease was reassuring and they felt less isolated. They were also felt more empowered to talk to health professionals about their arthritis (Ryan et al., 2003). There are also other health benefits from health education programmes, which are usually run for groups of patients. It is frequently observed, for example, that they often socialise amongst themselves and exchange advice concerning management of their disabilities. This must be considered a desirable consequence, contributing to the social life and possibly motivation and self-management skills of the person with arthritis.

In recent years more innovatory health promoting programmes have been successfully developed. For example, cognitive behavioural treatment has been offered to newly diagnosed patients in a randomised controlled trial and significant differences were found between the groups in terms of improvement in joint function and depression. Interestingly, improvements appeared to increase after a further short psychological treatment (Sharpe et al., 2003).

Perhaps with chronic disabling conditions like RA it is necessary to constantly repeat interventions in order to maintain effect. Like the rest of the population the person with RA is likely to forget certain management strategies in a bid to maintain normality, particularly with other aspects of their condition to monitor. With behavioural programmes constant repetition of facts and practices would be in order to preserve efficacy.

Other more specific health education programmes such as joint protection programmes are offered in some areas. Instruction is provided on the disease process and possible deformities of RA, methods of reducing the stress on the affected joints are discussed along with devices and gadgets to protect vulnerable areas. These groups aim to reduce pain and inflammation but also preserve joint integrity and improve function. In a randomised controlled trail lasting one year consisting of a joint protection programme, significant improvements were made in adherence to recommended treatment, pain, disease status and functional ability. These became more apparent with time (Hammond and Freeman, 2001). Reduction in pain levels is clearly an enabling concept and one that would be of significant interest to patients. Perhaps this suggests that joint protection can help slow the effects of RA. It is also worth considering that maybe the effects and changes in behaviour require learning and practicing, in order to be effective. Revision sessions may have value since the use of joint protection has been shown to tail off after 12 months (Hammond and Freeman, 2001).

Every consultation involving physiotherapists and people with arthritis can include a health education component. A perception of control over the management of their arthritis has been shown to have a positive effect on their wellbeing (Tennan et al., 1992). In one study with a sample of 40 patients, four major categories were identified as influencing control in people living with RA (Ryan et al., 2003). These were the reduction of physical symptoms, social support matching need, provision of information and the medical consultation. The authors concluded that the medical consultation could play an effective enabling role if used to its full potential. An important finding was that participants in the study enjoyed being asked their opinion and viewed the interaction as a partnership.

Exercise

Aerobic exercise in inflammatory and non-inflammatory arthritis at levels recommended for cardiovascular health is suitable for people with OA. However for those with advanced disease and those unable to participate in weight bearing activities, non-weight bearing activities such as swimming and cycling could be substituted (Hussey and Wilson, 2003). It is possible that repeated loading of joints with OA could precipitate further changes (Kujala et al., 1994; Spector et al., 1996).

For people with RA, aerobic exercise has been found to be effective in improving aerobic capacity, muscle strength and joint mobility; it does not increase inflammatory activity (van den Ende et al., 1998).

As well as the improvements listed the effects of aerobic exercise include mood elevation and a feeling of wellbeing (Kamwendo et al., 1999). In the person with arthritis who may be feeling low and perceive difficulty in coping with daily activities, this improvement in wellbeing is highly desirable. Exercise has long been one of the major forms of intervention prescribed by physiotherapists for those with arthritis (van den Ende et al., 1998). The aims of this form of management are to increase muscle power and maintain and improve joint mobility whilst promoting awareness of body mechanics and disease patterns. Recommendations for exercise should always be relevant and tailored to the needs of the patient. Individual goals should be set with the patient and monitored regularly; this way compliance can be maximised. Exercise should be reviewed for correct performance and updated frequently. By assuming responsibility for continuation of their exercise programme, people with arthritis are exercising self-management and promoting their own health. It is the expert instruction which empowers them to do this. In addition, it has been demonstrated that interest in exercise by all members of the multidisciplinary team (MDT) is important for its continuity, in particular the beliefs and attitudes of the rheumatologist concerning the effectiveness of the exercise programme (Iverson et al., 1999). In addition the communication skills of the health professional and all the MDT are crucial to the success of any intervention.

Hydrotherapy

Exercise in water has traditionally been used as an adjunct to land based exercise for people with arthritis. There is however little objective evidence available to support this development. A recent study comparing hydrotherapy and land based exercise regimes showed that both equally improved physical function and the gym based activity improved muscle strength (Foley et al., 2003). Exercise in water could be most beneficial for people with arthritis of the lower limbs, since reducing loading on these joints may reduce pain and therefore motivation to exercise could be increased.

In addition, for people with active RA and lengthy early morning stiffness, exercise in warm water assists in reducing the stiffness and enables a more active life (Foley et al., 2003). It must be remembered however that some of these people may require assistance from others to prepare for hydrotherapy or swimming, including assisted entry to the water.

Support

Along with other members of the multiprofessional rheumatology team, notably the occupational therapist, the physiotherapist may be involved in promoting heath through assisting the person with arthritis to manage their daily activities. This might involve advice concerning suitable resting positions such as those that are inclined to minimise any possible deformity, advice on how to intersperse activity with rest and how much activity is suitable. Self-management knowledge will aid the person with arthritis to manage their lives in the most efficient manner and also empower them to engage in the fullest possible activity levels and enjoyment. Physiotherapists should enable their clients to realise their full health potential. This will require effective partnerships and coordination across all sectors of health provision from the acute service in hospitals following recent diagnosis, to community and domiciliary support. It is important that the communication through all sectors is seamless and professional in order to achieve this objective.

People with RA who become severely disabled may require a partner or a spouse or another person to be their main care provider. In this case the health of the care giver also requires consideration (see Chapter 15 for further discussion of care giver wellbeing and health needs). It has been established that people derive high levels of self-esteem from giving care, but nevertheless support for them is required. It is suggested that this support may focus on maintaining the current scheduling of support and on emphasising the positive aspects of care giving (Jacobi et al., 2003).

The support required for people with arthritis is likely to fluctuate with the course of the condition. A recent study has indicated that the perception that support is present on a daily basis and is flexible enhances the sense of control of the person with arthritis (Ryan et al., 2003). Sometimes this support may be from a third party and may not be face to face with the patient. Many rheumatology departments, for example, use telephone help lines as an additional source of advice for the patient. Evaluation of phone links has suggested a 95 per cent satisfaction when the phone is used as an adjunct to the existing rheumatology service (Hughes et al., 2002). It may also further provide an empowering influence to support or confirm the decisions already taken by the patient.

Enabling a person with RA to maintain employment is a powerful empowerment strategy. Work disability is an adverse outcome of the disease and relates to physical health and quality of life (Young et al., 2002). The Young et al.

study found, unsurprisingly, that manual workers were more likely to quit their work early. Health promotion strategies such as education, exercise and empowerment should be designed and implemented early in the disease in order to maintain work status. A more radical approach would be to engage in more political endeavour and for physiotherapists to work as advocates in influencing employers, economists and policy makers in understanding the occupational health needs of people living with arthritis (see Tones and Green, 2004 and Chapter 1 for further discussion of the suggestion that health promotion is the militant wing of public health).

It is evident that people with arthritis wish to lead a full and active life. Many of these people are relatively young or in middle years and as such they need to feel able to contribute to all aspects of life. They also wish to have and to make choices, yet often due to the disease process these choices are removed. Occasionally when options are presented, the patient feels ill-equipped to make a rational decision. It is the duty of all health professionals to present the alternative regarding treatment interventions, but also to facilitate people with RA and OA to be able to make rational informed decisions regarding their own future. In order to achieve this, physiotherapists and health provision legislators need to move towards a more health promoting service rather than a service dominated by a medical view of the patient. One positive feature of the current NHS provision for people with arthritis is that it is team led and this enables the person to access many different professionals. Regular assessment of the person with arthritis should be arranged and a review of needs made in order for the physiotherapist to effectively engage in health promoting practice and support the person with arthritis to manage the changing nature of their condition.

References

American College of Rheumatology, Subcommittee on Rheumatoid Arthritis Guidelines (2002) Guidelines for the management of rheumatoid arthritis: 2002 update. *Arthritis Rheumatism* **46**: 328–46.

Buckley, C. D. (1997) Science, medicine and the future: treatment of rheumatoid arthritis. *British Medical Journal* **315**: 236–8.

Callahan, L. F. (1998) The burden of rheumatoid arthritis: facts and figures. *Journal of Rheumatology* **25** (supplement 53): 8–12.

Department of Health (1999) *Saving Lives: Our Healthier Nation*. London: The Stationery Office.

Donovan, J. L. and Blake, D. R. (2000) Qualitative study of interpretation of reassurance among patients attending rheumatology clinics: 'just a touch of arthritis, doctor?'. *British Medical Journal* **320**: 541–4.

Dickens, C., Jackson, J., Hay, E. and Creed, F. (2003) Association of depression and rheumatoid arthritis. *Psychosomatics* **44**: 209–15.

Dickens, C., McGowan, L., Clark-Carter, D. and Creed, F. (2002) Depression in rheumatoid arthritis: a systematic review of the literature with meta-analysis. *Psychosomatic Medicine* **64**: 52–60.

Emery, P., Breedveld, F. C., Dougados, M., Kalden, J. R., Schiff, M. H. and Smolen, J. S. (2002) Early referral recommendation for newly diagnosed rheumatoid arthritis: evidence based development of a clinical guideline. *Annals of the Rheumatic Diseases* **61**: 290–7.

Felson, D. T. (2000) Osteoarthritis: new insights. Part 1: the disease and its risk factors. *Annals of Internal Medicine* **133**: 726–97.

Foley, A., Halbert, J., Hewitt, T. and Crotty, M. (2003). Does hydrotherapy improve strength and physical function in patients with osteoarthritis: a randomised controlled trial comparing a gym based and a hydrotherapy based strengthening programme. *Annals of the Rheumatic Diseases* **62**: 1162–7.

Hallert, E., Thyberg, I., Hass, U., Skagren, E. and Skogh, T. (2003) Comparison between women and men with recent onset rheumatoid arthritis of disease activity and functional ability over two years (the TIRA project). *Annals of the Rheumatic Diseases* **62**: 667–70.

Hammond, A. and Freeman, K. (2001) One year outcomes of a randomised controlled trial of an educational-behavioural joint protection programme for people with rheumatoid arthritis. *Rheumatology* **40**: 1044–51.

Hart, R. P., Wade, J. B. and Martelli, M. F. (2003) Cognitive impairment in patients with chronic pain: the significance of stress. *Current Pain and Headache Reports* **7**: 116–26.

Hughes, R. A., Carr, M. E., Huggett, A. and Thwaites, C. E. (2002) Review of the function of a telephone helpline in the treatment of patients with rheumatoid arthritis. *Annals of the Rheumatic Diseases* **61** (4): 341–5.

Hussey, J. and Wilson, F. (2003) Measurement of activity levels is an important part of physiotherapy assessment. *Physiotherapy* **89** (10): 585–93.

Iverson, M. D., Fossel, A. H. and Daltroy, L. H. (1999) Rheumatologist–patient communication about exercise and physical therapy in the management of rheumatoid arthritis. *Arthritis Care Research* **12** (3): 180–92.

Jacobi, C. E., Van der Berg, B., Boshuizen, H. C., Rupp, I., Dinant, H. J. and van den Bos, G. A. M. (2003) Dimension-specific burden of care giving among partners of rheumatoid arthritis patients. *Rheumatology* **42**: 1226–33.

Jansen, L. M., van Schaardenburg, D., van der Horst-Bruinsma, I. E., Bezemer, P. D. and Dijkmans, B. A. (2000) Predictors of functional status in patients with early rheumatoid arthritis. *Annals of the Rheumatic Diseases* **59**: 223–6.

Kamwendo, K., Askenbom, M. and Walgren, C. (1999) Physical activity in the life of the patient with rheumatoid arthritis. *Physiotherapy Research International* **4** (4): 278–92.

Kuettner, K. and Goldberg, V. M. (eds) (1995) *Osteoarthritic Disorders.* Rosemount, IL: American Academy of Orthopaedic Surgeons.

Kujala, U. M., Kaprio, J. and Sarna, S. (1994). Osteoarthritis of the weight bearing joints of lower limbs in former elite male athletes. *British Medical Journal* **308**: 231–4.

Minnock, P., Fitzgerald, O. and Bresnihan, B. (2003) Women with established rheumatoid arthritis perceive pain as the predominant impairment of health status. *Rheumatology* **42**: 995–1000.

Neville, C., Fortin, P. R., Fitzcharles, M. A., Baron, M., Abrahamowitz, M., Du Berger, M. and Esdaile, J. M. (1999) The needs of patients with arthritis: the patient's perspective. *Arthritis Care and Research* **12** (2): 85–9.

Peat, G., McCartney, R. and Croft, P. (2001) Knee pain and osteoarthritis in older adults; a review of community burden and current use of health care. *Annals of the Rheumatic Diseases* **60**: 91–7.

Pincus, T. (1996) Rheumatoid arthritis. In Wegener, S. T., Belzer, B. I. and Gall, E. P. (eds) *Clinical Care in the Rheumatic Diseases*. Atlanta, GA: American College of Rheumatology.

Riemsma, R. P., Kirwan, J. R., Taal, E. and Rasker, J. J. (2003) Patient education for adults with rheumatoid arthritis. Cochrane Review. In *The Cochrane Library 1*. Oxford: Update Software.

Ryan, S., Hassell, A., Dawes, P. and Kendall, S. (2003) Control perceptions in patients with rheumatoid arthritis: the impact of the medical consultation. *Rheumatology* **42**: 135–40.

Sharpe, L., Sensky, T., Timberlake, N., Ryan, B. and Allard, S. (2003) Long term efficacy of a cognitive behavioural treatment from a randomised controlled trial for patients recently diagnosed with rheumatoid arthritis. *Rheumatology* **42**: 435–41.

Solomon, D. H., Warsi, A., Brown-Stevenson, T., Farrell, M., Gauthier, S., Mikels, D. and Lee, T. H. (2002) A controlled trial in a primary care physician network. *Journal of Rheumatology* **29** (2): 362–8.

Spector, T. D., Harris, P. A., Cicuttini, F. M., Nandra, D., Etherington, J., Wolman, R. L. and Doyle, D. V. (1996) Risk of osteoarthritis with long term weight bearing sports: a radiologic study of the hips and knees in female ex-athletes and population controls. *Arthritis and Rheumatism* **39**: 988–95.

Stuifbergen, A. K. and Rogers, S. (1997) Health promotion: an essential component of rehabilitation for persons with chronic and disabling conditions. *Advances in Nursing Science* **19** (4): 1–20.

Taal, E., Rasker, J. J. and Wiegman, O. (1997) Group education for rheumatoid arthritis patients: review. *Seminars on Arthritis Rheumatism* **26**: 805–16.

Tennan, H., Affleck, G., Higgins, P. M., Modola, R. and Urrows, S. (1992) Perceiving control, constructing benefits and daily processes in rheumatoid arthritis. *Canadian Journal of Behavioural Science* **24**: 186–203.

Tones, K. and Green, J (2004) *Health Promotion: Planning and Strategies*. London: Sage.

van den Ende, C. H. M., Vlieland, T. P. M., Munneke, M. and Hazes, J. M. W. (1998) Dynamic exercise therapy in rheumatoid arthritis: a systematic review. *British Journal of Rheumatology* **37**: 677–87.

van der Heide, D. N. F. M. (1995) Joint erosions and patients with early rheumatoid arthritis. *British Journal of Rheumatology* **34** (supplement): 74–8.

Young, A., Dixey, J., Kulinskaya, E., Cox, N., Davies, P., Devlin, J., Emery, P., Gough, A., James, D., Prouse, P., Williams, P. and Winfield, J. (2002) Which patients stop working because of rheumatoid arthritis? Results of a five years' follow up in 732 patients from the Early RA Study (ERAS). *Annals of the Rheumatic Diseases* **61**: 335–340.

PART IV
THE HEALTH PROMOTION CONTRIBUTION OF OTHER ALLIED HEALTH PROFESSIONALS

CHAPTER 17

Promoting Health: the Role of the Specialist Podiatrist

ALAN BORTHWICK AND SUSAN NANCARROW

The profession of podiatry, formerly known as chiropody, has been broadly depicted in the international literature as a healthcare specialty devoted to the treatment and prevention of afflictions of the foot (Skipper and Hughes, 1983; Dagnall and Page, 1992). However, such a broad, all embracing definition does little to illuminate the range of roles, skills and knowledge that inform modern podiatric practice. The role of the podiatrist has developed significantly in recent years, expanding in scope and breadth to include foot surgery, diabetes care and an embryonic role in rheumatology (Clements, 2001; Graham, 2000; Bowen, 2003a).

This chapter outlines the emerging specialist foci within podiatry and the reshaping of the therapeutic role in the context of the United Kingdom (UK) National Health Service (NHS) modernisation, manifest in a new, policy driven culture of multiprofessionalism emphasising interprofessional collaboration and changing professional boundaries (Department of Health (DoH), 2000a, 2000b, 2001a). Indeed, the central premise of this chapter, that increasing specialisation will demand a deep reconfiguration of podiatric services and roles and a fundamental shift in professional identity, has clear implications for the capacity of the profession to engage in comprehensive foot health promotion.

On the one hand, expanded specialist role development provides new opportunities for professional advancement in terms of professional status and patient health promotion. On the other hand, role restratification may be accompanied by professional fragmentation and a loss of core skills and identity. Developments in specialist care will be placed in the context of both patient demand and role boundary change in influencing and ensuring the promotion of foot health.

Feet are an overworked and undervalued part of the human anatomy. Population based health surveys show that between 15 and 25 per cent of the general public suffer from foot problems at any one point in time (Greenberg, 1994; Greenberg and Davis, 1993; Nancarrow, 1999). This rate increases threefold to nearly 75 per cent of those over 65 years (Munro and Steele, 1998). The presence of chronic illness, most notably diabetes, further increases the likelihood of severe lower limb complications including ulceration and amputation (Malgrange et al., 2003; see also Chapter 4 of this text for further discussion of diabetes and the health promoting role of the diabetes nurse).

Foot disorders in older people are associated with reduced balance capacity and people with multiple foot problems are at higher risk of falling than those with single foot conditions (Menz and Lord, 2001). The presence of corns and bunions is an independent risk factor for falling (Dolinis et al., 1997). In spite of these facts indicating a real need for health promoting action, podiatry has been slow to engage in health promotion (O'Boyle and Fleming, 2000). Nevertheless, the recent trend in the UK towards preventative care and patient empowerment reflects a growing specialisation in practice and hint at a profound reconstruction in professional roles, boundaries and identity.

The evolution of the role of the podiatrist

Podiatry remains a relatively unusual healthcare profession in that it is defined by a focus on a discrete body part, rather than a specific role, philosophy or approach to treatment. In this respect podiatry shares common ground with optometry and dentistry (Larkin, 1980, 1981; Nettleton, 1992). Indeed, podiatry and dentistry share common roots, emerging from the dual corn cutter and tooth drawer role of the 17th and 18th centuries (Seelig, 1953; Dagnall, 1995a, 1995b; Mandy, 2000). Since the separation of these occupational roles, podiatry has often been presented as a specialism in itself, a derivative branch of scientific medicine (Dagnall, 1970). It has also been construed as a natural branch of surgery; early surgeon chiropodists were often medically qualified practitioners with an exclusive interest in feet, an interest that was not to survive the specialisation of medicine into distinct role discrete branches such as orthopaedic surgery (Dagnall, 1956; Klenerman, 2002). By the mid 20th century medical power constrained the therapeutic role of the podiatrist, which was carefully circumscribed within the terms of membership of the UK Board of Registration of Medical Auxiliaries (Larkin, 1983, 1988, 1993, 1995). Scope of practice was limited to the treatment of the superficial excrescences of the foot, and in particular forbade the use of local analgesic procedures that would breach the true skin (Larkin, 1983). Today, by contrast, podiatry spans a wide field of practice, ranging from maintenance care of the elderly to elective surgical intervention and specialist care of the diabetic foot (Borthwick, 2000; Clements, 2001). Nevertheless, a new trend is emerging that will have a significant impact on the role of the podiatrist. The specialisation of podiatry in the key areas of foot surgery, diabetes and rheumatology care may increasingly isolate the maintenance role identified with the traditional practitioner, thus reshaping the core function of the profession. Already, a retreat from simple footcare is in evidence, with the inception of empower-ment projects, designed to promote self-care by patients and carers, and an increasingly complex intraprofessional division of labour involving the estab-lishment of tiered grades, ranging from assistant practitioners and aides to extended scope practitioners (Farndon and Nancarrow, 2003; Moore et al., 2003). Specialisation has also advanced preventative and educational health promotional approaches in diabetes care, whilst aiding the release of routine footcare tasks through educational programmes in self care (Nancarrow, 2003; Moore et al., 2003).

Development of the role of the specialist podiatrist

In retrospect, it is possible to identify the UK Professions Supplementary to Medicine Act 1960 as a watershed in the transition of podiatric scope of practice. Although little in the way of innovations in practice was evident through the decade that followed, the redefined scope of practice developed by the new regulatory body promised change (Dagnall, 1962, 1981; Bradley, 1965; Smedley, 1976; Borthwick, 1997). Medical authority was still assured through the vehicle of the Chiropodists Board, preventing unchecked expan-sion in scope, but the Act tacitly assumed role boundaries would remain largely intact, based on preexisting patterns of occupational jurisdictions (Larkin, 2002). This was not to be the case. Change resulted initially from a dispute over access to medicines, and in particular parenterally administered local anaesthetics, under the terms of the Medicines Act 1968, which became a professional cause célèbre (Borthwick, 2001a). More than a decade elapsed before the profession was able to secure an exemption order ensuring legal access to local anaesthetics, although Chiropodists Board approval in 1972 enabled the technique to be legitimately developed and scope of practice to expand into the domain of invasive foot surgery (Dagnall and Page, 1992; Lorimer, 1995; Borthwick, 2001a). These developments signalled the intention of the profession to reconstitute itself as a healthcare specialism with overall foot expertise, challenging the stereotypical image of the corn cutter and creating a new identity modelled on the notion of the foot doctor (Dagnall, 1995a, 1995b; Lorimer, 1995; Borthwick, 2001a).

The specialist podiatric surgeon

Lack of orthopaedic interest in the foot has been held responsible for the emergence of podiatric surgery (Klenerman, 1991; Grace, 1997). Recent esti-mates suggest only one in 20 orthopaedic consultants undertake a significant amount of foot surgery (Grace, 1997). The British Orthopaedic Foot Surgery Society boasts only 60 practising UK orthopaedic surgeons, of which some devote less than 30 per cent of their working time to the foot (Grace, 1997).

Indeed, a relatively recent British Orthopaedic Association census revealed that only 2 per cent of members listed the foot and ankle as their main sub specialty interest. Within orthopaedics it has been common for foot surgery to be delegated to junior staff, and to be regarded with less status than hip, knee or hand surgery, creating a hierarchy of esteem ensuring disinterest in the management of foot problems (Graham, 1982). In addition, the integration of podiatric surgery within mainstream NHS healthcare was also facilitated by the political ideology of Thatcherite Conservatism. The Conservative government of Margaret Thatcher (1979–90) firmly adhered to a neoliberal agenda espousing the values of the free market, open competition and minimal state intervention (Ham, 1994; Dorey, 1995). It was also gravely concerned at the monopolistic powers of the medical profession and the profligate use of resources for which medicine was held, in part, responsible (Cox, 1991). In a bid to reverse this trend, it introduced a series of radical health service reforms, most notably involving general management and a particular brand of marketisation characterised by an internal or managed market encompassing a re-emphasis on primary care through general practitioner (GP) fund holding (Webster, 2000). General managers were empowered to manage services across professional boundaries and GP fund holders were encouraged to adopt business values to secure best value for money (Cox, 1991; Ham, 1994; Flynn, Williams and Pickard, 1996). These measures provided the level playing field upon which the emergent and competitive specialism of podiatric surgery could thrive. Under GP fund holding and general management, podiatric surgery rapidly became an efficient, cost effective and accessible service (Borthwick, 1999, 2000; Foot and Ankle Surgery Editorial, 2002). Today, podiatric surgery involves a wide range of surgical options, ranging from procedures such as digital, bunion and metatarsal corrections, osteotomies and fusions, which deploy triplane concepts of function, to rear foot calcaneal osteotomies, neuroma excisions, fasciotomies, and digital or ray amputations (Tollafield, 1993; Hood et al., 1994; Kilmartin, 2000; Laxton, 1996; Milsom, 1995; Price and Tasker, 2000). Most cases are managed under local anaesthesia on a day care basis, although some procedures require hospitalisation (Borthwick, 2000; Wilkinson and Prior, 2000). Perhaps the most significant reflection of the degree to which podiatric surgery has achieved a firmly legitimate role within UK NHS healthcare has been the acquisition of medical consultant and associate specialist grade contracts (MC21 and MC01) for the highest ranking podiatric surgeons (Graham, 2000).

Many podiatrists would stress that podiatric surgery does not simply equate to orthopaedic foot surgery (Graham, 1982; Bell, 1983). It may be tempting to assume that this specialty has nothing new to offer therapeutically, and simply reflects a successful usurpation of orthopaedic territory. This would imply that orthopaedic care of the foot has simply been taken over by podiatrists and is not a new specialism so much as a borrowed or stolen one. However, there are clearly identifiable differences in the forms of theoretical knowledge that underpin the practices, and this has led to further interdisciplinary dispute over the best procedures to select and how to justify them (Graham, 1982; Bell, 1983; Borthwick, 2003a). Nevertheless, podiatric surgery can be wholly regarded as a specialty that contributes to patient health and wellbeing through the adoption and development of new approaches to surgical care of the feet (Kilmartin, 2003).

Currently, podiatric surgery probably constitutes the foremost subspecialty within podiatry. Its practitioners uniquely enjoy consultant level status in the NHS and Faculty level status within the College of Podiatrists of the Society of Chiropodists and Podiatrists. No other subspecialty has attained comparable status or rights within either the NHS or the professional body. Nor do their practices constitute such a radical departure from the natural order of professional roles, or the result of such a clearly successful usurpationary closure strategy (Parkin, 1979; Borthwick, 2001a, 2003a). In addition, as yet no other subspecialty requires a specific, formal, structured, postgraduate training to ensure uniform standards of practice or eligibility for appointment to specialist roles. Podiatric specialists in diabetes care, podiatric biomechanics and rheumatology care do exist, but with much less well defined routes for training and subsequent recognition. Within podiatric surgery, a new route for education and training has recently been proposed that should, it is claimed, underpin the creation of new podiatric surgical posts in the NHS in Scotland, where currently none exist (Podiatry Now, 2002).

The diabetes specialist podiatrist

The emergence of podiatric specialists in diabetes care can be traced back to the mid 1980s, although the presence of podiatrists working in diabetic foot clinics precedes these more formal appointments by several years (Edmonds et al., 1986; Rayman et al., 2000). As yet, the exact scope, role and training of diabetes specialist podiatrists remain undefined (Young, 2002). Many podiatrists do adopt the title of diabetes specialist podiatrist, but few share a common pathway in pursuit of this distinction and are often appointed and remunerated at variable NHS grades in recognition of their advanced roles (Farndon and Nancarrow, 2003). Indeed, hospital appointments for diabetes specialist podiatrists (DSPs) are dependent upon an interview and an assessment of the applicant's relevant experience and qualifications, whilst the title may in some instances even be self-conferred by community based podiatrists (Rayman et al., 2000).

At the time of writing, 81 per cent of NHS podiatry services claim to employ diabetes specialist podiatrists (Farndon and Nancarrow, 2003). However, a recent survey undertaken by Young (2003) of delegates at a conference revealed many of the current difficulties facing the development of this specialist health promoting role. Importantly, relatively few specialist diabetic foot clinics enjoy sufficient resources to employ specialist podiatrists, relying instead upon a system of purchasing from community services; and the lack of a competency based system of specialist diabetes training and education for podiatrists in this field has been contrasted critically with the clinical examinations required of specialist diabetes nurses (ENB928) (Young, 2002, 2003; see also Chapter 4 for an examination of the diabetes nurse's health promoting role). However, many professional experts within the multidisciplinary diabetic footcare team also have little uniform, structured specialist training in the care of the diabetic foot, including physicians, orthotists and surgeons as well as podiatrists (McInnes et al., 1998). Nevertheless, the need for specialist diabetes foot care is beyond dispute. It has been estimated that 10 to 15 per cent of patients diagnosed with diabetes are at risk of developing foot ulceration (Steed, 1998; McPherson and Binning, 2002). In spite of these concerns, a new initiative recently introduced by the Department of Health does acknowledge the utility of accessing informal expertise in diabetes care and other specialist areas by encouraging the development of networks of nurses and allied health professionals with special interests (AHPwSI), which may complement the current informal system in operation in diabetes footcare (DoH, 2003a). Not all specialists are in favour of pursuing the route of formal qualifications and acknowledge the immense contribution made by those whose expertise is derived from long experience of working in the field (McInnes, 2002). The evidence to support current interventions in the care of the diabetic foot is, surprisingly, quite sparse, and further research is required (Edmonds et al., 2001; Young, 2002). The key areas of care with which the specialist podiatrist is concerned centre on wound care, wound debridement, dressings, footwear and orthotic therapy, alongside a crucially important role in the monitoring and assessment of vascular and neurological status, with an eye on the rate of subtle change that might herald a phase of ulceration or gangrene (Gadsby and McInnes, 1998; McCormick and Young, 1999). Some diabetologists suggest the health promoting role of the podiatrist might conceivably and safely be expanded to include the measurement and treatment of hypertension, the alteration of patient insulin dosages and the provision of patient health education in the monitoring of blood glucose (Kerr and Richardson, 2000). Health education is already a key feature of the podiatrist's secondary health promoting role in diabetes. Foot care health education programmes for people with diabetes have been shown to be effective in improving knowledge and adaptation, and in preventing ulceration and limb loss in a high risk population (Barth et al., 1991). Indeed the identification and determination of risk, alongside the early introduction of preventative foot health education advice, are viewed as crucial to the reduction of amputation rates in diabetes, and form a natural focus for the DSP (Bild et al., 1989; Robbie, 2002). Moreover, novel diabetic foot screening programmes, focussed around preventative foot care and health promotion, have begun to emerge in response to the National Service Framework for Diabetes (Robbie, 2002). These involve annual physical screening for lower limb complications, one-to-one health education packages and improved treatment and referral options (Nancarrow, 2000, 2003; Robbie, 2002). Podiatry services remain best placed to provide these health promoting functions, as a recent study comparing GP and podiatry services concluded (Williams and Ridgway, 2002). However, the delivery of health education alone is regarded as insufficient in modifying behaviour in diabetes, and change demands innovative patient centred educational skills on the part of the DSP (Ashford et al., 2000; Stuart and Wiles, 2000). Skills in health promotion and prevention are, therefore, likely to feature prominently in any future training requirement for appointment to the role of DSP.

The independent prescriber

The Crown Report (DoH, 1999) signalled a profound change in the status and regulation of prescribing in UK healthcare. Since the deregulation of healthcare began in the Thatcherite era, indicative prescribing, deregulation of medicines from prescription only (POM) and pharmacy only categories and the introduction of nurse prescribing legislation have followed steadily. Most recently, supplementary prescribing has been introduced for nursing and pharmacy, and the government has identified ambitious targets for expanding new independent prescriber numbers (DoH 2003b, 2003c). At the time of the Crown Report (DoH, 1999), podiatry had been in consultation with the Medicines Control Agency (MCA) and its predecessor, the Medicines Commission, for more than 30 years in an almost continuous cycle of negotiations designed to improve practice through greater access to restricted medicines. In 1981, and again in 1997, state registered podiatrists attained extensions in access and administration rights for a range of POM and pharmacy only agents, including local anaesthetics with adrenalin, anti-inflammatory agents and antifungal agents, but they have consistently been denied rights to antibacterial antibiotics and adrenaline for emergency use (Borthwick, 2001c). The novelty of the Crown recommendations was the recognition of new independent prescribers capable of rendering a diagnosis and independently managing a patient caseload, to include the prescribing of medicines. Under the Health and Social Care Act 2001, clause 68 enabled prescribing by healthcare professionals other than doctors, dentists and nurses, who have their own primary legislation, and the Crown Report recommended podiatrists, optometrists and extended scope physiotherapists as potential independent prescribers. Podiatric surgeons were initially intended to be the recipients of this privilege, although the author of the report agreed to reinterpret the recommendations to include all podiatrists as specialists (Borthwick, 2001b). Since the year 2000 the use of patient group directions (PGDs) has served to enable access to medicines in the absence of full implementation of the Crown recommendations, although this has the disadvantage of regional disparity in practice (Ashcroft, 2002). The Society of Chiropodists and Podiatrists Medicines Committee again forwarded to the MCA a new submission in 2003, but evidence suggests that the Department of Health is intent on receiving submissions from all the AHPs, many of whom have no history of access or administration practices and have no clear vision as yet of how to approach such an opportunity. Independent prescriber status would enhance a wide range of podiatry roles, although it presently remains uncertain if the government is fully committed to implementing AHP independent prescribing (Borthwick, 2003b).

The podiatric biomechanics specialist

Intriguingly, it remains debateable whether the practice of podiatric biomechanics can credibly be regarded as a specialism distinct from general podiatric practice, although the knowledge base that constitutes the fabric of biomechanics has been widely accepted as a new contribution to the understanding of foot function (Root et al., 1971; Sgarlato, 1971; Schuster, 1974; Spencer, 1978; Anthony, 1990; Harradine et al., 2003). Although there are, to date, a number of practitioners working as lead clinicians in this field, the lack of formalised and structured access to specialist levels coupled with the widespread use of biomechanical knowledge in general podiatry practice render this area problematic when assigning specialist status (Farndon and Nancarrow, 2003). At the time of writing over two thirds of NHS podiatry service managers currently claim to provide a podiatric biomechanics specialty service (Farndon and Nancarrow, 2003). However, even a cursory glance through the job advert webpage of the professional body reveals a variable range of available specialist lead biomechanics posts at Senior Grade 1 or Chief Grade 3 level, alongside basic grade posts requiring a good working knowledge, experience in or even requiring work at advanced level in biomechanics (Society for Chiropodists and Podiatrists (SCP), 2003). Indeed, even at the level of Senior Grade 2, applicants are not uncommonly required to undertake specialist work in several specialist areas (SCP, 2003).

Theoretical elaborations continue to transform the knowledge base underpinning podiatric practice and provide increasingly sophisticated models informing therapeutic care. However, contradictory evidence continues to hamper the development of the specialism and undermine confidence in the viability and validity of the practice (McPoil and Cornwall, 1996; Kidd, 1997; Nester, Findlow and Bowker, 2001). It also ensures an ongoing controversy over the therapeutic value of orthoses, the in-shoe devices that are presumed to realign and normalise foot function (Kilmartin, 1991, 1994; Kilmartin and Wallace, 1994; Prior, 1994). Refinements in theory have led to the construction of three key frameworks, each of which is in some way contested: the subtalar joint neutral paradigm, which gave rise to the very construct of podiatric biomechanics and continues to inform most biomechanical practices; the more recent sagittal plane facilitation theory espoused by Dananberg (Dananberg, 1986, 1993a, 1993b; Dananberg and Guiliano, 1999); and the tissue stress theory associated with the work of Kirby and further elaborated by Fuller (Kirby, 1987, 2000; Fuller, 2000a, 2000b). In spite of these challenges, modern theorists continue to seek a unifying theory that would support a single explanatory model (Harradine, Bevan and Carter, 2003). However elusive, the promise of a robust model built upon a unified theory remains a tantalising prospect, one that might, in time, open new avenues of both care and preventative health promotion in the management of foot and lower limb disorders.

The rheumatology specialist podiatrist

Rheumatology probably represents the newest specialist domain within podiatry and one where there is much scope for a health promoting role. At present the status of the specialism is that of a special interest group of the professional body. Rheumatoid patients are commonly encountered by podiatrists although currently there are no available data on their podiatric needs (Woodburn and Helliwell, 1997). A small number of practitioners have secured NHS positions as lead clinicians in rheumatology, but few are able to devote their time exclusively to rheumatological work. Indeed, Farndon and Nancarrow's (2003) national study of specialty services has revealed that up to 15 per cent of NHS podiatry services claim to provide a podiatric rheumatology specialty service. Perhaps more revealingly, a recent conference organised by the podiatric rheumatology special interest group, the Podiatric Rheumatic Care Association, devoted time to considering strategies for developing consultant level posts in the NHS, largely through the standardisation of advanced practitioner qualifications, credentials that do not yet exist (Bowen, 2003a). At present the range of disorders that is referred for specialist podiatry care within rheumatology clinics encompasses heel pain, a variety of sports injuries, acute inflammatory arthritic conditions, bursitis and tibialis posterior tendon dysfunction (Bowen, 2003b). The link between rheumatic disorders and foot disability is clear, although paradoxically, few data exist to support claims for either the clinical or fiscal advantages of foot interventions (Minaker and Little, 1973; Woodburn and Helliwell, 1997). Nevertheless, rheumatologists have spoken out enthusiastically in favour of a specialist role for podiatrists in this discipline (Dickson, 1996). Evidence suggesting the benefits of early, preventative orthoses intervention in rheumatoid disease is promising, further enhancing the case for a recognised podiatric specialism within the NHS (Woodburn et al., 2002). Early use of orthoses may help to reduce foot pain and prevent deformity, and the prescription, fabrication and distribution of rigid foot orthoses clearly falls within the domain of the podiatrist (Woodburn et al., 2002). Unfortunately, evidence for the effectiveness of orthoses and other interventions is equivocal (Conrad et al., 1996; Hodge, Bach and Carter, 1999). Debridement of foot plantar calluses, although providing significant short term benefits in patients with rheumatoid disease, may also involve an elevation in peak plantar pressures following debridement (Woodburn et al., 2000). Nevertheless, research evidence which promotes an understanding of foot function in rheumatoid disease is gradually being assimilated, which may well help to underpin more effective therapeutic developments and interventions by podiatrists and encourage the establishment of increasing numbers of podiatric rheumatology specialist posts (Keenan et al., 1991; Budiman-Mak et al., 1995; Woodburn and Helliwell, 1996).

Specialisation, health promotion and patient empowerment

For many years demand for NHS podiatry services has outstripped capacity (Kemp and Winkler, 1983; Cartwright and Henderson, 1986). Disinvestment and case reprofiling measures have also, in recent years, reduced access to podiatry services (Campbell et al., 2002; Tippens, 1998). The greatest demand stems from older people, who account for up to 70 per cent of podiatry caseloads (Age Concern, 1998). However, the emergence of National Service Frameworks has also placed greater demands on services involving an enhanced role for specialist care, most notably in screening and education in diabetes care (DoH, 2001b). Innovative strategies designed to reduce service dependency have begun to emerge in parallel with increasing specialisation, profoundly reshaping service orientation and role identity (Farndon et al., 2002a, 2002b). The notion of patient empowerment permits a streamlining of services through a process by which patients identified by podiatrists as being at low risk are empowered to actively participate in their own footcare in line with current government policy (Moore et al., 2003). Although introduced as a practical necessity, the new vanguard empowerment scheme in operation in Sheffield reflects a major role revision, in which the podiatrist becomes a specialist concerned with managing patients defined as being at high risk, leaving lesser needs to be addressed either by care assistants or via self-care (Moore et al., 2003). Moore et al. (2003) describe empowerment talks designed to enlighten patients as to new eligibility criteria, revisions in the role of the podiatrist and the acquisition of new skills to self-manage or enhance carer support have been used and followed up in subsequent audits, resulting in an effective elimination of waiting lists (Moore et al., 2003). The success of the programme from a service perspective is likely to ensure a wider, national application of the scheme and accelerate the transition towards preventative care.

The future

The focus of podiatry care and service provision appears to be shifting direction in the manner anticipated in the *Feet First* report (DoH, 1994). Greater emphasis on specialist care in the areas of foot surgery, diabetes and rheumatology is emerging and new roles evolving. Government health reforms continue to encourage an expansion in role boundaries and promote the development of health professionals with distinctive interests that reflect these boundary changes (DoH, 2003a). The skills of health promotion, facilitation and preventative care are intimately linked to the new roles being shaped in each specialty field and also inform the changing nature of practice, where patient empowerment and self-care steadily replace basic footcare interventions. In this respect, podiatry is entering a new era, one centred on advice giving and task delegation for more routine forms of care, and specialist skill acquisition for new roles. This path forward presents the profession with both opportunities and challenges. More integrated models of care, grounded in multidisciplinary working environments, may offer greater professional status, broader skill recognition and enhanced therapeutic credibility. Specialist podiatrists in these circumstances may be less likely to be regarded as mere corn cutters engaged in routine, labour intensive, skill limited tasks as they increasingly adopt more glamorous, curative, virtuoso roles (Hugman, 1991). Of course, this is being accompanied by a parallel trend towards delegation, ditching the real or metaphorical dirty work, and restratification, which may yet have far reaching consequences for professional identity, workforce capacity and effective health promotion (Hugman, 1991; Farndon and Nancarrow, 2003).

References

Age Concern (1998) *On Your Feet! Older People and NHS Chiropody Services.* London: Age Concern.

Anthony, R. (1990) *The Manufacture and Use of the Functional Foot Orthoses.* London: Karger.

Ashcroft, D. (2002) Patient group directions: adrenaline and anaphylaxis. *Podiatry Now* 5 (6): 320.

Ashford, R. L., McGee, P. and Kinmond, K. (2000) Perception of quality of life by patients with diabetic foot ulcers. *The Diabetic Foot* 3 (4): 150–5.

Barth, R., Campbell, L. V., Allen, S., Jupp, J. J. and Chisholm, D. J. (1991). Intensive education improves knowledge, compliance, and foot problems in type 2 diabetes. *Diabetes Medicine* 8 (2): 111–17.

Bell, D. R. C. (1983) Personal correspondence. *British Chiropody Journal* 48 (53): 99–100.

Bild, D. E., Selby, J. V., Sinnock, P., Browner, W. S., Braveman, P. and Showstack, J. A. (1989) Lower extremity amputation in people with diabetes: epidemiology and prevention. *Diabetes Care* 12 (1): 24–31.

Borthwick, A. M. (1997) *A Study of the Professionalisation Strategies of British Podiatry 1960–1997.* Unpublished doctoral thesis, University of Salford.

Borthwick, A. M. (1999) Challenging medical dominance: podiatric surgery in the National Health Service. *British Journal of Podiatry* 2 (3): 75–83.

Borthwick, A. M. (2000) Challenging medicine: the case of podiatric surgery. *Work, Employment & Society* 14 (2): 369–83.

Borthwick, A. M. (2001a) Occupational imperialism at work: the case of podiatric surgery. *British Journal of Podiatry* 4 (3): 70–9.

Borthwick, A. M. (2001b) Predicting the impact of new prescribing rights. *The Diabetic Foot* 4 (1): 4–8.

Borthwick, A. M. (2001c) Drug prescribing in podiatry: radicalism or tokenism? *British Journal of Podiatry* 4 (2): 56–64.

Borthwick, A. M. (2003a) The changing character of medical dominance: co-equal partnerships or the annexation of podiatric surgery? Views from orthopaedic surgeons. Conference presentation, Society of Chiropodists & Podiatrists Annual Conference, Royal Horticultural Hall, London, 17 October.

Borthwick, A. M. (2003b) Prescribing rights for the Allied Health Professions: temporary lull or quiet abandonment? *Podium* 1 (4): 4–6.

Bowen, C. (2003a) Podiatric Rheumatic Care Association Conference Report. *Podiatry Now* 6 (6): 18.

Bowen, C. (2003b) The Podiatry Rheumatic Care Association. *Podiatry Now* 6 (11): 32.

Bradley, T. P. (1965) Educational developments in chiropody. *The Chiropodist* 20 (3): 58–63.

Budiman-Mak, E., Conrad, K. J., Roach, K. E., Moore, J. W., Lertratanakul, Y., Koch, A. E., Skosey, J. L., Froelich, C. and Joyce-Clark, N. (1995) Can foot orthoses prevent hallux valgus deformity in rheumatoid arthritis? A randomised controlled trial. *Journal of Clinical Rheumatology* 1: 313–21.

Campbell, J. A., Patterson, A., Gregory, D., Milns, D., Turner, W., White, D. and Luxton, D. E. A. (2002) What happens when older people are discharged from NHS podiatry services? *The Foot* 12: 32–42.

Cartwright, A. and Henderson, G. (1986) *More Trouble with Feet: a Survey of the Foot Problems and Chiropody Needs of the Elderly*. London: Institute for Social Studies in Medical Care.

Clements, D. J. (2001) Providing a diabetic foot care service: establishing a podiatry service. In Boulton, A. J. M., Connor, H. and Cavanagh, P. R. (eds) *The Foot in Diabetes*, third edition. London: Wiley.

Conrad, K. J., Budiman-Mak, E., Roach, K. E. and Hedeker, D. (1996) Impacts of foot orthoses on pain and disability in rheumatoid arthritis. *Journal of Clinical Epidemiology* 49 (1): 1–7.

Cox, D. (1991) Health service management – a sociological view: Griffiths and the non-negotiated order of the hospital. In Gabe, J., Calnan, M., and Bury, M. (eds) *The Sociology of the Health Service*. London: Routledge.

Dagnall, J. C. (1956) Pioneers of chiropody – Monsieur La Forest and D. Low. *British Chiropody Journal* 21 (4): 245–7.

Dagnall, J. C. (1962) Durlacher and 'the nail growing into the flesh'. *British Chiropody Journal* 27 (10): 263–7.

Dagnall, J. C. (1970) The origins of the Society of Chiropodists. *The Chiropodist* 25 (9): 315–23.

Dagnall, J. C. (1981) The history, development and current status of nail matrix phenolisation. *The Chiropodist* 36 (9): 315–24.

Dagnall, J. C. (1995a) The origins of the Society of Chiropodists and Podiatrists and its history, 1945–1995, part 1. *Journal of British Podiatric Medicine* 50 (9): 135–41.

Dagnall, J. C. (1995b) The origins of the Society of Chiropodists and Podiatrists and its history, 1945–1995, part 3. *Journal of British Podiatric Medicine* 50 (11): 174–80.

Dagnall, J. C. and Page, A. L. (1992) A critical history of the Chiropodial profession and the Society of Chiropodists. *Journal of British Podiatric Medicine* 47 (2): 30–4.

Dananberg, H. J. (1986) Functional Hallux limitus and its relationship to gait efficiency. *Journal of the American Podiatric Medical Association* 76 (11): 648–52.

Dananberg, H. J. (1993a) Gait style as an etiology to chronic postural pain, part 1: functional Hallux limitus. *Journal of the American Podiatric Medical Association* **83** (8): 433–41.

Dananberg, H. J. (1993b) Gait style as an etiology to chronic postural pain, part 2: postural compensatory processes. *Journal of the American Podiatric Medical Association* **83** (11): 615–25.

Dananberg, H. J. and Guiliano, M. (1999) Chronic low back pain and its response to custom made foot orthoses. *Journal of the American Podiatric Medical Association* **80** (3): 109–17.

Department of Health (1994) *Feet First: Report of the Joint Department of Health and NHS Chiropody Task Force.* London: DoH.

Department of Health (1999) *Final Report of the Review of Prescribing, Supply & Administration of Medicines (Crown Report).* London: DoH.

Department of Health (2000a) *A Health Service of All the Talents: Developing the NHS Workforce.* London: DoH.

Department of Health (2000b) *Meeting the Challenge: a Strategy for the Allied Health Professions.* London: DoH.

Department of Health (2001a) *Investment and Reform for NHS staff: Taking Forward the NHS Plan.* London: DoH.

Department of Health (2001b) *National Service Framework for Diabetes: Standards.* London: DoH.

Department of Health (2003a) *Practitioners with Special Interests: Bringing Services Closer to Patients.* London: DoH.

Department of Health (2003b) *Nurse Prescribers Extended Formulary: Proposals to Extend the Range of Prescription Only Medicines.* Consultation paper MLX 293. London: DoH.

Department of Health (2003c) *Supplementary Prescribing by Nurses and Pharmacists Within the NHS in England: a Guide to Implementation.* London: DoH.

Dickson, D. J. (1996) What do general practitioners expect from rheumatology clinics? *British Journal of Rheumatology* **35**: 920.

Dolinis, J., Harrison, J. E. and Andrews, G. R. (1997) Factors associated with falling in older Adelaide residents. *Australian and New Zealand Journal of Public Health* **21** (5): 462–8.

Dorey, P. (1995) *British Politics Since 1945.* Oxford: Blackwell.

Edmonds, M. E., Blundell, M. P. and Morris, H. E. (1986) Improved survival of the diabetic foot: the role of the specialised foot clinic. *Quarterly Journal of Medicine* **60**: 763–71.

Edmonds, M., McIntosh, C., Foster, A. and Munro, N. (2001) An initiative to widen the evidence base for the diabetic foot. *The Diabetic Foot* **4** (3): 108–11.

Farndon, L. and Nancarrow, S. (2003) Employment and career development opportunities for podiatrists and foot care assistants in the NHS. *British Journal of Podiatry* **6** (4): 103–8.

Farndon, L., Vernon, W., Potter, J. and Parry, A. (2002a) The professional role of the podiatrist in the new Millennium: an analysis of current practice, paper 1. *British Journal of Podiatry* **5** (3): 68–72.

Farndon, L., Vernon, W., Potter, J. and Parry, A. (2002b) The professional role of the podiatrist in the new Millennium: is there a gap between professional image and scope of practice?, paper 2. *British Journal of Podiatry* **5** (4): 100–2.

Flynn, R. Williams, G. and Pickard, S. (1996) *Markets and Networks: Contracting in Community Health Services.* Buckingham: Open University Press.

Foot and Ankle Surgery Editorial (2002) Chiropody, podiatry and orthopaedics. *Foot and Ankle Surgery* **8**: 83.

Fuller, E. A. (2000a) The Windlass mechanism of the foot: a mechanical model to explain pathology. *Journal of the American Podiatric Medical Association* **90** (1): 35–46.

Fuller, E. A. (2000b) Centre of pressure and its theoretical relationship to foot pathology. *Journal of the American Podiatric Medical Association* **89** (6): 278–91.

Gadsby, R. and McInnes, A. (1998) The at-risk foot: the role of the primary care team in achieving St Vincent targets for reducing amputation. *Diabetic Medicine* **15** (supplement 3): S61–4.

Grace, D. L. (1997) The problem of foot surgery. *British Journal of Podiatric Medicine and Surgery* **9** (3): 41–2.

Graham, R. B. (2000) Chiropody and podiatry. Conference presentation, *Developing the Therapy Professions*, Royal College of Surgeons, London, 10 May.

Graham, R. G. (1982) Display of arrogance in orthopaedics. *Therapy Weekly* **9** (4): 6.

Greenberg, L. (1994). Foot care data from two recent nationwide surveys: a comparative analysis. *Journal of the American Podiatric Medical Association* **84** (7): 365–70.

Greenberg, L. and Davis, H. (1993) Foot problems in the US: the 1990 National Health Interview Survey. *Journal of the American Podiatric Medical Association* **83** (8): 475–83.

Health and Social Care Act 2001, part 5, clause 68. London: The Stationery Office.

Ham, C. (1994) *Management and Competition in the New NHS*. Oxford: Radcliffe Medical Press.

Harradine, P. D., Bevan, L. S. and Carter, N. (2003) Gait dysfunction and podiatric therapy, part 1: foot-based models and orthotic management. *British Journal of Podiatry* **6** (1): 5–11.

Hodge, M. C., Bach, T. M. and Carter, G. M. (1999) Orthotic management of plantar pressure and pain in rheumatoid arthritis. *Clinical Biomechanics* **14**: 567–75.

Hood, I. S., Kilmartin, T. E. and Tollafield, D. R. (1994) The effect of podiatric day care on the need for NHS chiropody treatment. *The Foot* **4** (3): 155–8.

Hugman, R. (1991) *Power in Caring Professions*, Basingstoke: Macmillan (now Palgrave Macmillan).

Keenan, M. A. E., Peabody, T. D., Gronley, J. K., Perry, J. and California, D. (1991) Valgus deformities of the feet and characteristics of gait in patients who have rheumatoid arthritis. *Journal of Bone and Joint Surgery* **73-A** (2): 237–47.

Kemp, J. and Winkler, J. T. (1983) *Problems Afoot: Need and Efficiency in Footcare*. London: Disabled Living Foundation.

Kerr, D. and Richardson, T. (2000) The diabetic foot at the crossroads: vanguard or oblivion? *The Diabetic Foot* **3** (2): 70–1.

Kidd, R. (1997) Forefoot varus: real or false, fact or fantasy? *Australasian Journal of Podiatric Medicine* **31** (3): 81–4.

Kilmartin, T. E. (1991) But you haven't proved that orthotic works. *Search News* **12**: 8–12.

Kilmartin, T. E. (1994) *The effect of Functional Orthoses on Juvenile Hallux Valgus*. Unpublished doctoral thesis, University of Nottingham.

Kilmartin, T. E. (2000) Podiatric surgery in a Community Trust: a review of activity, surgical outcomes and patient satisfaction over a 27 month period. *Podiatry Now* **3** (9): 350–5.

Kilmartin, T. E. (2003) Current concepts in podiatric surgery. Conference presentation, Society of Chiropodists & Podiatrists Annual Conference, Royal Horticultural Hall, London, 17 October.

Kilmartin, T. E. and Wallace, W. A. (1994) A controlled prospective trail of a foot orthoses for juvenile Hallux valgus. *Journal of Bone and Joint Surgery* 74-**B** (2): 250–7.

Kirby, K. A. (1987) Methods for determination of positional variations in the subtalar joint axis. *Journal of American Podiatric Medical Association* 77 (5): 228–34.

Kirby, K. A. (2000) Biomechanics of the normal and abnormal foot. *Journal of the American Podiatric Medical Association* 90 (1): 30–4.

Klenerman, L. (2002) Development of foot and ankle surgery. In Klenerman, L. (ed.) *The Evolution of Orthopaedic Surgery.* London: Royal Society of Medicine Press.

Klenerman, L. (1991) Podiatry. *Bone and Joint Surgery* 73-**B**: 1–2.

Larkin, G. V. (1980) Professionalism, dentistry and public health. *Social Science and Medicine* 14a: 223–9.

Larkin, G. V. (1981) Professional autonomy and the ophthalmic optician. *Sociology of Health and Illness* 3 (1): 15–30.

Larkin, G. V. (1983) *Occupational Monopoly and Modern Medicine.* London: Tavistock.

Larkin, G. V. (1988) Medical dominance in Britain: image and historical reality. *Millbank Quarterly* 66 (supplement 2): 117–32.

Larkin, G. V. (1993) Continuity in change: medical dominance in the United Kingdom. In Hafferty, F. and McKinlay, J. (eds) *The Changing Medical Profession: an International Perspective.* Oxford: Oxford University Press.

Larkin, G. V. (1995) State control and the health professions in the United Kingdom: historical perspectives. In Johnson, T., Larkin, G. and Saks, M. (eds) *Health Professions and the State in Europe.* London: Routledge.

Larkin, G. V. (2002) Regulating the Allied Health Professions. In Saks, M. and Allsop, J. (eds) *Regulating the Health Professions.* London: Sage.

Laxton, C. (1996) Clinical audit of forefoot surgery performed by registered medical practitioners and podiatrists. *Journal of British Podiatric Medicine* 51 (4): 46–51.

Lorimer, D. L. (1995) A short history of the Society of Chiropodists 1945–1995. *The Journal of British Podiatric Medicine* 50 (5, supplement): 1–28.

Malgrange, D., Richard, J. L. and Leymarie, F. (2003) Screening diabetic patients at risk for foot ulceration: a multi-centre hospital based study, France. *Diabetes Metabolism* 29 (3): 261–8.

Mandy, P. J. (2000) *The Nature and Status of Chiropody and Dentistry.* Unpublished doctoral thesis, University of Sussex.

McCormick, K. G. and Young, M. J. (1999) A clinical audit of the diabetic foot ulcer clinic. *British Journal of Podiatry* 2 (3): 95.

McInnes, A. (2002) Are podiatrists qualified for the job? *The Diabetic Foot* 5 (2): 62–7.

McInnes, A., Booth, J. and Birch, I. (1998) Multidisciplinary diabetic foot care teams: professional education. *The Diabetic Foot* 1 (3): 109–15.

McPherson, M. V. and Binning, J. (2002) Chronic foot ulcers associated with diabetes: patients' views. *The Diabetic Foot* 5 (4): 198–204.

McPoil, T. G. and Cornwall, M. W. (1996) Relationship between three static angles of the rearfoot and the pattern of rearfoot motion during walking. *Journal of Orthopaedic and Sports Physical Therapy* 23 (6): 370–4.

Menz, H. and Lord, S. (2001) The contribution of foot problems to mobility, impairment and falls in community dwelling older people. *Journal of the American Geriatric Society* 49 (12): 1651–6.

Milsom, P. (1995) Foot surgery: the podiatric option. *The Practitioner* 239: 396–402.

Minaker, K. and Little, H. (1973) Painful feet in rheumatoid arthritis. *Journal of the Canadian Medical Association* 109: 724–30.

Moore, M., Farndon, L., Macmillan, S., Walker, S., Story, H. and Vernon, W. (2003) Patient empowerment: a strategy to eradicate podiatry waiting lists: the Sheffield experience. *British Journal of Podiatry* 6 (1): 17–20.

Munro, B. J. and Steele, J. R. (1998) Foot-care awareness: a survey of persons aged 65 years and older. *Journal of the American Podiatric Medical Association* 88 (5): 242–8.

Nancarrow, S. A. (1999) Reported rates of foot problems in rural south-east Queensland. *Australasian Journal of Podiatric Medicine* 32 (2): 56–73.

Nancarrow, S. A. (2000) First do no harm (editorial). *Australasian Journal of Podiatric Medicine* 34: 4.

Nancarrow, S. A. (2003) Stakeholder consultation in the development of 'high risk' foot care services in the Australian Capital Territory. *The Diabetic Foot* 6 (4): 190–200.

Nester, C. J., Findlow, A. and Bowker, P. (2001) Scientific approach to the mid-tarsal joint. *Journal of the American Podiatric Medical Association* 90 (7): 377–9.

Nettleton, S. (1992) *Power, Pain and Dentistry*. Buckingham: Open University Press.

O'Boyle, P. E. and Fleming, P. (2000) Health promotion in podiatry: podiatrists' perceptions and the implications for their professional practice. *British Journal of Podiatry* 3 (1): 21–8.

Parkin, F. (1979) *Marxism and Class Theory: a Bourgeois Critique*. London: Tavistock.

Podiatry Now Editorial (2002) Podiatric surgery in Scotland: a historic agreement. *Podiatry Now* 5 (10): 526.

Price, M. and Tasker, J. (2000) Putting the knife to the test: an audit of podiatric surgery services provided by First Community Health. *Podiatry Now* 3 (11): 455–61.

Prior, T. (1994) Editorial. *British Journal of Podiatric Medicine and Surgery* 6 (4): 65.

Rayman, G., Baker, N. and Barnett, S. (2000) Diabetes specialist podiatrists: time for recognition. *The Diabetic Foot* 3 (2): 38–40.

Robbie, J. (2002) Developing a diabetic foot screening service in primary care. *The Diabetic Foot* 5 (4): 191–7.

Root, M. L., Orien, W. P., Weed, J. H. and Hughes, R. J. (1971) *Biomechanical Examination of the Foot, Vol. 1*. Los Angeles: Clinical Biomechanics Corporation.

Schuster, R. O. (1974) A history of orthopaedics in podiatry. *Journal of the American Podiatry Association* 64 (5): 332–45.

Seelig, W. (1953) Studies in the history of chiropody – the beginnings of chiropody in England. *The Chiropodist* 8 (11): 381–97.

Sgarlato, T. E. (1971) *A Compendium of Podiatric Biomechanics*. San Francisco: Californian College of Podiatric Medicine.

Skipper, J. K. and Hughes, J. E. (1983) Podiatry: a medical care specialty in quest of full professional status and recognition. *Social Science and Medicine* 17 (20): 1541–8.

Smedley, R. (1976) *The History of Appliance Making in Chiropodial Education*. Unpublished study, Northern College of Chiropody, Manchester.

Society for Chiropodists and Podiatrists (2003) Jobs Directory webpage. www.members.feetforlife.org/cgi-site/jobs.cgi

Spencer, A. M. (1978) *Practical Podiatric Orthopaedic Procedures*. Cleveland, OH: College of Podiatric Medicine.

Steed, D. L. (1998) Foundations of good ulcer care. *American Journal of Surgery* 176 (supplement 2A): 5S–10S.

Stuart, L. and Wiles, P. (2000) Patient education and the diabetic foot: a panacea for prevention? *The Diabetic Foot* 3 (4): 118–19.

Tippens, M. (1998) Re-profiling a chiropody department. *Podiatry Now* 1 (9): 301–2.

Tollafield, D. R. (1993) Podiatric surgical audit: impact on foot health: results from a five year study. *Journal of British Podiatric Medicine* **48** (3): 89–92.

Webster, C. (2000) The history of the National Health Service. In Merry, P. (ed.) *Wellard's NHS Handbook.* Wadhurst: JMH Publishing.

Wilkinson, D. L. and Prior, T. (2000) Podiatrist – friend or foe? *Anaesthesia News* **151**: 1–6.

Williams, L. and Ridgway, S. (2002) Lower limb screening: GP mini-clinic vs. podiatry clinic. *The Diabetic Foot* **5** (2): 90–9.

Woodburn, J., Barker, S. and Helliwell, P. S. (2002) A randomised controlled trail of foot orthoses in rheumatoid arthritis. *Journal of Rheumatology* **29**: 1377–83.

Woodburn, J. and Helliwell, P. S. (1996) Relation between heel position and the distribution of forefoot plantar pressures and skin callosities in rheumatoid arthritis. *Annals of the Rheumatic Diseases,* **55**: 806–10.

Woodburn, J. and Helliwell, P. S. (1997) Foot problems in rheumatology. *British Journal of Rheumatology* **36** (9): 932–4.

Woodburn, J., Stableford, Z. and Helliwell, P. S. (2000) Preliminary investigation of debridement of plantar callosities in rheumatoid arthritis. *Rheumatology* **39**: 625–54.

Young, M. (2002) When is a diabetes specialist podiatrist not a DSP? *The Diabetic Foot* **5** (1): 5–7.

Young, M. (2003) Generalists, specialists and super-specialists. *The Diabetic Foot* **6** (1): 6.

CHAPTER 18

Speech and Language Therapists: Their Role in Health Promotion

James Law, Karen Bunning and Michelle Morris

Allied health professionals (AHPs) in general and speech and language therapists (SLT) in particular have not been explicitly associated with health promotion. This is not due to a lack of involvement in the area, merely that their activity has tended to be construed as clinical, working with the patient to alleviate the effects of illness or disability rather than promoting good health practice in the population as a whole. In an attempt to redress this balance the recently launched *Ten Key Roles for the Allied Health Professions* (DoH, 2003) describes the broad range of health promotional activities carried out by the allied health professions emphasising their central role in the promotion of health and wellbeing.

This chapter takes as its focus the interaction between speech and language therapy and health promotion. At face value this is something of an invidious task because speech and language therapists work with so many different client groups that it is difficult to distil any general messages that are not particular to a single group. Nevertheless the chapter begins by highlighting the central role of communication in the whole process of health promotion and goes on to highlight a number of specific contexts in which speech and language therapists work. Although reference will be made to specific client groups, in each case it is the interaction between the context and the person that will be of major interest. The second section looks at the relationship between communication and empowerment and its specific function in primary care. The chapter goes on to examine the interaction between health promotion and public health with regard to speech and language therapy. Finally, there is critical assessment of the future and whether there is a case for further shifting the balance from treatment to health promotion.

Speech and language therapists occupy an interesting place in the promotion of health and wellbeing. Although generally employed by health services in the United Kingdom (UK), for many this is an administrative convenience that does not fully represent the educational and social contexts in which they work. To reflect this a broad definition of health promotion is employed in the present chapter that concentrates on the mutual relationship between health, wellbeing and living with a communication disability (Naidoo and Wills, 2000). Interestingly this is almost what was originally intended in the WHO definition of health as being not just the absence of disease but the inclusion of mental, physical and social wellbeing (World Health Organisation (WHO), 1946; see also Chapter 1 of this text for further discussion of definitions of health promotion). Even for those speech and language therapists who work in a specialised medical area, such as special care baby units, child development centres or in dysphagia work with elderly people, health promotion does not restrict itself to the medical matters in hand. The person's physical condition is not the sole target of an intervention. Attention would always be paid to developing the individual's psychological resources to deal with difficulties experienced. This naturally links to the prevention of ill health in the longer term. It is the living with a communication disability, for whatever length of time, which is key to promotional activity (Bunning, 2004).

Speech and language therapists, probably more that any other allied health profession, have sought to pass on their expertise to others, by developing training and emphasising skill mix. In part this is simply a pragmatic response to the increasing number and range of clients for which speech and language therapists have a duty of care and the need to spread themselves thinly but effectively. It is also recognised that communication is not something that happens between a person's ears. It is a highly context specific skill and training in it separate from that context is often not appropriate.

In the case of environmental modifications, examples would include improving access to communication and health information for groups of people, such as translating the Patients' Charter or health education leaflets for people who are not literate using photographs, simplified language or symbol systems, introducing communication passports to facilitate the communication access of people with communication disabilities into primary care (Law et al., 2003). In the case of political modifications this would include raising the needs of the communication impaired at a local level within health provider, local education authority and other organisations or at a national level with ministers, Members of Parliament, but also lobbying for the rights of individual client groups in conjunction with specific charitable groups.

The role of communication in health promotion

Health promotion, in the main but particularly through the health education approach, assumes that the service user and the practitioner are able to understand one another. It is not simply a case of speaking the same language where messages are encoded and decoded. A one-to-one correspondence between word and meaning does not exist. Communication in daily life involves the joint construction of meanings between interactants (Fogel, 1993; Grove et al., 1999). Just as this is true of personal interactions that occur on a daily basis, so it is true of the health consultation. When it comes to accessing written information, the reader is reliant on his or her ability to deal with conventional linguistic code in the form of text. You cannot negotiate meanings with a printed leaflet. The linguistic demands of health promotion materials may place their key messages out of the reach of people with communication disability. Confusion, disengagement and abandonment amongst such consumers are possible outcomes. The key concern for health promotion is not just the message, but also the way in which that message is conveyed. Speech and language therapy views the format and content of the message as intrinsically linked and concerns itself with preparing literature that is appropriate for communication disabled clients and providing explanations that are accessible and meaningful given the individual's circumstance. In effect the medium becomes the message.

Client groups and contexts

Speech and language therapists work with people of all ages with physical and cognitive difficulties that may have an impact on their communication skills. This goes well beyond speech to the formation of sentences and the understanding of the spoken word and fostering communicative independence. Because of their training in anatomy and physiology, speech and language therapists are also well qualified to work with the swallowing mechanism and for this reason have become increasingly involved with clients with swallowing disorders or dysphagia in both children and adults. Table 18.1 summarises the client groups that are commonly seen and the type of health promotion activities associated with them.

The process of speech and language therapy inevitably places therapist and client in a situation where information needs surface. The medical explanation for current circumstances may elude the survivor of stroke or the person preparing for surgical intervention to remove a diseased larynx. The parents of the infant newly diagnosed with Down's syndrome may feel confused in their attempts to appreciate what such a condition means in the context of family life. In this context the maintenance of health and wellbeing is at least as important as its initial promotion.

It is important to stress that the health promotion examples cited in the right hand column of Table 18.1 relate to specific aspects of communication that are primary to the SLT consultation. However, consideration should also be given to secondary aspects involving the maintenance of psychological health and wellbeing. People with restricted communication may be at risk of psychological stresses simply because they cannot talk about what they are feeling or find answers to their questions. Therefore the prevention of mental health difficulties and the positive support for moves towards active citizenship become critical to health promotion.

Table 18.1 Client groups, stakeholders, contexts and types of health promotional activities covered by speech and language therapists

Client group (primary beneficiaries of activity)	Stakeholders (significant others to be involved with primary beneficiary, i.e. client)	Contexts (location of activity)	Health promotional activities (topical advice provided to service users on positive ways of addressing difficulties, for the enhancement of physical/psychological health and wellbeing)
Premature babies	Parents	Special care baby units and child development centres	Optimal feeding techniques and early interaction skills
Babies and young children with hearing impairment	Parents and siblings	Community	Early signing behaviours
Toddlers with early language delays	Parents and siblings	Community	Ways of encouraging interaction and language development
Young children with delayed or disordered speech or language in childcare facilities	Parents, early years educational staff	Community and childcare facility	Communication techniques, coping strategies for parents and ways of modifying context for childcare workers
School-aged children with delayed or disordered speech or language	Parents, teachers and learning support assistants	School and community	Advice to teachers on ways of optimising child's potential and differentiating the curriculum. Advice to parents on reducing child's anxiety and frustration
Young adults with communication impairments following head injury	Parents, partners, family members, significant others, support staff	Community and special facilities	Appropriate methods of facilitating communication and addressing psychosocial effects
Adults with learning disability	Family members, residential staff, day services support staff	Social education/resource centres and supported residential services	How to modify environment to maximise communicative independence, supported eating and drinking and maintenance of hearing
Adults with aphasia following stroke	Partner, family members, nursing staff, rehab. staff	Community and rehabilitation centres	How to manage acquired communication difficulty: how to maximise individual's potential
Adults with degenerative neurological conditions	Partner, family members, nursing and support staff	Hospital and community	Maximising communication potential and maintaining functional use of skills, e.g. communication, swallowing
Adults who have had head and neck surgery/laryngectomy	Partner, family members and nursing staff	Hospital and community	Safe eating/drinking practice
Elderly people with communication difficulties associated with dementia	Partner, family members, nursing and support staff	Hospital and community, residential and nursing home	Appropriate modifications to the environment to extend potential for as long as possible

Four particular areas are discussed in greater detail below by way of example, the social inclusion agenda and the promotion of good communication skills in socially disadvantaged children, the prevention of voice difficulties in teachers, improving better access to health for communication disabled people in primary care and the special case of the learning disabled population and their particular need for appropriate health promotion.

The social inclusion agenda

In recent years there has been increasing focus on the relationship between communication, psychosocial factors and the social inclusion agenda. In particular poor educational attainment is one of the critical features linked to social exclusion and subsequent depressed educational outcomes and employment prospects. The association between communication skills and social disadvantage is fully documented (Locke et al., 2002). Similarly the link between communication and mental health and behavioural difficulties has been effectively described (Benner et al., 2002) all of which, if unresolved, almost certainly increase the risk of poor educational achievement and unemployment and thus social exclusion. Speech and language therapists work alongside teachers in improving the communicative competence of children in the classroom. This need not be focussed on individual children, directing attention instead to the skills of the whole class in active listening, working on comprehension skills and drawing appropriate inferences, and presenting a good working model of health promotion in practice. There are many other examples: speech and language therapists working with young people who have offended, speech and language therapy work in pupil referral units (PRUs) where the focus is not on remediation of the communication impairment but on supporting the development of coping strategies and emphasising the power of communication over less appropriate non-verbal means.

One area in which speech and language therapists have become closely involved over recent years is Sure Start, a government initiative designed to alleviate the poverty of socially disadvantaged communities and improve their life chances. The aim is to do this by transforming involvement in communities at a local level, by increasing the readiness of young children from 0–4 years of age to benefit from school and to participate in other health promoting activities such as improving dental care and diet. This project effectively started in 1999 and by 2003 the number of programmes in England had risen to 524. The effectiveness of Sure Start is to be measured against a series of government targets or public service agreements. One specific target relates to the language development of young children. The achievement of this target has been tackled at a national level in two ways. On the one hand there is the production of specific guidance on how Sure Start programmes might develop their interventions and health promotional activities (Law and Harris, 2000). On the other hand the outcomes will be monitored at a national level and on an annual basis (Harris et al., 2004). By contrast, it is difficult to prescribe specific activities at a local level and to monitor the outcomes from individual programmes at any meaningful level.

The teacher's voice

In the preceding sections reference has been made to groups that are considered to be at risk of various health problems. A group who would not normally be considered to be at risk of communication difficulties but who all too commonly come under the remit of speech and language therapy services are teachers in general and more specifically teachers who misuse their voices in the classroom (Mattiske et al., 1998; Morton and Watson, 1998). They are not ill in any formal sense but if they misuse their voices over an extended period they may be at risk of losing their voices completely, which may have a significant effect on their professional functioning, their self-esteem in the classroom, their job prospects and their overall quality of life. At one level this could be considered a matter for traditional primary prevention in so far as teachers need to be aware of what is known as vocal hygiene, which represents sensible use of the voice. This involves avoiding talking loudly in noisy environments, drinking more water, not talking or singing at an inappropriate pitch or taking drinks that are likely to dehydrate, such as coffee or alcohol. Interestingly it is becoming increasingly apparent that some of the problems occur because of excessive ambient noise and can be dealt with in a truly preventive manner by restructuring the built environment, modifying acoustically poor classrooms (Canning and Street, 1999). In other words structural modifications often provide the best method of primary prevention. But intervention may also extend to secondary prevention as teachers with damaged voices receive speech and language therapy.

Communication and empowerment in primary care

It is one thing to give advice to promote better healthy behaviours but for many clients with communication disabilities what they need is less the healthy behaviours than the abilities to seek advice from others. Here again the medium and the message merge into one. For example, an individual may be ill with influenza. What they need most is to be able to go to the doctor and ask for the relevant treatment. They know what to do but are reluctant to do it because they had a stroke six months ago and find it difficult to think and communicate. The last time they visited their GP they received the statutory seven minutes' consultation time and received a prescription that they did not really want. They were left with a deep sense of frustration following the consultation because there were things they meant to communicate, but because they had became confused, were unable to ask.

There have been considerable attempts to improve the communication skills of practitioners working in primary care but, as Law and colleagues have indicated it requires more than just providing simple training programmes to doctors or other staff (Law et al., 2004). Communication works and the consultation is successful when both parties enter into a dialogue, a negotiated position about the best outcome for the client whose health seeking behaviours may be determined by their conversation skills. It is not simply a matter of saying one should have such a dialogue but of demonstrating how this can be achieved. This may even involve changing the way parties think of the consultation process. The definition of primary care has changed significantly in recent years, moving from a narrow definition largely involving a GP and a practice nurse and a health visitor, to the wider team who provide services to a general practice population. This now includes AHPs and many other health professionals.

Learning disability and health promotion

One of the real challenges of health promotion is the effective provision of health related information to people who are not able to understand the messages or at least readily confuse them. Adults with learning disabilities represent a constituency of health service users who have greater healthcare needs (Kerr, 1998). The government white paper *Valuing People: a New Strategy for Learning Disability for the 21st Century* (DoH, 2001) asserts the importance of collaboration between all agencies if inclusion of people with learning disabilities is to be achieved. Speech and language therapists have contributed to the range of activities that has been instigated in response to this directive. Fransman (2004) describes setting up hearing services with the dual aims of raising awareness of hearing related issues, including the importance of aural hygiene and wax removal, as well as providing information and services that are accessible to those with a learning disability.

Timely access to information is critical to the uptake of health promotional activities. For this purpose, people with learning disabilities are generally reliant on significant others. Staff training initiatives and augmentative communication strategies have been invoked to support the sharing and dissemination of information, which is considered crucial to good health promotion and maintenance. *Talking Mats* (Cameron and Murphy, 2002) is a light technology augmentative framework for soliciting the views of people who have communication difficulties associated with a learning disability. Its potential has been explored in the realms of option appraisal and choice making in person centred planning and schools transition and as such lends itself to the promotion and maintenance of health.

Health promotion is predicated upon good communication skills. Conventionally the emphasis has been placed on the communication skills of the practitioner and this has been reflected in the modifications made in recent years to professional training (Silverman et al., 1997; Charles et al., 2000). This presupposes that the key to the transmission of messages is the communication skills of the member of the healthcare team, that it is simply a matter of giving health promotional or other messages clearly. While this may be a prerequisite of the process of interacting with service users, the evidence above shows clearly that due consideration must be given to the communication skills of the client. People who have communication needs are going to need a carefully customised form of interaction if they are to respond to health promotion messages. All too often these messages need to be made available not only to the service user but also to carers and others who mediate the message on a daily basis for them.

Conclusion

In this chapter, the assumption has been made that there is a distinction between treatment of a client in the sense of training specific behaviours and the giving of meaningful advice that will change people's behaviour, such as in parent and child interaction. In reality the gap between the two may be narrower than suggested. However, there probably is a difference and this is that the former takes as read the level of engagement of the client. If they do not engage in the intensity and duration of the intervention it is clear that the treatment is not likely to work. The therapist will pay particular attention to fostering that commitment to the treatment programme. The health promotion model is more open ended in the sense that it involves the giving of advice rather than the training of behaviours, but the way in which that advice is provided is as subject to the principles of evidence based practice as traditional treatment. It is questionable whether a health education model is ever likely to be sufficient to bring meaningful changes in behaviour. But, of course, the issue of involvement and compliance is also critical. It is well documented that patients do not take all the advice that they are offered, but in health promotion the giving of advice may be an outcome in itself whereas the treatment model presupposes a client specific outcome. This approach is likely to mean little if it does not pay due regard to the individual's circumstances and this means tailoring the message to the individual.

References

Benner, G. J., Nelson, J. R. and Epstein, M. H. (2002) Language skills of children with EBD. *Journal of Emotional and Behavioural Disorders* **10** (1): 43–59.

Bunning, K. (2004) *Speech and Language Therapy Intervention: Frameworks and Processes*. London: Whurr.

Cameron, L. and Murphy, J. (2002) Enabling young people with a learning disability to make choices at a time of transition. *British Journal of Learning Disabilities* **30**: 105–12.

Canning, D. and Street, A. (1999) Classroom acoustics: listening and speaking. Presentation made to the NASUWT Health and Safety Representative Meeting, Birmingham.

Charles, C., Gafni, C. and Whelan, T. (2000) How to improve communication between doctors and patients. *British Medical Journal* **320**: 1220–1.

Department of Health (2001) *Valuing People: a New Strategy for Learning Disability in the 21st Century*. London: DoH.

Department of Health (2003) *Ten Key Roles for Allied Health Professionals*. London: DoH.

Fogel, A. (1993) Two principles of communication: co-regulation and framing. In Nadel, J. and Camaioni, L. (eds) *New Perspectives in Communication Development*. London: Routledge.

Fransman, D. (2004) Loud and clear. *RCSLT Bulletin* **621**: 16–18.

Grove, N., Bunning, K., Porter, J. and Olsson, C. (1999) See what I mean: interpreting the meaning of communication by people with severe and profound intellectual disabilities. *Journal of Applied Research in Intellectual Disabilities* **12**: 190–203.

Harris, F., Law, J., Roy, P. and Kermani, S. (2004) *Report of the Second Implementation of the Sure Start Language Measure*. Nottingham: DfES, Sure Start.

Kerr, M. (1998) Primary health care and health gain for people with a learning disability. *Tizard Learning Disability Review* **3**: 6–14.

Law, J., Byng, S., Bunning, K., Farrelly, S., Heyman, B. and Bryar, R. (2004) *Making Sense in Primary Care: Facilitating Communication between Primary Care Practitioners and People with Communication Disability*. Report available from the first author at Department of Language and Communication Science, City University, Northampton Square, London EC1V OHB.

Law, J., Garrett, Z. and Nye, C. (2003) Speech and language therapy interventions for children with primary speech and language delay or disorder. Cochrane Review. In *The Cochrane Library 3*. Oxford: Update Software.

Law, J. and Harris, F. (2000) *Promoting Language Development in Sure Start Areas*. Nottingham: DfES, Sure Start.

Locke, A., Ginsborg, J. and Peers, I. (2002) Development and disadvantage: implications for early years and beyond. *International Journal of Language and Communication Disorders* **37** (1): 3–15.

Mattiske, J. A., Oates, J. M. and Greenwood, K. M. (1998) Vocal problems amongst teachers: a review of the prevalence, causes, prevention and treatment. *Journal of Voice* **12**: 489–99.

Morton, V. and Watson, D. R. (1998) The teaching voice: problems and perceptions. *Logopedics Phoniatry Vocology* **23**: 133–9.

Naidoo, J. and Wills, J. (2000) *Health Promotion: Foundations for Practice*, second edition. London: Baillière Tindall.

Silverman, J., Kurtz, S. and Draper, J. (1997) *Skills for Communicating with Patients*. Oxford: Radcliffe Press.

World Health Organisation (1946) *1946 Constitution: Basic Documents*. Geneva: WHO.

CHAPTER 19

Promoting Better Nutrition: the Role of Dietitians

PAUL SCOTT, JULIA VERNE AND CHRISTINE FOX

Dietitians are graduates, trained in diet and nutrition who are competent in taking scientific information relating to food and health and translating it into terms that the general public can understand (British Dietetic Association (BDA), 2004). Most dietitians work in the National Health Service (NHS) in one or more specialist areas, such as diabetes or paediatrics. Although the majority are in acute clinical roles, there are also many NHS dietitians in community settings, providing health promotion and/or clinical services as time, resources and opportunities allow (BDA, 2004). About 20 per cent of dietitians work outside of the NHS (Fox, 1999) in a variety of roles, such as the food industry, sports, media or private practice. The term dietitian is used here to refer only to those individuals who have gained registration as a dietitian through the Health Professions Council. This requires an undergraduate degree, or a Masters/postgraduate diploma, in dietetics as a basic educational requirement completed by professional entry examinations in order to practice.

In this chapter the roles of dietitians in promoting better nutrition will be examined, including advocacy and mediation; empowering individuals or groups and facilitating the development of environments conducive to healthy eating. The limits of their role will be explored and an assessment made of the potential and possible tensions for multidisciplinary partnership working across professional boundaries. Finally, current opportunities will be gauged for individual dietitians and the profession to fulfil their potential in promoting health through better nutrition.

Nutrition and health

In terms of broad scientific agreement, there has never been such a good time to promote better nutrition. There is consensus in the international scientific community that certain nutritional factors affect the likelihood of developing chronic diseases. These factors particularly include a high intake of sugar, salt and saturated fat and a low intake of fruit, vegetables and fibre, a dietary pattern known to contribute to the development of obesity, diabetes, cardiovascular disease and some cancers (World Health Organisation (WHO), 2004). Good nutrition affects not only an individual's current state of wellbeing but, particularly during gestation and childhood, is also an important predictor of future health (Barker, 1998). The Department of Health's (DoH) *Food and Health Problem Analysis* (DoH, 2003) cites work by the British Heart Foundation (BHF) (BHF, 1998) estimating the cost to the NHS of treating ill health caused by poor diet as at least £2 billion each year.

In response to global changes in patterns of food production, preparation and consumption the World Health Organisation is formulating a global strategy on diet, physical activity and health. However, the WHO recognises that persuading people to change dietary habits is extremely difficult and that in addition to providing food education and skills to people, social and environmental support will also be necessary. Moreover, the WHO suggests that for effective implementation, significant resource should be invested in improving nutritional intake, and that compared to the costs of treatment of nutrition related disease, early intervention is a far more cost effective approach to improving a nation's health (WHO, 2004).

Determinants of food choice

Leach (2002) outlines several key social factors in determining an individual's food choices. For structured meals these particularly include family norms and cultural or religious traditions. For more unstructured meals, or snacks, these influences are more likely to be peers, social networks and the media. Indeed, as James and Ralph (2000) point out, there is a hundredfold greater amount spent on advertising of food and drink than on government health education, and given the profits at stake, it is no surprise that the food industry promotes a model of individual choice rather than a socially driven one. Leach proposes that the key to bringing about dietary change is to substitute unhealthy elements of existing meals without threatening the overall structure. Others have suggested that the increased consumption of snacks and soft drinks may be a more important problem, particularly in relation to obesity (Sharpe, 2004).

Socioeconomic circumstances also undoubtedly affect food choice. National surveys in the UK show that the dietary intake of people on low incomes exhibits a pattern more likely to lead to chronic disease than the intake of higher income groups (DoH, 2003). This includes a lower intake of fruit and vegetables, salads, oily fish and wholegrains; and more fat, sugar and processed meat products.

The reasons for this are complex. Households on low income spend a greater proportion of their available household income on food than higher income households. However, because of the smaller absolute amount available to them, shoppers from low income households tend to be more efficient shoppers. This means choosing affordable items that are generally high in energy, such as those high in fat and sugar, and low in protective nutrients such as antioxidants, fish oils, wholegrains, rather than healthier foodstuffs, which tend to be lower in energy and more expensive (James et al., 1997). Research by the Food Commission (Davey, 2001) has shown that the cost of a regular basket of food is cheaper than a basket of healthier equivalents.

In addition to this financial issue, there are also more structural barriers to a healthy diet. In urban areas communities often rely on convenience stores, with limited availability of fresh produce sold at relatively high prices. Many grocers shut down in the 1990s, due to competition from supermarkets which in turn moved to out of town locations and left what have been termed food deserts in many areas (James et al., 1997).

Although some cooking skills appear to have been lost in the younger generation, this appears to have impacted more on the poorest, as they are unable to afford to experiment with new recipes or buy fresh produce that may deteriorate quickly, displease the family or not be used at all (Lang and Rayner, 2002). Similar difficulties exist for some minority ethnic communities, where available income may be low and there is little access to familiar produce.

The effects of food poverty contribute not only to the health inequalities statistics relating to obesity, diabetes and heart disease seen throughout the UK population (James et al., 1997) but also to a wider sense of social exclusion (Leather, 1996).

There has been growing recognition that action to tackle these inequalities must address the range of factors that influence food choice, rather than focus on individualised approaches and health education which have been shown to be relatively ineffective in reducing disease risk factors and may even increase inequalities in health (Ebrahim and Davey Smith, 1997; Lang and Rayner, 2002).

The health policy context: new emphasis on nutrition and public health

In 1999, *Saving Lives: Our Healthier Nation* (DoH, 1999) put forward a plan for improving the nation's health, with an emphasis on a stronger public health function, working in partnership across professional boundaries, reducing inequalities and tackling social or environmental barriers to health. It also stated targets for reducing deaths from heart disease and cancer. There has been an emphasis, too, on tackling those diseases with high morbidity and mortality rates, coronary heart disease and cancers, and supporting people to adopt healthy diets in *The NHS Plan* (DoH, 2000a), *The NHS Cancer Plan* (DoH, 2000b), the National Service Frameworks for Coronary Heart Disease (DoH, 2000c) and Diabetes (DoH, 2001a) and the Department of Health Public Service Agreements (See www.dh.gov.uk for copies of these policy documents).

The NHS Plan (DoH, 2000a) also announced the creation of extended roles and new career opportunities for nurses and therapists and *Saving Lives: Our Healthier Nation* (DoH, 1999) announced the new post of public health specialist, which enabled appropriately qualified individuals from non-medical backgrounds to take a lead on public health programmes, which had until that point always been medically led. This was followed by *Shifting the Balance of Power within the NHS* (DoH, 2001b), which heralded the creation of Primary Care Trusts, integration of community healthcare services and new opportunities for multidisciplinary working at a local level.

The Department of Health consulted on a *Food and Health Problem Analysis* (DoH, 2003). In preparation for a final report, the *Food and Health Action Plan*, they produced a discussion paper (DoH, 2004), which identified three broad areas that it will support and influence. These include the way food is produced, manufactured and prepared; the ease with which consumers can purchase or obtain healthy foods; and the provision of information to consumers about healthy eating, as well as acquisition of skills and behaviours necessary for good nutrition.

Contributing to the strategic aim of improving public health in England through better nutrition, the discussion paper highlighted four objectives:

- increase access to the wider range of food choices contributing to a healthy diet
- improve the availability and awareness of nutritional and dietary information
- increase fruit and vegetable consumption to at least five portions a day
- reduce the levels of salt, fat and added sugar and increase fibre in the diet.

The paper further stated that several important themes would permeate the action plan, including:

- addressing the specific needs of disadvantaged groups
- promoting appropriate healthy eating at all stages of the life course, including among children, expectant mothers and older people
- considering the drivers of food production, supply and consumer demand
- linking in with existing work
- ensuring effective evaluation and monitoring of success.

Existing action in promoting health through better nutrition

The discussion paper identifies key settings and issues for promoting better nutrition and examples of existing work in each of these. These are listed in the table below with the potential roles of dietitians highlighted.

There have been several useful reviews of the evidence to promote healthy eating and prevent related chronic diseases (Health Development Agency

(HDA), 1997, 2001), however there has been very little work by dietitians themselves in publishing studies on their role in promoting nutrition. This is in contrast to the wide literature available on the more clinical roles of dietitians. There is also a large volume of work that has not been included in reviews, either due to the poor methodological quality of the individual studies or because many innovative food projects simply never get written up and published. This is an area that needs attention from everyone involved in promoting health through good nutrition.

Evolution of the community and health promotion role of dietitians

In 1974, NHS reorganisation created districts as new work areas, leading to posts for district dietitians. Amongst these dietitians, a group with particular interest in community nutrition emerged, which grew from 14 members in 1974 to 195 members in 1985 (Briscoe-Sayer, 1990). This growth mirrors an international shift from high technology hospitals to preventive, primary healthcare. It also coincided with nutritional recommendations for the population published by the National Advisory Committee on Nutrition Education (NACNE) (1983) and the Committee on the Medical Aspects of Food Policy (COMA) (1984).

Much of this early development in community dietetics was characterised by intraprofessional conflict between community and hospital based dietitians, as well as interprofessional conflict with, for example, generalist nurses (Briscoe-Sayer, 1990). Additionally, the nutritional guidelines being created and the new posts being funded were under the dominant control of the medical profession.

In trying to establish its own territory the Community Nutrition Group (CNG) of the BDA was perhaps overly protective, excluding, for example, professionals with an interest in community nutrition who were not dietetically qualified, such as graduate nutritionists. Moreover, the study by Briscoe-Sayer (1990: 229) suggested that part of this protectionism, and the perceived need for a clinical aspect to dietetic work, may have been to maintain a medical mystique that distinguishes dietitians as the authority on food and distances them from the general public or other professionals. Indeed, a possible threat to dietetic territory was perceived as the growth in non-dietetic community nutrition work, such as nurses offering preventive nutrition advice, health promotion specialists running community food initiatives and commercial organisations running slimming clubs. The study also found that colleagueship with other dietitians in clinical settings was greater than amongst dietitians in the community, perhaps due to the large diversity of community roles and their host organisations, such as the health authority, local authority, industry and private practice. There was little cohesion amongst dietitians working in the community and territorial threats were often tolerated as they were either sanctioned by a powerful medical administration or felt to be only subject to influence at national level and therefore the responsibility of the national body, the BDA.

It was clear that dietitians in the community lacked institutional support, had not identified a clear mission and could not therefore decide on the best methods for achieving their aims. The study concluded by highlighting the need for clearer strategic development for the community role of dietitians, as well as redefinition of their particular expertise.

In 1993, the BDA and its specialist interest Community Nutrition Group produced the report *Dietitians in the Community: Opportunities for the Future* (BDA, 1993), based on consultation with a wide group of both dietitians and non-dietitians from many areas of work. The report set out a vision for the year 2000 for the speciality of dietetics in the community. This involved a clear cross sector niche, not just the NHS; a mix of traditional clinical work with a newer non-clinical nutrition facilitation function to promote healthier eating through a range of strategies; and an evaluation role to improve practice and potentially increase the numbers of posts.

The report recommended changes to pre and post registration training for dietitians, to equip them with better understanding of community issues and skills. This needed to include access to postregistration training opportunities through modular study for Masters degrees in community nutrition and dietetics.

In clarifying the nutrition facilitation function of community dietitians, the report cited several key work areas:

- teaching/training
- advice/support
- media work/communication
- community development work
- liaison/networking.

Examples given for these areas concentrate on a group or population approach, rather than work with individuals. The report also identified the knowledge and skills needed to perform this role. These include:

- needs assessment
- population dietary assessment
- community development
- programme planning and implementation
- policy
- advocacy
- epidemiology
- health education and promotion.

An interesting reflection from one respondent to the consultation process was to compare the situation of dietitians in the community to that of public health physicians, and the suggestion that public health medicine training could be used as a model comparison. This point will be revisited later in the chapter.

By the end of the 1990s, job roles had developed further into more specialised posts such as health promotion dietitians, community development dietitians and public health dietitians. A study by Fox (1999), on all dietitians in the BDA with an interest in community work, found that there was still huge variation in practice between dietitians working in the community. Many worked in multiple workplaces, with no clear links to colleagues. Most reported doing a mixture of clinical and health promotion functions, a picture consistent with previous work (BDA, 1993), and this mixed function was seen as a way of surviving market forces. A further finding was that posts appeared to be becoming more differentiated with nutrition promotion work being done by, for example, community development dietitians, and more traditional community dietetic posts focussing very much more on clinical work in primary care. More than two thirds of community dietitians were not responsible for budgets, a key factor in determining their actual and potential role.

Work in the South West of England showed that dietetics services lacked capacity and were under enormous pressure even to provide basic support to patients with clinical needs. It also found that practice nurses and health visitors were playing an important role in nutrition promotion, as were health promotion specialists who were generally responsible for planning food and health work (South West Public Health Observatory (SWPHO), 2002). This is likely to be a picture reproduced in the other regions of England and highlights the need for all professionals working on food and health to collaborate. Interestingly, a study by Ravenscroft (2000) found that due to a shortfall in appropriately qualified staff, many of the professionals taking a lead on public health nutrition issues in health authorities lacked qualifications in nutrition.

Following *Shifting the Balance of Power within the NHS* (DoH, 2001b) there has been a growth in integrated primary care teams and the disintegration of previous professional groupings. It is likely that some specialist skills within former dietetic or health promotion departments have been lost as the small workforce is spread thinly across Primary Care Trusts (PCTs) and forced to adapt to a generalist health promotion role, where promoting health through nutrition may only be a small component. This may mean that the capacity of PCTs to deliver food and health work is lower than was previously the case.

Looking back to the BDA and CNG vision for the year 2000, it seems that a small amount of progress has been made. This is particularly the case for the expansion of dietetic roles in local authorities, disadvantaged communities and other public health settings, such as school and work place catering, 5 a Day community initiatives and Sure Start. However, Fox (1999) has shown that there is still great diversity in the community dietetic role, poor intraprofessional cohesion and much training still occurs experientially, a finding replicated elsewhere (Hughes, 2003a). There is still much that could be done.

Given the increased importance of promoting health through better nutrition, and the multiprofessional interest from nurses, doctors and therapists (see Chapter 10 for discussion of the occupational therapist role in eating disorders); health promotion and public health teams; teachers; caterers and restaurateurs; community workers, and the food industry, it appears that dietitians have many opportunities available to engage in significant health promoting roles. Many of these are outlined in Table 19.1 and complement or support the roles of the professionals outlined above. Indeed, working across sectors and with non-dietetic professionals is likely to be key for dietitians aiming to promote good nutrition in the community, and a clarification of roles at a local level will enable closer integration of practice and a more optimal skill mix in the workforce.

Table 19.1 Current action on nutrition and health

Setting	Existing work	Potential role of dietitians
Early years (Sure Start settings, nurseries, playgroups, mother and toddler groups and the home)	Healthy Start (reform of Welfare Food Scheme) Sure Start (infant feeding, weaning, healthy eating) Breastfeeding promotion Production of children's food ranges, low in salt, sugar or fat.	• Advise on foodstuffs included in the programme • Support nutrition training needs of professionals involved in Healthy Start, Sure Start and breastfeeding promotion • Work in or with industry to create healthy food ranges targeted for children
Schools and colleges	National Healthy Schools Standard Food in Schools (breakfast clubs, tuck shops, vending, cookery clubs, water provision, growing projects) OfSTED assessment of food education and provision Sustainable procurement	• Work with DfES to ensure adequate nutrition component of national curriculum • Work with schools or educational organisations to create nutrition resources • Support teachers in running food projects • Support caterers to promote healthy eating and sustainable procurement
NHS (as an agent and as a setting)	Catering Sustainable procurement Advice and support on nutrition to patients Community initiatives Sharing best practice	• Support caterers to promote healthy eating and sustainable procurement • Support nutrition training needs of primary care nurses, doctors and other professionals • Support planning and evaluation of community initiatives

Continued

Table 19.1 Continued

Setting	Existing work	Potential role of dietitians
		• Create opportunities for sharing best practice (networks,conferences, resource packs)
Food chain	Food production (healthier ranges, low fat, salt or sugar versions) Food supply and access to food	• Work in or with industry • Support needs assessment and food mapping work • Support health impact assessment of new retail developments • Work strategically with retailers and planners to ensure adequate accessibility
Local communities and local authorities (as an agent and as a setting)	Improve access to healthy food in disadvantaged areas (such as '5 a Day' programmes) Improved access to retailers, by planning powers and local transport policies Growing projects	• Support nutrition training needs of community workers and volunteers • Support planning stages of food projects • Support needs assessment and food mapping work • Support health impact assessment of new retail developments • Work strategically with retailers and planners to ensure adequate accessibility • Support evaluation
Two further issues were also identified: **Cross cutting issues**		
Communicating with consumers	Increasing public awareness and knowledge of healthy eating Advertising and promotion Sponsorship and support for consumer health education Food labelling and health claims	• Work with media professionals to promote consistent messages • Contribute to Food Standards Agency work on food advertising • Work with, or for, industry, to improve labelling • Lobby UK and EU policy makers to improve food labelling
Monitoring and evaluation	National surveys, such as the National Diet and Nutrition Survey National programmes (such as the School Fruit Scheme) Local programmes, such as community initiatives	• Contribute to the design, delivery and interpretation of evaluation work, at national and local level

Source: Adapted from information in DoH (2004)

Potential developments for dietitians

In order to maximise their opportunities and achieve their full potential, dietitians working in the community will need to work collaboratively with the broad range of professionals now involved in food work. Dietitians can strengthen their knowledge and skills through training, and provide key functions in public health nutrition work, alongside non-dietetic colleagues. These functions were well described in the BDA document in 1993, including training, advocacy, planning, needs assessment, community empowerment and evaluation. These functions are going to be essential in delivering the Department of Health's *Food and Health Action Plan*, the first national strategy for improving nutrition in England. However, in order to fulfil this potential, dietetic training must progress to include a sufficient amount of the broader public health and health promotion competencies previously identified. At this point, it is worth referring to two separate professional groups who have recently undergone a change in their training and/or remit. This has enabled them to play new roles and maximise their knowledge and skill base. Dietitians wishing to play more nutrition promoting roles could embrace similar developments.

The first group are public health nutritionists. Until the 1990s, nutrition posts in the NHS were almost exclusively limited to professionals with state registration in dietetics. Through professional lobbying at a national level, and possibly due to a limited capacity or capability amongst dietitians, the Nutrition Society now provides NHS recognised professional accreditation to nutritionists with appropriate qualifications and experience, to undertake nutrition promotion work. These are generally termed public health nutritionists, but they may also be qualified dietitians.

The BDA and Nutrition Society produced a guidance document clarifying the role of appropriately qualified nutritionists in NHS nutrition and dietetic departments (BDA/Nutrition Society, 2002). The main differences between nutritionists and dietitians are clarified in Table 19.2.

It is worth reiterating that some of these public health nutritionists will be dietitians, who may perceive the role and title change as a good opportunity to do nutrition promotion work and access career development. This also questions the need for initial dietetic, rather than nutrition, training.

Table 19.2   Role differences between nutritionists
and dietitians

Dietitians	Nutritionists
Both therapeutic and preventative role	Mainly preventative
Work with ill people and healthy people	Work with healthy people
Mainly work on a one to one basis	Mainly work with groups

Source: Reproduced from BDA/Nutrition Society (2002)

The BDA paper outlines the role that nutritionists can play, which as can be seen above, is more in line with the vision statement described earlier. This is different to the view of the American Dietetic Association, which produced a position paper on the role of dietetics professionals in health promotion and disease prevention (Hampl et al., 2002). It outlines the clinical and economic case for promoting healthy nutrition and strongly advocates that dietetics professionals have valuable knowledge and skills and should become more involved in this line of work, which they perceive as becoming increasingly important. They point out that dietitians playing this health promotion role will require a shift in their training from a clinical focus to an emphasis on population based public health practice.

Nonetheless, there is agreement in essence that promoting better population nutrition will involve core specialist knowledge and skills, whoever does it. Once gained, perhaps it will be a moot point whether they call themselves public health nutritionists or public health dietitians?

There is a second group recently undergoing a momentous change. Until the late 1990s, senior public health posts in the NHS were open only to medically qualified professionals. In 1999, *Saving Lives: Our Healthier Nation* (DoH, 1999) announced the new post of public health specialist, open to individuals with appropriate experience and qualifications, both medical and non-medical, and equivalent to the medical consultant grade. This was in recognition of the many non-medical professionals playing important roles in public health but without access to structured training and career opportunities. It may also have been partly due to limited capacity amongst the medical community to deliver the expanding public health agenda. As such, access to specialist registrar training schemes has been opened to non-medics, and more experienced professionals can gain specialist accreditation by meeting clearly laid out competency requirements of the Faculty of Public Health (FPH). There was great debate about the merits of allowing non-medically qualified professionals to play leading public health roles (McPherson et al., 2001) and there has also most likely been debate among many public health physicians regarding their own separation from clinical roles and colleagues. The parallels with dietitians in the community are clear. However, the identification of clear, standardised job aims, along with core competency requirements, provides a strong base for a new multidisciplinary public health function in which professionals from different backgrounds can operate equally. Indeed, these discussions have already been held internationally in the public health nutrition field (Hampl et al., 2002; Hughes, 2003b, 2003c) and in the UK (www.nutritionsociety.org/misc/publicHealthNutrition.htm).

The BDA is represented on the Faculty of Public Health's tripartite steering group for the registration of defined groups of specialists; however it is only nutritionists at present, represented by the Nutrition Society, who are being considered for inclusion in these specialist groups. The BDA's Faculty of Public Health representative is likely to recommend to the central BDA board that aspects of the competencies for general public health training be incorporated in to pre and postregistration dietetic training, particularly the courses run by the Community Nutrition Group (Cristofoli, 2004, personal communication). Concurrently, the CNG is working, with the education leads in the BDA, to reformulate their current courses into modules that can be taken as part of a BDA accredited Masters degree in Advanced Dietetic Practice. It is proposed that non-dietetic professionals could also attend this course. Other options also exist for Masters level training in public health nutrition, at universities in the UK.

Whether dietitians and the BDA embrace these opportunities will be seen over the coming years. Whatever the outcome, the previously mentioned need for clarification of different public health and health promoting roles and good cross sector collaboration will still be crucial.

Dietitians can play a wide range of potential roles in achieving public health targets by implementing health promotion strategies outside of their clinical, therapeutic roles. There are difficulties, such as sharing dietetic territory with other professions involved in population nutrition work and a lack of leadership and pathways for professional development. However, there are also opportunities, including new integration of professional roles in primary care and the forthcoming *Food and Health Action Plan*. The new multidisciplinary focus for public health, with clear competencies that can be incorporated in to existing nutrition and dietetic training, will provide new opportunities for advanced level practice in community or public health nutrition, for a range of professionals.

In summary, there are many roles to play in promoting better nutrition. Dietitians cannot play them all, and promoting the need for clinical qualifications to do this work risks constraining them to a therapeutic niche role. Opportunities for public health nutrition training and practice exist and are continually being strengthened, as are chances for cross sector collaborative work. Whether dietitians grasp these opportunities will depend on strategic leadership from the BDA and from individuals moving beyond old professional boundaries.

References

Barker, D. J. P. (1998) *Mothers, Babies and Health in Later Life*, second edition. Edinburgh: Churchill Livingstone.

Briscoe-Sayer, C. (1990) *Dietitians in the Community: an Emerging Profession? Vol. 1.* Unpublished Masters thesis, Cranfield University.

British Dietetic Association (1993) *Dietitians in the Community: Opportunities for the Future.* Birmingham: BDA.

British Dietetic Association/Nutrition Society (2002) *The Employment of Nutritionists in NHS Nutrition and Dietetic Departments: a Professional Development Guidance Document.* www.nutritionsociety.org/!Docs/NewDocs/Nutritionists%20in%20nhs.pdf (accessed 14 February 2003)

British Dietetic Association (2004) *The Work of Registered Dietitians.* www.bda.uk.com/Downloads/work%20of%20dietitians.pdf (accessed 20 January 2003)

British Heart Foundation (1998) *Coronary Heart Disease Statistics: Economics Supplement.* Cited in Department of Health (2003) *Food and Health Action Plan: Food and Health Problem Analysis for Comment.* www.dh.gov.uk/assetRoot/ 04/07/25/43/04072543.pdf (accessed 20 January 2003)

Committee on the Medical Aspects of Food Policy (COMA) (1984) *Diet and Cardiovascular Disease.* London: Department of Health and Social Security.

Cristofoli, A. (2004) BDA representative to Faculty of Public Health. Personal communication with author.

Davey, L. (2001) Shopping for healthier foods can cost you a packet. *Food Magazine* **55** (October/December): 17.

Department of Health (1999) *Saving Lives: Our Healthier Nation.* London: The Stationery Office.

Department of Health (2000a) *The NHS Plan: a plan for investment. A plan for reform.* London: The Stationery Office.

Department of Health (2000b) *The NHS Cancer Plan.* London: The Stationery Office.

Department of Health (2000c) *National Service Framework for Coronary Heart Disease.* London: The Stationery Office.

Department of Health (2001a) *National Service Framework for Diabetes: Standards.* London: The Stationery Office.

Department of Health (2001b) *Shifting the Balance of Power within the NHS: Securing Delivery.* London: The Stationery Office.

Department of Health (2003) *Food and Health Action Plan: Food and Health Problem Analysis for Comment.* www.dh.gov.uk/assetRoot/04/07/25/43/04072543.pdf (accessed 20 January 2003)

Department of Health (2004) *Towards a Food and Health Action Plan: Discussion Paper.* London: DoH.

Ebrahim, S. and Davey Smith, G. (1997) Systematic review of randomised controlled trials of multiple risk factor interventions for preventing coronary heart disease. *British Medical Journal* **314**: 1666–74.

Fox, C. (1999) *Community Dietetics: Supporting the Future.* Leeds: BDA.

Hampl, J. S., Anderson, J. V. and Mullis, R. (2002) The role of dietetics professionals in health promotion and disease prevention. *Journal of the American Dietetic Association* **102**: 1680–7.

Health Development Agency (1997) *Health Promotion Interventions to Promote Healthy Eating in the General Population: a Review.* Health Promotion Effectiveness Reviews. www.hda-online.org.uk/html/research/effectivenessreviews/ ereview6.html

Health Development Agency (2001) *Coronary Heart Disease: Guidelines for the Implementation of the Preventive Aspects of the National Service Framework.* www.hda-online.org.uk/downloads/pdfs/chdframework.pdf (accessed 20 January 2003)

Hughes, R. (2003a) Competency development needs of the Australian public health nutrition workforce. *Public Health Nutrition* **6** (8): 830–47.

Hughes, R. (2003b) Public health nutrition workface composition, core functions, competencies and capacity: perspectives of advanced-level practitioners in Australia. *Public Health Nutrition* **6** (6): 607–13.

Hughes, R. (2003c) Definitions for public health nutrition: a developing consensus. *Public Health Nutrition* **6** (6): 615–20.

James, W. P. T., Nelson, M., Ralph, A., and Leather, S. (1997) Socioeconomic determinants of health: the contribution of nutrition to inequalities in health. *British Medical Journal* **314**: 1545–8.

James, W. P. T. and Ralph, A. (2000) National strategies for implementing changes in dietary patterns. In Garrow, J. S., James, W. P. T. and Ralph, A. (2000) *Human Nutrition and Dietetics*, tenth edition. Edinburgh: Churchill Livingstone.

Lang, T. and Rayner, G. (eds) (2002) *Why Health Is the Key to the Future of Food and Farming*. London: UK Public Health Association, Chartered Institute of Environmental Health, Faculty of Public Health Medicine, National Heart Forum and Health Development Agency.

Leach, H. (2002) Food habits. In Mann, J. and Truswell, A. S. (eds) *Essentials of Human Nutrition*, second edition. Oxford: Oxford University Press.

Leather, S. (1996) *The Making of Modern Malnutrition: an Overview of Food Poverty in the UK*. London: Caroline Walker Society.

McPherson, K., Taylor, S. and Coyle, E. (2001) Public health does not need to be led by doctors. *British Medical Journal* **322**: 1593–6.

National Advisory Committee on Nutrition Education (NACNE) (1983) *A Discussion Paper on Proposals for Nutritional Guidelines for Health Education in Britain*. London: Health Education Council.

Ravenscroft, N. (2000) *An Assessment of Public Health Nutrition Practice at Health Authority Level in England*. Unpublished Masters thesis, University of Wales College of Medicine.

Sharpe, R. (2004) Health. www.racetothetop.org/indicators/module7/ (accessed 20 January 2003)

South West Public Health Observatory (2002) Mapping dietary services provided in the South West Region. Personal communication.

World Health Organisation (2004) *Nutrition and NCD Prevention*. www.who.int/hpr/nutrition/index.shtml (accessed 18 January 2004)

CHAPTER 20

Promoting Health through Community Pharmacies

MIRIAM ARMSTRONG, CLAIRE ANDERSON, ALISON
BLENKINSOPP AND RUTH LEWIS

Pharmacists work in a number of settings including hospitals, primary care
and industry. In the United Kingdom (UK) the general public are most
likely to come into contact with community or retail pharmacists who work in
over 12,000 pharmacies (Royal Pharmaceutical Society of Great Britain
(RPSGB), 2003) and serve an estimated six million customers a day (RPSGB,
1993). Community pharmacists make a significant contribution to improving
the public's health through their day-to-day activities around the sale of medicines and their supply via National Health Service (NHS) Patient Group
Directions. Pharmacists also provide invaluable information and advice,
facilitate self-care, visit the homes of housebound people and advise on health
topics such as smoking cessation and emergency hormonal contraception.
Based in the heart of communities they create an informal network of drop-in
access points for healthcare services, medicines and advice on health and
wellbeing.

Community pharmacy is unusual in that it straddles both public and private
sectors. Community pharmacies are independent contractors to the health
service, giving advice and dispensing medicines for the NHS, but also have to
survive as a small business in a local community or as a major retailer in the
high street. The dual health and commercial role of pharmacy offers a unique
opportunity to target activities towards healthy people, as well as those with
health problems, and pharmacy users' experiences are often more consumer
orientated that patient orientated.

Visitors to pharmacies come from all sectors of the population and research
has found that the use of community pharmacies for general health advice is
higher among women, respondents with young children, older people and
lower socioeconomic groups (Anderson et al., 2003a, 2003b) and people
without easy access to a car or public transport (RPSGB, 1996). Community
pharmacy could therefore be used to improve access to and quality of primary
care services in deprived areas.

Current policy context

The UK government's focus on promoting the public's health is considerable and is primarily directed at developing capacity within the public health workforce and reducing inequalities in health (Department of Health (DoH), 2001, 2002a, 2002b). Often the potential contribution that pharmacists can make to achieve these stated aims are omitted. However, in recent years, a number of key policy documents have outlined the areas in which the public health role of pharmacists should be developed further. For example, the House of Commons Health Committee (2001) inquiry into public health recommended that the government take steps for community pharmacists to play a more active role in public. The government strategy document for outlining the future direction of pharmacy, *Pharmacy in the Future* (DoH, 2000) recognised that the skills and expertise of the pharmacist could be further utilised. According to the strategy this could be achieved through pharmacy becoming more integrated with the NHS, through working more flexibly as part of a multidisciplinary healthcare team and through playing a greater role in supporting self-care. *Tackling Health Inequalities: a Programme for Action* (DoH, 2003a) highlights the importance of community settings and services in addressing health inequalities, including community pharmacies. *Tackling Health Inequalities* goes on to state community pharmacists have a vital role to play in improving the public's health by giving advice, specifically on how to quit smoking, offering exercise on prescription, identifying patients at risk of heart disease and providing services for substance misusers. *A Vision for Pharmacy in the New NHS* (DoH, 2003b) recognises the untapped contribution that pharmacists can make to the public health agenda. This document outlines the public health component in the new national pharmacy contract and the need to develop a pharmacy public health strategy for England that is fully integrated with the wider public health agenda and workforce. The strategy paper *Building on the Best; Choice, Responsiveness and Equity in the NHS* (DoH, 2003c) also set out how NHS services will be more responsive to patients, by offering more choice across the spectrum of healthcare, including increased choice of where, when and how to get medicines.

The evidence for community pharmacy's contribution to public health

The Royal Pharmaceutical Society of Great Britain and the charity Pharmacy Health Link commissioned a review of the UK and international evidence base relating to the contribution of community pharmacy to improving the public's health. The first report was a systematic literature review of the published evidence relating to the contribution of community pharmacy to public health and health promotion, both in the UK and internationally for 1990–2001 (Anderson et al., 2003a, 2003b). The report covered 35 trials or experimental studies reported in 40 papers. Of these, 18 were UK studies, 14 were from the United States or Canada and eight from Europe. There were also 34 descriptive studies, of which 14 were from the UK, 12 were from the US or Canada and eight from Europe. The second report examined non-peer reviewed literature and unpublished work, sometimes referred to as grey literature. It included 37 studies, which comprised Masters and doctoral research at schools of pharmacy, independent research reports of government and other bodies and expert consensus documents. The findings of the first two reports in this series highlighted the significant contribution that community pharmacy can make to improve the public's health at a local level. The following two sections describe some key findings from this evidence based review.

Health topics

Smoking cessation

Community pharmacy smoking cessation services, run by trained pharmacy staff, are both effective and cost effective. Training, especially in behaviour change methods, was found to be essential to the success of pharmacy smoking cessation services. Without training pharmacists were more likely to respond reactively to smokers' requests for advice rather than to initiate opportunistic conversations about smoking, for example, when a client buys cough medicine.

Healthy eating, obesity and weight reduction

Community pharmacy can contribute to reducing the number of people who are obese and overweight by running pharmacy based weight reduction programmes and promoting healthy eating and physical activity. Pharmacies, both in the UK and internationally, have initiated weight loss programmes, and there are examples of pharmacy weight monitoring as part of heart disease risk factor identification programmes; however there were few studies found. Given the relevance of obesity to heart disease and cancer, further research into the potential contribution of pharmacy to weight reduction is urgently needed with a view to extending and expanding successful programmes in the future.

Coronary heart disease screening and management

The evidence based review found that community pharmacists are effective in supporting secondary prevention for heart disease. Using pharmacy medication records to identify patients at risk of heart disease was found to be an effective method of identifying those most at risk and targeting health promotion measures, as appropriate. Pharmacists can also provide advice and information on maintaining healthy blood pressure and the use of medicines such as, aspirin, statins, ACE inhibitors, beta blockers and warfarin to control risk factors. Pharmacy is a valuable source of advice on the appropriate use of prophylactic aspirin to the public, and can intervene to minimise potential harm from self-initiated aspirin treatment in people with contraindications to its use.

Skin cancer

Pharmacies are a valuable source of information about sun protection and also sell a range of related products. Pharmacy based information on skin cancer prevention raises public awareness of the risks, but more research is needed to see whether this heightened awareness has a positive effect on behaviour patterns.

Diabetes

The evidence based review found that community pharmacy based monitoring and information giving on diabetes shows promise in improving diabetic control, as does group education for people with diabetes through pharmacy (for further discussion of diabetes control see Chapter 4).

Sexual health

The evidence suggests that there is a desire by the public for easy access to information on both contraception and safer sex and that they would be willing to receive this advice from pharmacists. Pharmacists appear to want an expanded advisory role in sexual health, but access to training that incorporates and encourages networking with other local service providers is likely to be crucial in increasing pharmacists' confidence in dealing with these issues appropriately and effectively. The vast majority of service users report sufficient privacy to discuss these topics in a pharmacy, but a consistent minority, up to 20 per cent, has residual concerns.

Community pharmacy has already made a considerable and well documented contribution to reducing teenage pregnancy through over the counter provision of emergency hormonal contraception (EHC). The evidence points to this service having high levels of user satisfaction and that pharmacists are positive about their experience of providing emergency hormonal contraception. The review also found that the supply of EHC through pharmacy enables most women to receive EHC within 24 hours of unprotected intercourse and that pharmacy is highly rated by women as a source of EHC.

It is hoped that this service will be developed further in order to meet young women's needs at a local level, particularly through increased use of Patient Group Directions to supply under 16 year olds. This will need to be done in conjunction with existing services and linked to other youth support programmes. It is also hoped that pharmacy supply of EHC will be free to people from disadvantaged areas or on low incomes via Patient Group Directions.

Drug misuse

Community pharmacy based drug misuse services were found to be highly valued by drug misusers. Pharmacy based needle exchange schemes are cost effective and methadone administration services supervised by a community pharmacy achieve high attendance rates and are acceptable to most clients. Positive pharmacist attitudes are correlated with higher service provision for drug misusers, but training is needed to address translating technical terms into an appropriate language for drug misusers.

Immunisation

Studies from the United States of America (US) confirm that immunisation services for adults can be safely provided through pharmacies and that user satisfaction from these services is high. Community pharmacy could make a significant contribution to influenza immunisation targets by administering immunisation for the elderly and other groups. Older people are often in regular contact with their pharmacist, which provides opportunities for pharmacists to proactively approach, advise on and recommend immunisation. Patient medication records can be used to identify other at risk groups and invite them for immunisation either at the pharmacy, or elsewhere. Piloting of direct provision of immunisation in UK pharmacies and their role in meeting local targets is urgently needed.

Head lice

Considerable evidence was found to support the involvement of community pharmacy in head lice monitoring and treatment. Members of the public see pharmacists as an approachable source of advice and treatment for head lice and pharmacists and other health professionals are positive about the service and would like to see it continue. Pharmacists follow the protocol requirement for examination and proof of infection and where treatment is supplied, adherence to the local formulary appears to be extremely high, approaching 100 per cent. Further research to assess the effectiveness and cost effectiveness of these pharmacy based interventions is required together with the need for local planning and coordination of treatment services and messages. It may be necessary to have a private consultation area in the pharmacy to cater for members of the public who find this a very sensitive issue, as user feedback found that between 18 per cent and 34 per cent of users reported having concerns about privacy.

Accidental injury

Pharmacy contributes to reducing accidental injury in a number of ways, for example, through reducing medicines related injuries and through pharmacy based screening services for osteoporosis involving pharmacist and nurse input. This service was said to be valued by users and effective in identifying women at risk of osteoporosis in order to initiate health promotion interventions. Pharmacy could also contribute to reducing accidental injury by providing facilities for returning used medicine to reduce accidental poisoning and used needles and syringes to reduce disease transmission and needle stick injuries.

Public health information provision

The main source of pharmacy public health information is in the form of leaflets, which cover health issues such as folic acid, quitting smoking, oral health, and depression. Community pharmacists consider health information leaflets to be an important component of their health improvement toolkit and that pharmacy users who have received health advice are positive about the service and gained useful health information. Community pharmacy has been identified as a potentially promising setting for interventions to change health behaviours because of the frequency of contacts between the public and a health professional. There is evidence of the efficacy of brief interventions. A brief intervention is characterised as a time limited five to ten minutes' interaction between health professional and client with a focus on changing client behaviour. The method has been used in modifying a range of health behaviours including smoking, physical activity, adherence to diet in diabetes, weight control, alcohol moderation, domestic violence and safe sex. The use of this method in primary care by pharmacists has considerable potential to improve public health. The evidence suggests pharmacists could develop their advice giving role further by proactively offering advice and leaflets.

Although there is no doubt that leaflets are still the core communication device in many situations, there is mounting evidence to suggest that how patients received health information depended on their individual user preferences. So in order to appeal to a much wider audience other methods of communication need to be utilised. There is not currently sufficient evidence to suggest that one particular form of information presentation is more effective compared to any other. Instead it appears that different methods of receiving health information depend on individual user preferences and characteristics. When a pharmacist or member of pharmacy staff actively engages with patients about their health needs, it may be possible to determine what method of information provision might suit them best. For example touch screen kiosks in pharmacies seem more likely to appeal to and be used by younger people, particularly those under 40 years old.

Support for pharmacy public health role

Pharmacists are very positive about and attach a high degree of importance to public health activities in the pharmacy and their role in delivering these. However, at present their approach tends to be reactive rather than proactive and centred around the use of medicines rather than adopting a more holistic view of health. This is primarily due to the nature of the current contract with the NHS, which rewards pharmacists for the volume of NHS prescriptions dispensed rather than the quality of services provided. This is all set to change with the current discussions and the structure of the new NHS pharmacy contract, which will reward pharmacists more for quality and include public health as a core activity. In order for community pharmacists to carry out this extended public health function a comprehensive underpinning support infrastructure must be developed, that includes appropriate inservice training and continuing professional development, the provision of facilitators and information technology and the consideration of the redesign and use of pharmacy premises.

Training and facilitators

Training and facilitators have positive effects on the information giving behaviour of community pharmacy staff. They result in increases in the number and the length of consultations between pharmacists and pharmacy users on health issues and increase pharmacists' participation in local health improvement programmes. Appropriate training also increases user satisfaction with pharmacy health promotion interventions.

Information technology

Information technology can be a valuable tool in increasing the effectiveness and number of public health interventions provided by pharmacies. There is, for example, substantial evidence that pharmacy medication records can be used to identify clients at risk of certain illnesses, such as influenza and also for health promotion purposes. A common electronic patient record will also facilitate exchange of relevant information between different health professionals and patients. Data protection and confidentiality agreements will of course need to be followed.

Design and use of pharmacy premises

The design of pharmacy premises, in particular whether there is an obvious private area for consultation, is a key feature in facilitating the nature of discussions between the pharmacist and client. The review found that the vast majority of pharmacy users report satisfaction with privacy and confidentiality levels within community pharmacies. In addition, some clients choose to use a pharmacy to maintain their anonymity. However, a number of the areas in which pharmacists could potentially contribute to improving the public's health involve sensitive issues and users often emphasise the importance of confidentiality and privacy, for example, sexual health, head lice management, drug use management and mental health. Pharmacists must respond to these needs if they are to expand their involvement and provide a high level of user satisfaction. Facilities must be available to enable confidential consultations, especially when giving advice on sensitive topics, and the pharmacist's duty to preserve confidentiality should be clearly visible to pharmacy users.

Community pharmacy can and already does make an important contribution to improving the public's health and reducing health inequalities, due to the skills and experience of the pharmacy workforce and the location and accessibility of pharmacies. However the public health role of pharmacists and their staff could be expanded further and this is likely to happen with the introduction of the new national pharmacy contract and as training for pharmacists becomes more integrated with that of other health professionals. To do this effectively, an appropriate infrastructure support needs to be established. This infrastructure support must include training and education, appropriate reimbursement, information technology and development of pharmacy premises to enable confidential consultations, especially when giving advice on sensitive topics. Once the support infrastructure is in place pharmacists will be able to engage much more positively and effectively with the public health agenda.

Public awareness of the advice giving role of pharmacists is currently low but is likely to increase as pharmacists become much more engaged with the public health agenda. Information provided to the public must be evidenced based and consistent with that of other health professionals. Close working is needed between the pharmacy profession, the government and other healthcare professionals to achieve this.

References

Anderson, C., Blenkinsopp, A. and Armstrong, M. (2003a) *The Contribution of Community Pharmacy to Improving the Public's Health, Report 2: Evidence From The*

Non Peer-reviewed Literature 1990–2001. London: PharmacyHealthLink. www. rpsgb.org.uk/pdfs/phlevrep2.pdf

Anderson, C., Blenkinsopp, A. and Armstrong, M. (2003b) *The Contribution of Community Pharmacy to Improving the Public's Health, Report 1: Evidence from the Peer-reviewed Literature 1990–2001*. London: PharmacyHealthLink. www.rpsgb. org.uk/pdfs/phlevrep1.pdf

Department of Health (2000) *Pharmacy in the Future: Implementing the NHS Plan*. London: DoH. www.doh.gov.uk/pharmacyfuture

Department of Health (2001) *Report of the Chief Medical Officer's Project to Strengthen the Public Health Function*. London: DoH. www.doh.gov.uk/phfunction.htm

Department of Health (2002a) *Improvement, Expansion and Reform: the Next 3 Years: Priorities and Planning Framework 2003–2006*. London: DoH. www.doh. gov.uk/planning2003–2006

Department of Health (2002b) *Tackling Health Inequalities: 2002 Cross-cutting Review*. London: DoH. www.doh.gov.uk/healthinequalities/ccsrfinal.pdf

Department of Health (2003a) *Tackling Health Inequalities: a Programme for Action*. London: DoH. www.doh.gov.uk/healthinequalities/programmeforaction

Department of Health (2003b) *A Vision for Pharmacy in the New NHS*. London: DoH.

Department of Health (2003c) *Building on the Best: Choice, Responsiveness and Equity in the NHS*. London: DoH.

House of Commons Health Committee (2001) *Second Report on Public Health*. London: The Stationery Office. www.doh.gov.uk/phreport2.htm

Royal Pharmaceutical Society of Great Britain (1993) *Pharmaceutical Care: the Future for Community Pharmacy: a Report of the Joint Working Party on the Future Role of Community Pharmaceutical Services*. London: RPSGB.

Royal Pharmaceutical Society of Great Britain (1996) *Baseline Mapping Study to Define Access and Usage of Community Pharmaceutical Services*. London: RPSGB.

Royal Pharmaceutical Society of Great Britain (2003) *Statistics of Pharmacists and Registered Premises*. London: RPSGB. www.rpsgb.org.uk/pdfs/registerstats.pdf

CHAPTER 21

Orthoptists and their Scope in Health Promotion

FIONA ROWE AND VERONICA HENSHALL

The possession of good and adequate vision and ocular alignment is crucial to development, performance and attainment in both the child and adult populations. The psychosocial impact of poor ocular alignment can manifest itself in many ways and reduced visual capabilities can impact on general health, well-being and quality of life.

Knowledge of visual status is important to all health professions in the management aspect of care plans for the individual and dissemination of such information amongst the multidisciplinary team is therefore of importance. The multidisciplinary approach for orthoptists is varied with teamwork a feature of the acute ophthalmic unit, with additional liaising with other healthcare professionals as appropriate. Orthoptic practice has evolved from a purely hospital based service to include community clinic practice within Primary Care Trusts (PCTs) and school based assessment.

This changing face of orthoptic liaison is reflected in the education of orthoptic undergraduates and practitioners in relation to role boundaries, communication and holistic patient care. The expanded role of the orthoptist not only addresses specialist orthoptic areas of ocular alignment and movement, and associated vision defects, but also the investigation and care of patients with visual field abnormalities, cataract, glaucoma, stroke and neurological rehabilitation, specific literacy difficulties and low vision impairment.

The education and promotion of knowledge regarding the investigation and management of the varied aspects of orthoptic practice amongst orthoptic practitioners and health professionals is crucial to continued and further developments in quality patient care.

This chapter will address the health education aspect of orthoptic practice and the emerging health promoting role within extended practice and the multidisciplinary team.

The role and function of orthoptists

Orthoptists are allied health professionals registered with the Health Professions Council and practise under the professional term of orthoptist. The professional body is the British and Irish Orthoptic Society. The Society is also a charity and seeks to widen understanding of binocular vision problems and visual development in children and adults, and in other areas of eyecare such as low vision, reading difficulties, glaucoma and diabetic screening.

Orthoptists are primarily concerned with the assessment, diagnosis and management of defects of ocular motility and vision. Some examples of these problems are:

- amblyopia (lazy eye), which is a reduction in vision arising from a defect present in infancy or early childhood, which prevents the eye from receiving adequate visual stimulation
- defective binocular vision, which is the inability to use the two eyes together in the correct way; this can lead to impairment of depth perception and reading difficulties
- abnormal eye movements, arising from injury or disease affecting the eye muscles or the nerve supplying the muscles, or a physical obstruction to eye movement
- diplopia (double vision) resulting from abnormal eye movements or strabismus (squint) (Nolan, 2003a).

Orthoptists are skilled in the performance and interpretation of a variety of diagnostic procedures where an underlying ophthalmological condition exists. Examples of these diagnostic procedures include:

- perimetry (assessment of the field of vision), automated and non-automated
- tonometry (measurement of the pressure inside the eye)
- tomography (assessment of the optic disc appearance)
- topography (digital representation of corneal surface)
- fundus photography (photography of the retina)
- biometry (measurement of the length of the eye and the curvature of the cornea)
- electrodiagnosis (measurement of electrical potentials from the eye and/or brain in response to visual stimuli)
- low vision aids (assessment of the use of visual aids for partially sighted children and adults)
- paediatric contact lenses (insertion and removal of contact lenses, and the teaching of the procedure to parents/patients).

The importance of vision to health

The visual perception of an object is resolved according to light sense, form sense and colour sense (Rowe, 1997). Form sense may be divided into central vision (the ability to discriminate fine high contrast detail) and peripheral (the field of vision). Visual acuity (central form sense) is defined as the ability to discriminate detail. It is dependent upon the minimal discrimination an individual can make between the constituent parts of an object. The fovea (central visual area) is responsible for accurate daylight vision and is comprised of cones that also subserve colour vision. Vision relating to the peripheral visual area is comprised of rods that subserve black and white contrast and contribute to daylight vision but predominantly night vision.

Variables affecting vision include:

- retinal stimulation (central stimulation involves the fovea for higher acuity function and peripheral stimulation results in the perceived field of vision)
- luminance (brightness of target)
- contrast (sensitivity to shades)
- eye movements (even when looking steadily at targets there are constant refixation movements to maintain steady central fixation of an object)
- contour interaction (it is easier to identify a target presented singly than one with other surrounding stimuli).

The first 18 months to two years of life are most important in the development of normal binocular single vision and the first six months of life are a critical period for the development of binocularity (ability to use both eyes together as a pair) in humans. Results from normal infants show that response to stereopsis (3-D vision) begins at approximately four months of age (Bechtoldt and Hutz, 1979; Fox et al., 1980; Birch et al., 1983; Archer et al., 1986) with the development of the sensory capacity for stereopsis.

Orthoptists are recognised as the experts in childhood vision screening, and undertake primary screening of children aged four to five years, in line with the recommendations of the National Screening Committee (2000). Orthoptists may also undertake vision screening in younger children to detect defects such as a reduction in visual acuity in one or both eyes, and small angle or underlying strabismus that may be difficult for parents to detect which may have a significant effect on the development and function of the visual system (Donahue et al., 2003).

Secondary screening is still offered in some areas as well as or instead of primary screening. This is dependent on local arrangements. Secondary screening can apply to preverbal and verbal children, children with learning and/or physical disability, children with special needs and children with specific risk conditions, such as prematurity among babies and known genetic conditions. It is important to remember that while testing or screening for visual problems, the orthoptist can also identify and reassure those patients whose vision is good.

Sight, as one of the major senses, is of utmost importance to daily functioning and as such, to health, wellbeing and general quality of life. Quality of vision is an important factor in leading a full and useful life at all ages. It is crucial to infant development, to a child's education, to employment prospects, to the pursuit of leisure activities and to the enjoyment of retirement. An ocular disability, perhaps initially slight, can become a major visual handicap if not promptly identified and treated. Loss of vision or visual impairment impacts on career, driving ability and many other aspects of normal life.

Dependent on the type of visual impairment there are a number of treatment options available including the wearing of glasses to correct refractive errors such as long sight and short sight and patching for amblyopia to stimulate the affected eye without competition from the better eye (Wickham et al., 2002).

Strabismus (a deviation in one or both eyes) whether constantly present or intermittently may also impact on the individual's life with psychosocial implications of acceptance by peers, secondary involvement of vision, for example development of amblyopia, and self-awareness issues. The above treatment options of glasses and patching may be of relevance for associated visual impairment and specific types of strabismus. In addition appropriate referral for surgical correction of strabismus can dramatically improve lifestyle for patients of all age groups (Rowe, 2000). Proponents of early surgery state the increased chance of achieving binocular interaction and improved psychosocial implications (Taylor, 1963, 1972; Ing et al., 1966; Fisher et al., 1968; Ing, 1983; Deacon, 1998). Early surgery aids the normal development of parent and child relationships and the social and emotional development of the infant because of the impression of the general appearance of the child (Tolchin and Lederman, 1978). Early surgery may also improve the general performance of the child, an observation often made by parents and which has been quantified where improvement in fine motor skills and visually directed tasks has been noted with alignment to less than five degrees (Rogers et al., 1982).

Orthoptists' contribution to health promotion

Orthoptists need to have highly developed levels of manual, communicative and analytical skills. The orthoptist deals with patients of all ages but has a particular interest and expertise in the very young and the elderly as these age groups specifically have a higher incidence of ocular pathology. Orthoptists currently play an important role in many different multidisciplinary teams. Orthoptists also work closely with other professionals within the National Health Service (NHS), education, social services and the voluntary sector on a one-to-one basis. The orthoptist's expertise extends to patients of all age groups, including those with special needs, specific learning difficulties, maxillofacial injuries, oncology patients, endocrine abnormalities, stroke patients and those with low vision and neurological conditions.

Orthoptists undertake screening and assessment of the elderly population, in environments such as stroke units to assist with detecting and treating the symptoms of cerebrovascular accident (Freeman and Rudge, 1988; Freeman, 2003; MacIntosh, 2003). Many orthoptists participate in shared care glaucoma clinics for adults where the condition is diagnosed, the most appropriate treatment given and regular monitoring carried out (Blakey et al., 2003). Orthoptists investigate the state of the visual fields in all age groups of patients with head injury, intracranial tumours, and systemic conditions, monitoring and interpreting their fields on a regular basis for any subtle changes that may indicate a change in the systemic condition. Children and adults with special needs have a higher incidence of visual defect, and the caring and skilled approach of the orthoptist is vital with these patients.

The orthoptist's prime consideration must always be the interests of each individual patient, within the context of the general standard of the orthoptic service provided to the public as a whole.

The *Health for All Children* report (Hall and Elliman, 2003) states that disorders of vision can be subdivided into categories that include serious defects likely to cause a disabling impairment of vision ranging from partial sight to complete blindness, and the common and usually less incapacitating defects including refractive errors, squints, amblyopia, and defects of colour discrimination. These are individually and collectively uncommon with a combined prevalence of visual impairment of about 1 per 1000 population.

Early detection of serious visual impairment is important for several reasons. Ophthalmic symptoms or signs such as squint or progressive visual failure can be the presenting feature of serious systemic disease. Some conditions are sight or life threatening and are treatable. Many visual disorders have widespread and/or genetic implications, and developmental guidance and early educational advice by specialist teachers is much appreciated by parents and may reduce the incidence of secondary disabilities such as behaviour problems.

Health promotion pertains to a number of different areas in orthoptic practice. It must be encouraged amongst individual orthoptic practitioners starting at undergraduate level and continuing throughout professional life in clinical practice.

Undergraduate education primarily addresses the teaching and content of the programme to produce a clinician who is deemed to have achieved a certain level of theoretical and practical knowledge and is considered competent to practice. Core to the theoretical and practical aspects of the course content is the education in communication aspects, ethics of practice, professional practice guidelines, awareness of professional boundaries and the importance of other health professions, holistic patient care and its specific importance to the treatment of the individual patient to ensure the best possible outcome for the treatment and care. The concept of shared learning is advocated and promoted by the Department of Health.

Postgraduate education is available to all health professions and can take the form of structured learning programmes offered by higher education institutions but also smaller forums such as clinical meetings and conferences with shared learning across professions. This forms part of the orthoptist's continuing professional development that is an important aspect of clinical practice in order to maintain standards and best practice. Postqualification life-long learning has been addressed at national level and specifically the NHS University promotes such aspects amongst all health professionals (www.nhsu.nhs.uk). The United Kingdom (UK) government has stressed its commitment to lifelong learning for healthcare workers (Department of Health (DoH), 1999). Education and continuing professional development for allied health professionals in particular is part of plans for the NHS (DoH, 2000).

The British and Irish Orthoptic Society in addition to NHS acute hospital and primary care Trusts promotes clinical audit and research amongst its members to ensure best practice and evidence based practice, to encourage continuing professional development amongst its members and ultimately the best quality care for patients (British and Irish Orthoptic Society, 2003; Rowe and Clarke, 2003). The Society also encourages its members to take on health promoting roles and is active in ensuring health promotion among lay persons in the general community and other professions in the medical and education sectors. There is representation on multiple national committees for the latter but with provision of information for the general public either directly from the general office or via its website (www.orthoptics.org.uk).

Orthoptists undertake clinical audit and research on a regular basis and appreciate the need to practice evidence based orthoptics. The orthoptist must have regard to accepted clinical practice, take responsibility for their own clinical professional development, and be governed by the professional standards as laid down by the Council for the Professions Supplementary to Medicine and its successor, the Health Professions Council.

Health promotion with the lay community

Health education and health promotion with the lay community take many forms with provision of information via websites, leaflets or direct access through professional bodies. Orthoptists cannot prevent a primary visual abnormality or strabismus from occurring. However, with early detection significant loss of visual function is most often prevented through appropriate and early treatment regimes (Rahi and Stanford, 2001; Rahi and Dezateux, 2002). It is the early detection and treatment that are imperative. Health education and promotion which raise awareness of the importance of this early detection and early treatment can encourage attendance at screening appointments for young children to ensure that any potential problems can be picked up at the early stages. This is partly addressed by lay education events such as mother and baby talks during the early infancy period, educational talks to nursery and primary school teachers and pupils, educational talks to NHS Trust and high street optometrists, and patch clubs offering information and a supportive environment for children already undergoing treatment (Salisbury, 2003).

Health promotion activities once attending for a visual problem is advantageous and beneficial in improving compliance with follow up appointment attendance and any treatment regime that is implemented, such as occlusion for reduced vision. It has been shown clearly that early treatment improves visual outcome (Williams et al., 2003). Existing measures for health promotion within orthoptic departments include patient information leaflets that enhance patient and parent knowledge of the visual problem. This improved perception of their problem in turn allows informed consent to their treatment, improved compliance with the treatment required and ultimately better treatment outcomes (Newsham, 2000, 2002).

Health promotion interventions also target the prevention of accidents causing visual loss or impairment, such as with air guns, rifles and other sporting injuries. It has been shown in particular that those individuals who have already lost vision in one eye are particularly susceptible to injuries to their good eye, which would render them partially sighted or blind (Rahi et al., 2001, 2002a, 2002b; Rahi and Cable, 2003). The implications of this are great with regard to the individual's coping strategies and the support mechanisms subsequently required to enable them to continue with a standard of living appropriate to their visual ability. A number of organisations are involved with this aspect such as the Royal National Institute for the Blind, the Institute of Ophthalmology and blind or visual impairment voluntary groups. Such health promotion interventions can be provided at the community level or via the hospital eye services.

Health promoting partnership

Orthoptists work in partnerships with many other allied health professional groups. Traditionally they are part of the eyecare team that is comprised of ophthalmologists, optometrists, ophthalmic nurses, ophthalmic photographers and ophthalmic technicians (McCarry, 1999). The boundaries of professional practice have changed substantially in recent years and the recognition of holistic patient care has meant that new partnerships have been forged in many areas such as community practice, with health visitors; primary care practice, with GPs and teams; school nurses; neurology; endocrinology; stroke rehabilitation and low vision services; and services for those with specific literacy difficulties. The promotion of orthoptic practice amongst these professionals in addition to the lay public has ensured better working practice, better provision of care and ultimately better outcomes for the patients themselves.

Continued health promotion across professional boundaries is considered essential to this ongoing improvement in patient care as knowledge of visual disability can radically change the type of care and treatment being considered by other health professionals.

Targeting special needs

Individuals with special needs are predominantly composed of infants, such as those with delayed visual maturation or ex prematurity related visual problems, and children attending child development centres for assessment, those who attend special schools or those integrated into mainstream schools. Adults with special needs are generally assessed through routine referral to the hospital eye service. The elderly are known to be at particular risk where undiagnosed decline in vision can result in accidents and falls (Ivers et al., 2000; Wang et al., 2000; Rubin et al., 2001; West et al., 2002; Abdelhafiz and Austin, 2003; Chia et al., 2003; Smeeth et al., 2003).

Although the multidisciplinary team of orthoptists, ophthalmologists, optometrists and ophthalmic nurses and technicians exists in the hospital eye service the need to expand the sharing of information to other health professionals outwith these services is important, for example to GPs and health visitors and geriatric assessment units (Jack et al., 1995) to ensure that the elderly have appropriate vision screening to diagnose undetected visual impairment thereby aiding prevention of accidents with the associated large costs linked with such accidents in this population.

Multidisciplinary team assessment in child development centres and special schools is often well developed and established. Needless to say such working practices should always be monitored and improved and enhanced where appropriate.

There is a growing need for provision of assessment and care for individuals with specific literacy difficulties as the referrals for such cases continue to rise. The assessment of these cases is currently a random process across a number of professions but this issue has been recognised and collaboration between eye professionals with specific interest in this area has resulted in the development of minimum assessment recommendations. The impact of specific literacy difficulties can be devastating for the individual with profound difficulties experienced with education and career achievement. Early implementation of care by a multidisciplinary team is of paramount importance including a diverse range of professionals within education, orthoptics, optometry, occupational therapy, educational psychology and where appropriate, voluntary groups, such as the British Dyslexia Association. Optimising alternative coping strategies for education at the earliest stage possible can only serve to benefit the individual with specific literacy difficulties enhancing progression and potentially lowering cost implications for education at a later age.

Work in the acute sector

Within the acute sector there are a number of cross unit referrals. The volume of these referrals continues to rise with the recognition of the importance of input from other health professionals in terms of the overall care and eventual outcome for each individual patient. The orthoptist receives referrals from specialties such as maxillofacial and there is liaison with ophthalmologists, maxillofacial surgeons and dentists in the immediate care of the patient (Rowe and Crowley, 2003). This has proved necessary in ensuring that those patients requiring immediate surgical management of their fracture receive such prompt attention whereas those who are assessed as being in a less severe category are closely monitored to ensure improvement. However the multidisciplinary team involvement can extend further to general practitioners and even police and refuge centres in cases of abuse or other non-accidental injury (Beck et al., 1996; Hartzell et al., 1996).

Referrals are received from oncology units with mixed long term prognoses for these patients. In what is an extremely difficult time for the patient and where vision may not be considered to be an important issue, in view of general health and life expectancy, the correct assessment and diagnosis of any ocular condition and appropriate management is imperative to enhance the quality of life of the patient. The multidisciplinary team includes members of the ophthalmic team with feedback to the referring physician, Macmillan nurses and the voluntary sector where appropriate.

Endocrine referrals cover many conditions such as diabetes, thyroid dysfunction, pituitary and other gland abnormalities. The ocular consequences of endocrine pathology can vary from mild visual defects that may go unnoticed by patients and can remain undiagnosed, to severe defects that can render the patient partially sighted and severely visually disabled. Multidisciplinary team involvement in these cases is important encompassing radiology, neurosurgery, medical ophthalmology and ocular plastics specialists. Many ocular problems are preventable. Diabetes that is well controlled, for example, is associated with far fewer ocular problems than uncontrolled diabetes (Klein, 2002; see Chapter 4 for further discussion of health promotion interventions with diabetes patients). The education of the individual patient is therefore of importance in such instances in addition to the education of other health professionals to promote the background knowledge of such conditions. Education of patients and health professionals as to ocular signs of the condition can result in the earlier detection of potentially sight threatening events with appropriate preventative treatment applied.

Work in rehabilitation

A large area for multidisciplinary team working is stroke and neurological rehabilitation (see Chapter 13 for further discussion of client education and empowerment in neurological rehabilitation). Such services are in much demand and there is government recognition of the need for such services as stroke care. This forms part of the government National Service Framework (NSF) for older people (DoH, 2001; MacIntosh, 2003). Stroke and neurological conditions can impact on the visual system in a variety of ways such as

visual field impairment, impairment of central vision, inattention and disturbance of eye movement and alignment (Freeman and Rudge, 1988). A significant proportion of patients in stroke or rehabilitation units have visual
problems that often go unrecognised and these patients receive no advice or
management (Pollock, 2000).

The multidisciplinary team within the eye unit can address many of these
issues directly but paramount to the holistic overall care of the patient is the
timely feedback of such information to other health professionals involved in
the care of these patients including acute and primary care services, radiology,
neurology, ward staff, occupational therapy, physiotherapy, speech and language therapists and others (Nicolson et al., 2003). For example a patient
receiving treatment from an occupational therapist (see Part II of this text) as
part of their stroke rehabilitation will not perform certain tasks that require full
visual field function if they have lost half their vision as a result of the stroke.
Daily living and normal social function can be influenced by visual acuity level,
visual field and inattention. Speech and language therapists use recognition
and verbalisation of pictures as part of their treatment plan and therefore need
to be aware of any visual problems (see Chapter 18 for a further discussion of
the health promoting role of speech and language therapists). Physiotherapists
(see Part III of this text) need to know about double vision and nystagmus that
may affect mobility and if a compensatory head posture is required to maintain
single vision (Freeman, 2003). Equally feedback that a visual deficit is recovering is important in altering future management options to enhance a patient's
progress in rehabilitation.

Within the acute eye unit and primary care eye services there is specific liaison
between eyecare professionals for care provision of patients with conditions
such as glaucoma and cataract that are widespread. There may also be shared
care of defined paediatric ocular conditions (Nolan, 2003b). Eyecare professionals may work alongside clinicians in a semi autonomous unit (Hitchings,
1995). Such shared care results in reduced waiting times, standardised patient
care and improved referral pathways without the necessity for ophthalmologist
assessment at every visit (Edwards et al., 1999). Low vision can also be a
defined shared care practice among the eyecare team but the significance of the
impact of low vision must be shared out with the eyecare service system with
liaison amongst GPs, education providers, sensory support groups as appropriate and dependent on patient age groups. Making the best use of existing vision
is of utmost importance for these patients. When planning shared care within
the eye unit areas that need to be considered include patient selection, conditions involved, investigations, protocols, training, lines of communication and
referral, frequency of follow up and re referral (Burns-Cox, 1995; Royal
College of Ophthalmologists, 1996; Association of Optometry, 1998). Indeed
these principles apply to all multidisciplinary team approaches.

In summary, the primary role of orthoptists within the acute and primary
care sectors, individually and as part of a wider multidisciplinary team, is
essential to the correct provision of care to patients with visual impairment due

to a wide variety of causes. There is national recognition amongst orthoptists of the need for health promotion at all levels involving the lay community, patients and health professionals with endeavours at all levels from undergraduate to postgraduate to address this issue.

References

Abdelhafiz, A. H. and Austin, C. A. (2003) Visual factors should be assessed in older people presenting with falls or hip fracture. *Age and Ageing* 32: 26–30.

Archer, S. M., Helveston, E. M., Miller, K. K. and Ellis, F. D. (1986) Stereopsis in normal infants and infants with congenital esotropia. *American Journal of Ophthalmology* 101: 591–6.

Association of Optometry (1998) *Shared Care Information Pack*. London: Association of Optometry.

Bechtoldt, H. P. and Hutz, C. S. (1979) Stereopsis in young infants and stereopsis in an infant with congenital esotropia. *Journal of Pediatric Ophthalmology and Strabismus* 16: 49–54.

Beck, S. R., Freitag, S. L. and Singer, N. (1996) Ocular injuries in battered women. *Ophthalmology* 103: 997–8.

Birch, E. E., Gwiazda, J. and Held, R. (1983) The development of vergence does not account for the onset of stereopsis. *Perception* 12: 331–6.

Blakey, A., Moore, D. and Telfer, M. (2003) Integrated glaucoma services: the orthoptist's role. *Parallel Vision (British and Irish Orthoptic Society)* 57: 2–3.

British and Irish Orthoptic Society, Professional Development Committee (2003) *Research Document*. London: British and Irish Orthoptic Society.

Burns-Cox, C. J. (1995) Shared care, past and future. *Ophthalmic and Physiological Optics* 5: 379–81.

Chia, E. M., Mitchell, P., Rochtchina, E., Foran, S. and Wang, J. J. (2003) Unilateral visual impairment and health related quality of life: the Blue Mountains Eye Study. *British Journal of Ophthalmology* 87: 392–5.

Deacon, M. A. (1998) Social and psychological implications of strabismus. *British Orthoptic Journal* 55: 75–8.

Department of Health (1999) *Continuing Professional Development Quality in the New NHS*. London: DoH.

Department of Health (2000) *Meeting the Challenge: a Strategy for the Allied Health Professions*. London: DoH.

Department of Health (2001) *National Service Framework for Older People*. London: HMSO.

Donahue, S. P., Arnold, R. W., Ruben, J. B. and AAPOS Vision Screening Committee (2003) Preschool vision screening: what should we be detecting and how should we report it? Uniform guidelines for reporting results of preschool vision screening studies. *Journal of the American Association for Pediatric Ophthalmology and Strabismus* 7: 314–16.

Edwards, R. S., Davis, A. R. and Shilling, J. L. (1999) The role of orthoptists in biometry. *British Orthoptic Journal* 56: 19–21.

Fisher, N. F., Flom, M. C. and Jampolsky, A. (1968) Early surgery of congenital esotropia. *American Journal of Ophthalmology* 65: 439–43.

Fox, R., Aslin, R. N., Shea, S. L. and Dumais, S. T. (1980) Stereopsis in human infants. *Science* 207: 323–4.

Freeman, C. F. (2003) Collaborative working on a stroke-rehabilitation ward. *Parallel Vision (British and Irish Orthoptic Society)* 56: 3.

Freeman, C. F. and Rudge, N. B. (1988) Cerebrovascular accident and the orthoptist. *British Orthoptic Journal* 45: 8–18.

Hall, D. M. B. and Elliman, D. (2003) *Health for All Children,* fourth edition. Oxford: Oxford University Press.

Hartzell, K. N., Botek, A. A. and Goldberg, S. H. (1996) Orbital fractures in women due to sexual assault and domestic violence. *Ophthalmology* 103: 953–7.

Hitchings, R. (1995) Shared care for glaucoma. *British Journal of Ophthalmology* 79: 626.

Ing, M. R. (1983) Early surgical alignment for congenital esotropia. *Journal of Pediatric Ophthalmology and Strabismus* 20: 11–18.

Ing, M., Costenbader, F. D., Parks, M. M. and Albert, D. G. (1966) Early surgery for congenital esotropia. *American Journal of Ophthalmology* 61: 1419–22.

Ivers, R. Q., Norton, R., Cumming, R. G., Butler, M. and Campbell, A. J. (2000) Visual impairment and risk of hip fracture. *American Journal of Epidemiology* 152: 633–9.

Jack, C., Smith, T., Neoh, C., Lye, M. and McGalliard, J. (1995) Prevalence of low vision in elderly patients admitted to an acute geriatric unit in Liverpool: elderly people who fall are more likely to have low vision. *Gerontology* 41: 280–5.

Klein, R. (2002) Prevention of visual loss from diabetic retinopathy. *Survey of Ophthalmology* 47: S246–52.

MacIntosh, C. (2003) Stroke re-visited: visual problems following stroke and their effect on rehabilitation. *British Orthoptic Journal* 60: 10–14.

McCarry, B. (1999) Orthoptists current shared care role in ophthalmology. *British Orthoptic Journal* 56: 11–18.

National Screening Committee (UK) (2000) *Second Report of the UK National Screening Committee.* London: Department of Health.

Newsham, D. (2000) Parental non-concordance with occlusion therapy. *British Journal of Ophthalmology* 84: 957–62.

Newsham, D. (2002) A randomised controlled trial of written information: the effect on parental non-concordance with occlusion therapy. *British Journal of Ophthalmology* 86: 787–91.

Nicolson, A., Foreman, P. and Carpenter, J. (2003) Orthoptists within the stroke team. *Parallel Vision (British and Irish Orthoptic Society)* 56: 3.

Nolan, J. (2003a) *Role of the Orthoptist.* London: British and Irish Orthoptic Society.

Nolan, J. (2003b) Community child care: orthoptists and optometrists: working as partners. *Parallel Vision (British and Irish Orthoptic Society)* 55: 3.

Pollock, L. (2000) Managing patients with visual symptoms of cerebro-vascular disease. *Eye News* 7: 23–6.

Rahi, J. S. and Cable, N. (2003) British childhood visual impairment study group: severe visual impairment and blindness in children in the UK. *The Lancet* 360: 1359–65.

Rahi, J. S. and Dezateux, C. (2002) Improving the detection of childhood visual problems and eye disorders. *The Lancet* 359: 1083–4.

Rahi, J. S., Logan, S., Borja, M. C., Timms, C., Russell-Eggitt, I. and Taylor, D. (2002a) Prediction of improved vision in the amblyopic eye after visual loss in the non-amblyopic eye. *The Lancet* 359: 621–2.

Rahi, J. S., Logan, S., Timms, C., Russell-Eggitt, I. and Taylor, D. (2002b) Risk, causes and outcomes of visual impairment after loss of vision in the non-amblyopic eye: a population-based study. *The Lancet* 359: 597–602.

Rahi, J. S. and Stanford, M. (2001) Treatment of amblyopic eyes. *The Lancet* **357**: 902–4.

Rahi, J. S., Williams, C., Bedford, H. and Elliman, D. (2001) Screening and surveillance for ophthalmic disorders and visual deficits in children in the United Kingdom. *British Journal of Ophthalmology* **85**: 257–9.

Rogers, G. L., Chazen, S., Fellows, R. and Tsou, B. H. (1982) Strabismus surgery and its effect upon infant development in congenital esotropia. *Ophthalmology* **89**: 479–83.

Rowe, F. J. (1997) *Clinical Orthoptics.* Oxford: Blackwell Science.

Rowe, F. J. (2000) Long term postoperative stability in infantile esotropia. *Strabismus* **8**: 3–13.

Rowe, F. J. and Clarke, S. (2003) *Clinical Audit Document.* London: British and Irish Orthoptic Society.

Rowe, F. J. and Crowley, T. (2003) Outcome of ocular motility disturbances in orbital injuries. *Strabismus* **11**: 179–88.

Royal College of Ophthalmologists (1996) *Shared Care.* London: RCO.

Rubin, G. S., Bandeen-Roche, K., Huang, G., Muñoz, B., Schein, O. D., Fried, L. P. and West, S. K. (2001) The association of multiple visual impairments with self-reported visual disability: SEE project. *Investigative Ophthalmology and Visual Science* **42**: 64–72.

Salisbury, T. (2003) Patch party: Norfolk and Norwich University Hospital. *Parallel Vision (British and Irish Orthoptic Society)* **53**: 1.

Smeeth, L., Fletcher, A. E., Hanciles, S., Evans, J. and Wormald, R. (2003) Screening older people for impaired vision in primary care: cluster randomised trial. *British Medical Journal* **327**: 1027.

Taylor, D. M. (1963) How early is early surgery in the management of strabismus? *Archives of Ophthalmology* **70**: 752–6.

Taylor, D. M. (1972) Is congenital esotropia functionally curable? *Transactions of the American Optical Society* **70**: 529–76.

Tolchin, J. G. and Lederman, M. E. (1978) Congenital (infantile) esotropia; psychiatric aspects. *Journal of Pediatric Ophthalmology and Strabismus* **15**: 160–3.

Wang, J. J., Mitchell, P. and Smith, W. (2000) Vision and low self-rated health: the Blue Mountains Eye Study. *Investigative Ophthalmology and Visual Science* **41**: 49–54.

West, C. G., Gildengorin, G., Haegerstrom-Portnoy, G., Schneck, M. E., Lott, L. and Brabyn, J. A. (2002) Is vision function related to physical functional ability in older adults? *Journal of the American Geriatric Society* **50**: 136–45.

Wickham, L., Stewart, C., Charnock, A. and Fielder, A. (2002) The assessment and management of strabismus and amblyopia: a national audit. *Eye* **16**: 522–9.

Williams, C., Northstone, K., Harrad, R. A., Sparrow, J. M., Harvey, I. and ALSPAC Study Team (2003) Amblyopia treatment outcomes after preschool screening v. school entry screening: observational data from a prospective cohort study. *British Journal of Ophthalmology* **87**: 988–93.

Author Index

Subject Index

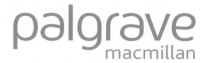

palgrave macmillan

More Health Promotion titles

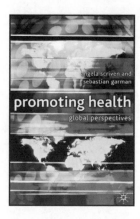 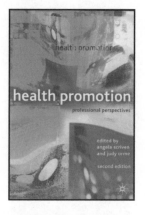

Promoting Health
Global Perspectives
explores many contentious
and debated issues
associated with the
promotion of health at a
global level and provides a
future orientation for
current practice.

Health Promotion
Professional Perspectives
looks at the different
professional domains in
health promotion and the
organisational and
policy contexts that can
influence the range and
nature of interventions.

2005

2001

PB 1-4039-2137-7
HB 1-4039-2136-9

PB 0-333-94834-3

www.palgrave.com/nursinghealth/healthpromotion.htm